2147

EVOLVING THOUGHT FIELD THERAPY

THE NORTON ENERGY PSYCHOLOGY SERIES

Fred P. Gallo, Ph.D., Series Editor

Energy Psychology includes therapies that address bodily energy systems. While traditionally chemical, neurologic, cognitive, and situational factors are seen as integral to psychological problems, energy psychology posits that bioenergy information or energy configurations also are involved. These therapies specifically target presenting problems and offer revolutionary techniques and methods for symptom alleviation. Titles in the Norton Energy Psychology Series will keep readers abreast of this burgeoning field and offer a wide array of perspectives, techniques, and methodologies in these exciting approaches to treatment.

A Norton Professional Book

EVOLVING THOUGHT FIELD THERAPY
The Clinician's Handbook of Diagnoses, Treatment, and Theory

JOHN H. DIEPOLD, JR.
VICTORIA BRITT
SHEILA S. BENDER

W. W. Norton & Company
New York & London

For information about permission to reproduce
selections from this book, write to
Permissions, W. W. Norton & Company, Inc.,
500 Fifth Avenue, New York, NY 10110

Production Manager: Leeann Graham
Manufacturing by Haddon Craftsmen, Inc.

Library of Congress Cataloging-in-Publication Data

Diepold, John H.
  Evolving thought field therapy : the clinician's handbook of diagnoses, treatment,
and theory / John H. Diepold, Jr., Victoria Britt, Sheila S. Bender.
      p.   cm. – (The Norton energy psychology series)
"A Norton professional book."
Includes bibliographical references and index.
ISBN 0-393-70405-X
1. Mind and body therapies—Handbooks, manuals, etc. 2. Acupuncture
points—Handbooks, manuals, etc. I. Britt, Victoria. II. Bender, Sheila S.
III. Title. IV. Series.

RC489.M53D525 2004
616.89'13—dc22   2003059721

W. W. Norton & Company, Inc., 500 Fifth Avenue, New York, N.Y. 10110
www.wwnorton.com

W. W. Norton & Company Ltd., Castle House, 75/76 Wells St., London W1T 3QT

1 3 5 7 9 0 8 6 4 2

Dedication

To our families

CONTENTS

Foreword   *Fred P. Gallo, Ph.D.*   ix
Acknowledgments   xi
Introduction   xv
1   In the Beginning   1
2   The Paradigm Challenge   11
3   The Acupuncture Meridian System and EvTFT   30
4   Accessing and Using the Human Psycho-Soma System   51
5   The Touch-And-Breathe Treatment Technique   80
6   System Disruptions and Treatment Blocks   94
7   Describing and Expanding the Theory/Model   115
8   The Structural Components of EvTFT   131
9   EvTFT Diagnostic Methods   145
10   The Basic Diagnostic and Treatment Protocols   161
11   Diagnosis and Treatment of Elaters   180
12   Supplementary and Modified Protocols   185
13   The Algorithm Approach   230
14   The Integration of EvTFT into Psychotherapy   239
15   Understanding the Effectiveness of EvTFT   281
Epilogue   303
Afterword   *William A. Tiller, Ph.D.*   312
Appendices   317
Notes   343
Glossary   353
Bibliography   359
Index   365

FOREWORD

Since the mid 1960s, my interest in human behavior and transformation has taken me on an exciting excursion of theories, methods, and techniques. This excursion has also afforded me the opportunity to meet some talented professionals. Thought field therapy (TFT) has been one of the approaches that has captured my attention, and John H. Diepold, Jr., Victoria Britt, and Sheila S. Bender are three such persons.

Thought field therapy is a mind-body approach that utilizes the mind's imaginative powers, the body, and intention to relieve suffering and promote positive change in an amazingly rapid process. Originated by Dr. Roger J. Callahan in the early 1980s, TFT has steadily evolved in theory, methodology, and technique. In addition to Dr. Callahan's own contributions, this evolution has been carried forward by several of his earliest students. For several years, I had the opportunity of studying with Dr. Callahan and offering my own interpretation of this viewpoint on psychological functioning and treatment. The result of my inquiry was two comprehensive approaches that I refer to as *energy diagnostic and treatment methods* (EDxTM) and *energy consciousness therapy* (ECT). I also had the privilege of coining the term *energy psychology*, which has been adopted by the field as a whole with its various permutations (Gallo, 1999, 2000, 2002; Gallo & Vincenzi, 2000; Furman & Gallo, 2000).

In the early 1990s it became my mission to proliferate TFT and some other approaches that have origins in energy theory as well as applied kinesiology—the brain child of Dr. George J. Goodheart, Jr. I found these methods of treatment so beneficial that I could not bring myself to limit their application to my clinical work with clients. I felt compelled to make these concepts available to as many people as would listen, learn, and have the willingness to participate in charting this new course. Therefore I developed a series of training seminars and published several articles, manuals, and books to communicate these findings. This is how I came to make the acquaintance of many of the clinicians and communicators who are advancing this field with their exciting contributions (Gallo, 2002).

Diepold, Britt, and Bender are among the first professionals who not only considered what I had to offer but also studied TFT with Dr. Callahan. In time they developed their own approach to this work, what is referred to as *evolving thought field therapy* (EvTFT). As I witnessed their personal and professional evolution, I became absolutely compelled to invite them to write a book on their approach. Thus, here we offer you the fourth book in the Energy Psychology Series, a forum for disseminating practical information and concepts in the field of energy psychology. In addition to this work on thought field therapy, presently the series includes an anthology of methods, *Energy Psychology in Psychotherapy: A Comprehensive Source Book* (Gallo, 2002), a volume on various aspects of the human vibrational matrix (*Creative Energies* by Hover-Kramer, 2002), and one that focuses on integrating energy psychology with eye movement desensitization and reprocessing (*Energy Psychology and EMDR* by Hartung & Galvin, 2003).

I'm sure that all therapists and communicators who take their craft seriously will discover in this handbook wonderful opportunities to significantly advance their understanding, skill, and impact with clients. This volume is an invaluable training manual that contains a wonderful balance of history, theory, and instruction in revolutionary methods and techniques for conceptualizing and treating a wide range of problems. Reading this book is the next best thing to personally studying with these master therapists and educators. Therefore I take great pleasure in welcoming you to this opportunity. So with that in body-mind, please sit back, read, study, practice, and enjoy!

Fred P. Gallo, Ph.D.
Energy Psychology Series Editor
May 2003

ACKNOWLEDGMENTS

In writing this book we have been privileged to share our journey with many wonderful people and would like to thank them for their individual contributions, insights, guidance, and expertise.

First we would like to thank Fred P. Gallo, our first teacher in thought field therapy. Fred sparked our interest and excitement about meridian-based psychotherapy and has continued to be an inspiration. It was his recognition and encouragement of our work that lead to the invitation to write this book as part of W. W. Norton's Energy Psychology series. We consider Fred a teacher, colleague, friend, and fellow pioneer in this developing new field of energy psychology.

We wish to acknowledge the earliest of the energy psychology pioneers, Roger J. Callahan and John Diamond whose writings and teaching have been profoundly influential in providing a basis for our evolving psychotherapeutic approach. We suspect that the insights and daring evidenced by these men in their pursuit of atypical mind-body-energy approaches to psychotherapy will be recognized in the very near future as the turning point in the development of many truly short-term and effective psychotherapy methods. The writings of George J. Goodheart, Jr. and David Walther have also contributed greatly to our understanding and practice of muscle testing and therapy localization in the facilitation of our EvTFT procedures.

And where would our fledgling field of energy psychology be without the brilliant research, insights, writing, inspiration, and teaching of William Tiller? Dr. Tiller is a scientist and true friend of energy psychology whose carefully controlled studies on intention and thought have built metaphors and models that aid in the understanding of the unseen energies that influence our very being. The mind-opening research and ideas presented in *Science and Human Transformation* has insured that he will remain a key person in the development of this paradigm-challenging psychotherapy.

We wish to acknowledge our patients whose trust, partnership in healing, and infinitely valuable feedback aided in so many of our discoveries and refinements.

Thanks to Charles Figley for his foresight in exploring emerging innovative psychotherapies and for supporting the initial publication of the Touch And Breathe treatment approach. Other colleagues we wish to acknowledge include: Lee Pulos, who sparked the curiosity that initiated this journey in meridian-based psychotherapy; Philip Friedman, whose boundless enthusiasm for original ways to heal patients provided an early example for the study and exploration of the emerging approaches in energy psychology; and James V. Durlacher for his friendship and the methods described in *Freedom From Fear Forever*.

Our close friends and relatives gave freely of their time and contributed valuable editorial and illustration services to us. For his time and meticulous work on reformatting our EvTFT protocol flow charts, as well as his excellent editorial advice, we thankfully recognize John De-Salvo. We very much appreciate the wonderful artwork contained in our training manual that was provided by John H. Diepold, Sr. and Angela Cali. A special thanks is also extended to Molly Cobb for the skillful artwork and computer graphics that grace the pages of this book, and to Judy Cobb who managed to obtain the hard to find references when needed.

Many thanks to all the members of our original study group in thought field therapy diagnosis who contributed time and expertise in furthering the understanding and application of this novel psychotherapeutic approach: Pam Altaffer, Tom Altaffer, Kurt Ebert, Marilyn Luber, William Pagell, Robert Pasahow, Ange Puig, Sandi Radomski, Robert Schwarz, David Tinling, and Thomas Tudor. Special thanks goes to long-time colleague and friend, Tom Tudor, for his enthusiasm and support of our evolving methods and for providing feedback on the modified EvTFT protocol when treating patients with dissociation. We also wish to acknowledge David Goldstein for his interest in our work and his expertise in QEEG neurofeedback used to quantify the rapid changes in brain wave patterns that are evident after treatment with EvTFT.

Other friends and colleagues provided assistance in numerous ways that influenced the development of procedures detailed in this book. Accordingly we wish to thank Sharon Toole for the opportunity to present many of the "evolving" concepts and procedures as they were developing via the annual Energy Psychology Conference in Toronto over the past several years. We are also grateful to Willem Lammers for inviting us to present training in EvTFT at the First European Energy Psychology Conference in Furigen, Switzerland in 2001. A warm thank you is also extended to head coach Gary Papa, his coaching staff, and to all the Fighting Irish wrestlers of Camden Catholic High School in Cherry Hill, NJ, for their willingness to use EvTFT procedures over the years; their participation aided enormously in developing our understanding of the application and effectiveness of EvTFT in competitive athletics and in the development of our Peak Performance protocol.

Many events happened behind the scenes that influenced our teaching as well as the writing of this book. Specifically, this book would not have been possible without the expert assistance of attorney Mitchell D. Kamarck. Gary Craig lent a gracious and guiding hand to us when we needed it most. Thanks also to Gregory Nicosia for his collaboration in our early algorithm workshops, and for recommending Mitchell Kamarck.

We relied on the advice and expertise of several allied professionals who furthered our understanding of traditional Chinese medicine and applied kinesiology. We are grateful to Loretta Imbrogno, Annalee Kitay, Robert Monokian, and Richard Reilly for their help.

A special acknowledgement is extended to Joan Hitlin who, after participating in our three-day basic workshop in Switzerland, suggested the term *evolving* in lieu of *evolved*. Thanks also to Elizabeth de Barros Barreto for bringing EvTFT to Brazil.

We have been able to refine EvTFT in large part because friends and colleagues generously provided their knowledge and support. In this regard we wish to acknowledge Uri Bergmann, Nancy Napier, and Larry Stoler for their sustained and sustaining interest in our work. We warmly acknowledge the friends and colleagues who have graciously sponsored our workshops over the past five years: Carol Forgash, Irene B. Giessl, Barbara Hensley, Deany Laliotis, Patti Levin, Daniel Merlis, Mel Rabin, Larry Stoler, and Trip Woodard. We are also grateful to Peter Balde and Ludwig Cornil for the opportunity to bring EvTFT training to Holland and Belgium.

Thank you to all of the psychotherapists who have studied with us and offered valuable feedback and suggestions. Their contributions have enhanced our workshops and enabled us to evolve our concepts and methodology reflected in this book. So too, we truly appreciate our consultees who have acted as sounding boards for our ideas and encouraged us to refine our work: Roger Cambor, Jay Kind, Nancy Napier, Susan Pines, Sheila Salama, Emily Schneider, Synnove Trier, and Albert Speranza in New York; and Barbara Folts, Richard Carroll, Robin Bilazarian, Stacy Hoffer, Elizabeth Bond, Jeanne Glowacki, Bob LoPresti, Joseph Gorman, and Roger Poire in Moorestown.

We are grateful and indebted to our administrative support staff, Kim McDermott and Patricia Carr Christiansen, for their help and calmness.

Although we worked countless hours to complete this text, we could not have done so without the love, support and, above all, understanding of our families. Our very special and deep thanks go to: Jackie, Julia, and Jeff Diepold; John, Jeremy, and Sebastian DeSalvo, Thomas Britt; and Michael and Joseph Bender. We greatly appreciate you allowing us the space and grace to complete this book.

Lastly we wish to thank the capable people at W. W. Norton, with special appreciation to Deborah Malmud and Michael J. McGandy for their continued support, assistance, patience, and encouragement.

INTRODUCTION

The BDB Group (Britt * Diepold * Bender) is the name we used when we began teaching thought field therapy algorithm workshops in 1997. It is the name we still use, but what we now teach and practice is considerably more advanced and effective. The focus has shifted from teaching recipe-like treatment prescriptions to presenting a comprehensive diagnostic and treatment approach of meridian-based psychotherapy, which we call Evolving Thought Field Therapy (EvTFT). The resulting integrative and evolving model draws from principles and procedures found in traditional psychotherapy, applied kinesiology, acupuncture, and quantum physics, as well as from our own clinical experiences and observations. Our workshop emphasis now mirrors our clinical work in private practice, which reflects the sum of our learning from teachers, colleagues, patients, reading, and our own innovations.

About The BDB Group

How we, The BDB Group, got together appears to reflect chance and choice as each of us independently sought improved ways to facilitate psychotherapy's transformation processes. We each learned, along our unique paths, to be open to new advances in psychotherapy, and to those who might lead us in a beneficial direction. In this regard we share the story of our beginning and the writing of this book.

John Diepold Begins

The chronology of our first learning about thought field therapy to the writing of this book entails some interesting twists. As a backdrop, the three of us independently possess a strong commitment to involvement in continued learning and integration of useful constructs into our respective clinical practices. In April 1995, I reported to my peer study group on trauma and dissociation about a weekend workshop I attended in which psychologist Lee Pulos demonstrated algorithm approaches in thought field therapy that could be used for anxiety and trauma. Intrigued by what I saw, I contacted Lee and received more information about this approach, and then shared with the study group what I had learned. In December 1995 the founding member of our study group, psychologist Tom Tudor, shared a flyer he received on thought field therapy training. In February 1996 the entire study group attended a weekend workshop in Philadelphia on thought field therapy algorithms (Level I) taught by Fred Gallo. In a fine display of synchronicity, we were snowed-in that weekend at the hotel, so our group spent most of the night talking with Gallo about thought field therapy, and watching videos of case studies he brought. That was it; I was hooked. The process and results of this therapy approach were unprecedented. I needed to learn more.

Upon returning from the weekend training in algorithms, I called Sheila Bender to tell her about this unusual and exciting psychotherapy. Sheila and I had co-chaired the student affiliate committee of the New Jersey Psychological Association for many years and shared an interest in studying innovations for psychology. When I first told Sheila about thought field therapy, she began to laugh and said "Here we go again!" I had done this sort of thing before when I called her two years prior to tell her about the workshops I'd completed with my study group on a psychotherapy called eye movement desensitization and reprocessing (EMDR). Following my suggestion, Sheila had taken the EMDR Level I training, and in a group of over 200 participants had sat near Victoria Britt. They had worked together at Catholic Charities ten years earlier and recognized one another.

Sheila Bender Continues

I knew from John's call early in 1996 that there was going to be another adventure. He had talked about thought field therapy in prior conversations but, fresh from the Gallo workshop, his conviction about the importance of what he had learned was contagious. He issued an invitation to come down to Moorestown, New Jersey, to see for myself what he was talking about. Acknowledging John's enthusiasm and being open to new concepts, I asked John if Victoria Britt could come along and he readily agreed. Little could we have predicted at this first meeting what we three would eventually get ourselves into studying thought field therapy.

Fortunately, most of it has been exciting for us and rewarding for our patients.

During the meeting John freely shared with us the material and learning from his first workshop with Fred Gallo. In May 1996 we three took the Level II workshop in thought field therapy from Fred Gallo. In June 1996, John completed the diagnostic level training in thought field therapy (the Callahan Techniques™) with the originator of the approach, psychologist Roger Callahan, in Indian Wells, California. This was the most money John had ever spent for three days of training ($5,000 for tuition alone), but he was determined to learn all he could about this unusual but highly effective psychotherapy. Victoria and I went to the desert in January 1997 to study the diagnostic approach with Callahan.

Victoria Britt Concludes

In the early 1980s Sheila and I worked, but not together, as family therapists in the same agency; interestingly, we made no real connection at the time and soon went our separate ways. Then in 1994, I read an article in the *Family Therapy Networker* on Francine Shapiro's EMDR. I immediately took the training and was astounded at the deep levels of change that occurred with my patients when using this intriguing approach to psychotherapy. It had the effect of further opening my mind to the idea of rapid yet profound psychological change. The training also gave me the wonderful opportunity to re-connect with Sheila and to then begin, some 15 years after our initial meeting, what has become an important and enduring partnership in all ventures and adventures therapeutic.

An EMDR colleague, psychologist Marilyn Luber, first introduced me to thought field therapy as a technique for treating trauma and anxiety. Soon after, I got the call from Sheila that John Diepold was willing to share his new workshop knowledge about thought field therapy with us in one mind-boggling day. I, too, became intrigued by this method of psychotherapy and joined the learning adventure that soon followed. After we had trained with Fred Gallo for the algorithms II workshop, and then with Roger Callahan for diagnosis, John began a study group, inviting therapists in the New Jersey, New York, and Pennsylvania area who had been trained by Roger Callahan in thought field therapy diagnostics. A group of 12 gathered once a month for three hours as a peer study group to study thought field therapy and related clinical issues. Because of distance and logistics, the group was short-lived (approximately 18 months), but it gave spark to the fire that ignited the teaching team of The BDB Group, which in turn fostered the explorations and development of EvTFT. Thus began another journey with creative and curious companions.

In Summary

We were intrigued and excited by the unusual diagnostic approach using thought, emotion, and the acupuncture meridian system, and found that it opened a door to accessing powerful information that could quickly arrest and help heal emotional disturbance. As we used thought field therapy daily in our clinical practices we observed and listened to our patients as they experienced the process. We also researched the source materials from which thought field therapy sprang, involving applied kinesiology (e.g., George Goodheart, D.C., David Walther, D.C.), acupuncture and traditional Chinese medicine, psychiatrist John Diamond's behavioral kinesiology, and readings in related topics and authors (e.g., Richard Gerber, M.D., William Tiller, Ph.D., James Durlacher, D.C.), which served to deepen our facility and understanding of the process. As a result, we experimented with variations and elaborations of the Callahan Techniques™ to "see what would happen" if we deviated from the originally learned methods.[1] After some of our variations in procedure achieved successful outcomes, but were accomplished more quickly or more comfortably, or were experienced as more profound, we began to introduce the changes into our early algorithm workshops.

In 1998, we developed our initial comprehensive manual to teach an affordable three-day workshop in thought field therapy diagnosis and treatment, incorporating our changes. In writing this manual we sought to bring clarity and organization to the instruction and to align the practice of thought field therapy more closely with traditional and accepted psychotherapy procedures. The BDB Group manual has since become an ever-evolving work that reflects our clinical experience and the enormously valuable feedback from workshop attendees and patients regarding the effectiveness, ease, and comfort of our alternative methods to fine-tune this psychotherapy approach. After many requests from our workshop attendees, and with the encouragement of the series editor, Fred Gallo, we made the decision to expand our teaching manual into the text that comprises this book.

ABOUT THIS BOOK

There is something special about writing a book for the first time, which is not to say that this book has not been written and rewritten by us hundreds of times in our minds and on computers in an effort to convey the passion we feel about this form of psychotherapy. We have been dedicated and driven in our quest, with a sense of obligation and destiny perhaps, to share with other psychologists, social workers, psychiatrists, and mental health professionals the power and ease of utilizing our mind-body-energy interface to comfort those who seek assistance with life's challenges.

This book is by no means a definitive work. It is instead a statement of where we stand currently in the evolving and unfolding process of using the mind-body-energy interface in psychotherapy. It is truly our expectation that our acupuncture meridian- and intention-based methods will continue to evolve for the enhancement of psychological healing and effectiveness for patients who seek our assistance.

In organizing this book, we have tried to keep some chapters independently readable. In this way we offer the clinician who is interested in method alone the opportunity and ease to go directly to those chapters. For example, Chapters 2, 7, and 15 contain more philosophical musings and historical anecdotes and perspectives. We also endeavored to arrange the chapters in a linear format, where a preceding chapter sets the historical, theoretical, or procedural stage for the next. In all, we offer 15 chapters and an epilogue that fortify the conceptual and practical aspects of using and integrating EvTFT into your clinical practice.

The chapters of the book are arranged as follows:

Chapter 1: In the Beginning

Here we give the history of the development of thought field therapy and EvTFT. Documenting the developmental history is important to us as it provides information about key figures and their contributions as this form of psychotherapy began to take shape. Controversies not withstanding, we owe these pioneering clinicians a great deal of gratitude for exploring, developing, and making available their findings and experiences regardless of the process used.

Chapter 2: The Paradigm Challenge

This chapter is for the reader interested in how the EvTFT model of psychotherapy naturally flows from Western philosophic and scientific traditions and is easily linked to traditional methods of psychotherapy. The EvTFT form of psychotherapy, however, poses challenges on several fronts for both professionals and patients. The methods and underlying hypotheses challenge traditional practices and conceptualizations about the nature and treatment of psychological issues. Our current professional paradigm in psychology and psychotherapy is now being challenged regarding causal factors, the role of thought and emotion, and treatment strategies that are "outside the box" of conventional protocol. This chapter presents a thought-provoking walk through history and philosophy as the minds of Eastern and Western thinkers and researchers begin to merge.

Chapter 3: The Acupuncture Meridian System and EvTFT

This chapter gives a brief overview of traditional Chinese medicine (TCM) and the acupuncture meridian system (AMS) as it is relevant to the practice of EvTFT. The 12 main meridians and the two vessels, constituting 14 info-energy pathways, are briefly described including location, alarm points, treatment points, and correlated emotional implications. The concept and procedure of therapy localization and its relation to the diagnostic methods is described. This chapter also includes some recent Western research on the AMS and evidence of its credibility.

Chapter 4: Accessing and Using the Human Psycho-Soma System

This chapter gives the reader the history and basis of muscle testing from applied kinesiology, and describes how it is used with the acupuncture meridian system in EvTFT. The mind-body-energy relationship becomes unmistakably clear when muscle testing is used to guide therapeutic interventions. Also evident are the interactive effects between patient and therapist, and thought and intention, on the muscle response of the patient. Procedural guidelines are offered in the various uses of muscle testing with EvTFT, as well as symptoms and treatments for a phenomenon known as neurologic(al) or polarity disorganization.

Chapter 5: The Touch-And-Breathe Treatment Technique

This chapter details the discovery and use of touch-and-breathe (TAB), the treatment procedure used in lieu of tapping, for all EvTFT treatments. It also reviews the history and limitations of the tapping treatment, and the hypothetical underpinnings of how TAB and tapping treatments differ relative to proposed meridian involvement.

Chapter 6: System Disruptions and Treatment Blocks

This chapter is a glimpse into what happens when psycho-energetic activity in the mind-body-energy interface is compromised. The reader who has prior knowledge of the concept of psychological reversal (PR) from algorithmic or other diagnostic trainings will recognize that the construct has been expanded and further delineated. Descriptions, procedural tests, and treatments for the varying forms of psychological reversal and belief related blocks, which interfere or block effective treatment, are offered with accompanying cognitive statements. The detection and treatment of unknown blocks to treatment is also introduced.

Chapter 7: Describing and Expanding the Theory/Model

This chapter defines and explains the basic terms and theoretical framework that originated in the Callahan Techniques™ pertaining to the concepts of thought fields, perturbations, active information, subsumption, and holons. In addition, this chapter introduces new concepts advanced by the authors (e.g., elaters, harmonizers, and the emotional signaling mechanism), which serve to enhance both the clinical application of EvTFT and the theoretical model.

Chapter 8: The Structural Components of EvTFT

In this chapter we begin to discuss the structural components of EvTFT in historical and current terminology and usage. Specifically, treatment points, the treatment sequence, therapy notation for treatment points, the integration sequence, use of the subjective units of distress (SUD) scale, the ground to sky eye-roll treatment, and therapy documentation are described.

Chapter 9: EvTFT Diagnostic Methods

This chapter defines and describes the term and concept of diagnosis as it is practiced in thought field therapy. We also present a historical overview of the three distinct diagnostic methods used in EvTFT: *Contact Directed Diagnosis-Patient (CDdx-p)*, *Contact Directed Diagnosis-Therapist (CDdx-t)*, and *Thought Directed Diagnosis (TDdx)*. In addition, the rationale of attunement to a thought field, and how to specify a thought field for clinical use, is presented.

Chapter 10: The Basic Diagnostic and Treatment Protocols

This chapter provides a step-by-step description of the EvTFT protocol, which is general to all three diagnostic methods. During the course of our workshop trainings we have found it beneficial to include a substantial level of detail in order to provide the beginning EvTFT therapist with a solid map of options to facilitate a successful diagnostic process. In addition to the detailed protocol, guidelines for establishing home-based treatment (i.e., homework, if needed) and for muscle-testing SUD levels are described. The curious phenomenon known as the apex problem is also described.

Chapter 11: Diagnosis and Treatment of Elaters

This chapter introduces an experimental method for diagnosis and treatment of positive emotions and thoughts that drive or contribute to unwanted and self-sabotaging behaviors. Not only are negative emotions apparent with problematic behaviors, which are hypothesized to be caused by perturbations in the thought field, but it is the positive emotions that sometimes sustain addictive and repetitive action, which we hypothesize are influenced by elaters. We therefore present a model that accounts for these positive emotional experiences and a method to diagnose and treat these elaters when they contribute to undesirable outcomes.

Chapter 12: Supplementary and Modified Protocols

This chapter describes nine supplementary and modified protocols that build on or modify the basic EvTFT diagnostic and treatment protocols. The specific protocols pertain to:

1. Diagnosis and treatment of known (e.g., psychological reversals) and unknown (e.g., belief or event) blocks,
2. The future performance imagery index,
3. Peak performance issues,
4. Issues of pain and pain management,
5. Diagnosis and treatment of patients with dissociative identity disorder and other dissociative disorders,
6. Use of a cluster technique to treat multiple thought fields,
7. Recognition and treatment of body-energy disrupters,
8. Ways to muscle-test and diagnose oneself, and
9. Use of surrogates for diagnosis or treatment.

These supplementary and modified protocols are for clinicians who are already proficient with the basic EvTFT protocol.

Chapter 13: The Algorithm Approach

Algorithms are preset, recipe-like sequences of thought field therapy treatment points that are used to treat a specified psychological trauma or negative emotions. We discuss the origin of these algorithms and the origin of the term as well. The use of algorithms in a clinical practice, and as a general self-help technique, is discussed and contrasted with the diagnostic methods. Examples of algorithm treatments are also presented and described.

Chapter 14: The Integration of EvTFT into Psychotherapy

This chapter is intended as a guide for practitioners who wish to incorporate EvTFT into their practices. Using case examples and procedural steps, this chapter presents a variety of clinical vignettes (25 in all) to illustrate the power and versatility of EvTFT. Ways to integrate EvTFT into one's everyday practice with adults, adolescents, children, families, and couples are also presented. Examples incorporate a full patient problem spectrum ranging from traumatic experiences to the use of surrogates, to phobia and athletic performance issues, and most everywhere in-between.

Chapter 15: Understanding the Effectiveness of EvTFT

This chapter serves to expand the hypothetical underpinnings of why and how EvTFT and other meridian-based psychotherapeutic methods achieve their rapid and robust effects. We are also reminded that hypotheses and model building must precede theory development. The concept of frequency resonance coherence (FRC) is presented as a metaphor to possibly explain the info-energy exchange, which ultimately leads to changes in feeling, thought, and behavior. Meridian activity with thought field influences, and the functions of chi, are elaborated. We also address the controversial issue of treatment sequence in algorithm and diagnostic approaches using the FRC metaphor to describe the process and explain the results. Hypothetical models of dynamical energy systems are shared as extensions of FRC to help understand the far-reaching scope of our synergistic mind-body-energy relationship. Lastly, this chapter explores the interface of EvTFT with consciousness and spirit, and illustrates how thought fields bridge the vast resources of a timeless unconscious. Our intention is to stimulate the reader's understanding and creative thoughts about this method of meridian-based psychotherapy.

Epilogue

We have chosen to make our research chapter an epilogue. It is only recently that the thought field diagnostic protocol has been taught at a price that would be affordable to those in academic or institutional environments. Despite the demands of the Boulder method on clinical education, we are still faced with financial considerations when it comes to integration of research and clinical practice. Exposure to these new methods is critical if not essential, either in the university as a student or at a workshop as a participant, to encourage those who might be unable to afford the high-priced trainings that are necessary before undertaking research. With the availability of our trainings, we have found a nexus of participants who have started to think about the important research that needs to be done. We also discuss research avenues in the study of EvTFT to facilitate its evolution, and we recommend that psychological researchers use the insights gleaned from the hard science of physics as a model to guide future research.

The preamble to the *Ethical Principles of the American Psychological Association* (1992) stated that a psychologist's goal "is to broaden knowledge of behavior and, where appropriate, to apply it pragmatically to improve the condition of both the individual and society." This said, we invite you to explore, study, and apply the EvTFT methods and procedures presented in this book to pragmatically assist those who seek your help in improving their psychological wellbeing.

EVOLVING THOUGHT FIELD THERAPY

Chapter 1

IN THE BEGINNING

We stand today on the edge of a New Frontier.
—John F. Kennedy

Evolving Thought Field Therapy (EvTFT) is a groundbreaking and paradigm challenging psychotherapy that utilizes the acupuncture meridian system to diagnose and treat psychological problems. We describe EvTFT as an integrated, meridian-based, mind-body-energy psychotherapy that includes diagnostic and treatment procedures performed while the patient is attuned to his or her problem. In EvTFT, disruptive[1] emotions are alleviated through gentle activation of designated acupuncture points, which neutralizes or eliminates the energetic cause of the experienced problem (Diepold, 2002; Britt, Diepold, & Bender, 1998).

EvTFT models and methodology build upon and expand the thought field therapy framework, which presents a paradigm shift for traditional psychotherapy, both in process and content. Two essential premises of thought field therapy are that thought is a part of mind and thought has parameters that go beyond traditional constructs. The propositions are as follows: Thought is contained in fields; fields can be tuned into or attuned; and problematic or disturbing thoughts or thought fields can be treated at the interface of mind and body. EvTFT is one of several innovative psychotherapies that have been developed since the late 1970s. Psychologist Fred Gallo (1998) has proposed the umbrella term *energy psychology* to categorize these diverse methods.

Energy Psychology is defined as the branch of psychology that studies the effects of energy systems on emotions and behavior. These systems include, but are not limited to, the acupuncture meridians and morphic

1

resonance. *Energy Psychotherapy* consists of approaches to psychotherapy that specifically address bioenergetic systems in the diagnosis and treatment of psychological problems. (p. xi)

THE ORIGINS OF EVOLVING THOUGHT FIELD THERAPY

The authors' search for more effective and efficient methods of psychotherapy that could more rapidly alleviate the pain and suffering of our patients has been a career-long endeavor. Our combined 70 years of clinical experience has led us to include a wide variety of traditional and innovative psychotherapeutic methods in both our practice and teaching. Thought field therapy, as we studied it and as it has evolved for us, has provided one of the most valuable shifts in our abilities to conceptualize and facilitate the resolution of emotional problems. Our experiences with the treatment effects of this therapy have had an immediate and profound impact on us as professionals and as people.

As we immersed ourselves in the study and practice of thought field therapy and its roots, we came to realize that more information was needed to further theoretical considerations and clinical application, and to construct a more seamless connection to traditional psychotherapy. We began by studying Fred Gallo's teachings about the techniques developed by psychologist Roger Callahan; we later studied directly with Callahan. The more we used this therapy and the more we read, the more we began integrating the ideas and concepts independently offered by John Diamond, David Walther, and William Tiller, to name just a few. Our colleagues and patients also provided valuable information that helped form the basis for the evolving process that led us to conceptualize the method and modeling as *Evolving Thought Field Therapy*. Before we detail our current evolving model, we believe it is important to describe our path of learning and its historical perspective.

In the 1960s, the developer of applied kinesiology, chiropractor George Goodheart,[2] noticed some interesting links between the strength of patients' muscles and what patients were thinking as they were muscle-tested. Because the workshops and conferences Goodheart taught in applied kinesiology were open to all health professionals, the muscle-testing component of applied kinesiology and its possibilities as a physical bridge to the mechanisms of thought captured the attention and imagination of those mental health professionals who were present. One such professional was John Diamond, a highly regarded and successful

Australian psychiatrist who came to New York to expand his repertoire of complementary and preventative medicine. Diamond described himself as the first mental health professional to study applied kinesiology with its innovator. (John Diamond & John Diepold, personal communication, January 13, 2001).

Building on Goodheart's discovery that nerve and muscle function are related to activity in the acupuncture meridian system, Diamond (1985) posited a connection between specific emotions (positive and negative) and meridians, and he set forth the idea that the meridian-emotion connection is quantifiable using the muscle-testing procedures from applied kinesiology. In *Behavioral Kinesiology* (1979), Diamond introduced muscle testing as a method to assess the flow of what he termed *life energy* or *chi* through the meridians. Just as needling or moxibustion are used in classic acupuncture as means to adjust the quality and quantity of chi necessary to restore health, Diamond experimented with additional methods of adjusting chi geared toward restoration of emotional wellbeing. These methods included affirmations, meditations, and nutritional supplements, as well as stimulation of the thymus gland, which Diamond is convinced "monitors and regulates energy flow in the meridian system" (1979, p. 28) and is influenced by stress, emotional attitudes, social environment, physical environment, food, and posture.

Diamond (1985) demonstrated how therapy localization, a diagnostic procedure in applied kinesiology, could be used to assess disruption in emotions, beliefs, and life energy, and he attempted to correlate specific emotions with individual meridians. Like Goodheart before him, Diamond observed that when a patient was making a positive statement, the patient's muscle would remain strong, and when making a negative statement, the patient's muscle would weaken. Diamond further observed that patients would sometimes muscle-test in a *reversed* manner, testing weak to a pleasant or positive statement and strong to an unpleasant or negative statement. Diamond called this phenomenon a "reversal of the body morality" (1988, p. 15), which forms part of the foundation of meridian-based psychotherapies and EvTFT.

Callahan, a former and brief associate of Diamond, studied applied kinesiology with chiropractors David Walther and Robert Blaich in the late 1970s. The motivation to do so came after undergoing a muscle-testing demonstration by psychiatrist and friend Harvey Ross, who had just returned from a weekend training in applied kinesiology with Goodheart and was eager to show Callahan what he had learned. Like Diamond, Callahan was impressed by Goodheart's work, and, after completing a 100-hour applied kinesiology course, he began clinical experimentation using acupuncture meridians with applied kinesiology techniques to treat psychological problems. This led to the development of the Callahan Techniques™ and thought field therapy.

THE CALLAHAN TECHNIQUES™ THOUGHT FIELD THERAPY

Despite their common ground in the study of applied kinesiology, Callahan's explanations and conjectures about the nature and treatment of psychological problems differ considerably from Diamond's. Callahan speculates that the root cause of all negative emotions stems from the bioenergetic influence of *perturbations* that are experienced when a person is thinking about or experiencing a problem. Further, Callahan began to look at the "container" for the contents of typical analytic interpretations. What was the role of thought and where was it held? From his readings in physics and biology, it began to occur to him that thought probably rested in some type of field and that the field in which thought rested could be manipulated. In contrast, Diamond remains grounded in his psychoanalytic training,[3] although he does incorporate applied kinesiology, meridian and thymus energy methods, and spirituality in his psychotherapy.

The idea of a *thought field* is a unique and essential aspect of the Callahan Techniques™ and of most of the meridian-based psychotherapy approaches that have evolved from this model. Building upon the concept of *field*, Callahan hypothesized that thought fields are psycho-energetic entities that serve as causative agents impacting human behavior, emotions, and experience. The concept that emotional disturbance is mediated by subtle energetic forces (e.g., perturbations) in a person's thought field, which can be identified and treated via the acupuncture meridian system, is also a novel paradigm-challenging notion posited by Callahan.

Callahan's methods of diagnosis and treatment constitute an intriguing mix of his exposure and experience in psychology, quantum physics, applied kinesiology, and the acupuncture meridian system.[5] The fundamental elements of the Callahan Techniques™ involve the assessment and correction (if needed) of psychological reversals, treatment of designated meridian points in a specific order, the 9-gamut treatments, the eye-roll treatment, and a collarbone breathing procedure (if needed).

Callahan presented two primary forms of treatment: diagnostic methods and algorithm methods. Callahan and Callahan (1996) described the diagnostic method as "causal," compared to descriptive, because specific causal information is uncovered through diagnosis, and then it is immediately treated. Using therapy localization procedures as gleaned from applied kinesiology, Callahan (1998) muscle-tested a subject using one of the fourteen meridian alarm points to ascertain if any perturbations, which serve to sustain the negative emotion in the targeted thought field, were detectable in the tested meridian. Once a perturbation-effected meridian was identified, it was treated at the designated acupoint along that meridian. The patient was then muscle-tested again while attuned to the problem thought field in order to determine if additional perturbation-effected meridians need to be diagnosed. This process of diagnose-treat-check continues until the patient muscle-tests strong to the thought field. Sometimes a single meridian treatment is all that is required; however, multiple treatment sites are more common.[6]

Callahan believes that the exact order in which the treatment points are revealed via diagnosis constitutes a natural code, which must be followed exactly for alleviation of the negative emotions corresponding to the targeted thought field.[7] In his first book, *Five-Minute Phobia Cure* (1985), Callahan introduced the method of using fingers to tap designated acupoints (e.g., 5 to 50 times) for the treatment of negative emotions. While acknowledging that there are numerous ways to engage meridian activity, he continues to exclusively use tapping as his sole treatment approach. Further, Callahan (1981) observed the same reversed muscle-testing phenomenon as Diamond did (testing weak to a pleasant or positive statement and strong to an unpleasant or negative statement). Callahan, however, described this as indicative of what he termed *psychological reversal*. The diagnosis and treatment of psychological reversals are an integral part of his techniques.

Based on reported observations using his diagnostic method, Callahan developed a simpler and more popularized version of thought field therapy: the algorithm method. Callahan claims that after diagnosing hundreds of patients, he noticed that particular patterns recur for specific life events or emotional disturbances. For example, he teaches a simple three-meridian-point recipe for several different types of anxiety. He taught these recipe-style algorithms to his students as part of the training in the Callahan Techniques™. These algorithms have been published and taught by his trainees, and even added to (unofficially) over time by others, including Gallo (1994a, 1994b) and Lambrou and Pratt (2000).

ADVANCES IN THEORY AND METHOD

The seeds planted by Diamond and Callahan in the use of the acupuncture meridian system to treat psychological problems have begun to germinate into other alternative and complementary models of energy psychotherapy. Since about 1990, new techniques and fresh approaches in energy psychology have slowly made their way to interested therapists and to the general public via the Internet, conferences, training workshops, and publications. As of 2003, the utilization of these potent psychotherapeutic methods in mainstream psychology and psychiatry, as well as recognition and acceptance by professional governing bodies, are goals to be achieved. It appears that the psychotherapy community views with amazement and skepticism the rapid and efficient way in which meridian-based psychotherapy can treat and resolve emotional problems. In a therapeutic world acculturated to the idea that psychological change is a necessarily slow and gradual process, these doubts are surely to be expected.

Thought field therapy introduces the concepts of thought fields and subtle energies as instrumental agents to affect change at what we believe to be a more fundamental level of experience than traditional psychotherapies. The psychotherapeutic interventions used in thought field therapies are truly different from those of other psychotherapy approaches, such as psychoanalytic, cognitive-behavioral, and hypnotic therapies; thought field therapies require a paradigm shift in the understanding of the cause and treatment of psychological problems.

EVOLVING THOUGHT
FIELD THERAPY

EvTFT is a next step in the evolution of thought field psychotherapy in that it expands the dimension of targeting the mind-body-energy interface that facilitates the process of how the mind and body work together. The EvTFT model presented in this book includes three energetically-related diagnostic methods, the touch-and-breathe treatment alternative to tapping (Diepold, 2000), diagnostic and treatment procedures that include positive emotions when they are instrumental in maintaining self-defeating and addictive behaviors, the hypothesis that attainment of *frequency resonance coherence* between and among meridians when attuned to a thought field accounts for the rapid relief experienced with meridian-based psychotherapies, and several conceptual models involving a *dynamical energy systems approach* to understanding this evolving paradigm-challenging method of psychotherapy.

EvTFT utilizes aspects of applied kinesiology, the acupuncture meridian system, and traditional psychotherapy to diagnose and treat psychological problems by engaging the body's subtle energy system and its electromagnetic and magnetic biofields. We hope to make clear that thought and emotions, the two fundamental resources of mainstream psychotherapies, are nontangible, subtle-energetic constructs of enormous influence on behavior and body function, and that treatment interventions that utilize and influence the body's subtle energies are highly relevant to the practice of psychotherapy.

Treatment procedures in thought field therapy and other meridian-based methods, such as the emotional freedom techniques (Craig & Fowlie, 1997) and the energy diagnostic and treatment methods (Gallo, 2000), have almost exclusively employed finger tapping on the treatment points. Finger tapping on or near the beginning or end points of specified meridians or vessels is hypothesized to restore energetic balance by transducing kinetic energy into the meridians (Callahan, 1985, 1990, 1992). Still others have used touch with inner awareness (e.g., Fleming, 1996) and tapping with subconscious processing (e.g., Nims, 2001). John Diamond (e.g., 1979, 1985, 1988) utilizes an even broader range of techniques. EvTFT, however, uses the touch-and-breathe (TAB) treatment alternative to tapping (Diepold, 2000), a method that has proved to be more client-friendly, more natural to the rhythms of the body, more mindful of the psychotherapy process, and perhaps more profound in its treatment application.

Unfortunately, the very reasons that make EvTFT such a powerful intervention are the reasons that make it difficult to enter as a legitimate method of psychotherapy. Remember, we speak of the body's subtle energy system, the rapid rate in which emotional problems can be resolved, hypothetical architecture and underpinnings, and treatment methodologies that are strikingly different from traditional ones, thus setting EvTFT apart from most other psychotherapies. We are mindful of the difficulties, yet so swayed by the power of the intervention that we, with many of our colleagues, have supported and encouraged research into the mechanisms that underlie the process. Traditional and nontraditional research strategies will be needed to document, scrutinize, and further develop the methods presented in this book. Successful application of learning from research and clinical study can provide the "proof" relative to what is known to advance the paradigm. In addition, the ability to identify unknown (currently undetectable or untestable) factors and to hypothesize, study, and incorporate the unknowns serves to further expand our understanding of that which is outside the box of traditional thought.

In a practical vein, EvTFT methods are well suited to managed-care providers for whom time-limited psychotherapy services are at a premium. Results using simplified thought field therapy treatments are comparatively quick (Figley & Carbonell, 1995), thorough, and lasting. Applications of EvTFT are versatile and, per our clinical experience and colleague reports, have been used to successfully treat the full spectrum of psychological issues, including traumatic experience, post-traumatic stress disorder, anxiety, panic, and phobias, among others. EvTFT is also useful in stress management, addictive behavior, pain management, and sports and performance issues.

EvTFT approaches can be used with patients of all ages and from all cultures. Young children and physically handicapped and bedridden patients can also benefit from the use of surrogate testing and treatment protocols.[8] As in all good psychotherapy, diagnosis and treatment proceeds solely on the basis of the patient's experiences, memories, thoughts, and feelings.

While EvTFT diagnosis and treatment may seem unusual compared to traditional talk therapies, they are meant to blend and integrate easily with mainstream psychotherapy methods. Regardless of therapist orientation and training, the EvTFT methods as presented in this book can be readily applied when the time is right for intervention on targeted issues. However, EvTFT therapies are not presented as stand alone treatments: They are meant to be integrated into the psychotherapeutic process when they are deemed clinically appropriate by the therapist and patient.

It is critical that practitioners who consider EvTFT for their patient populations not offer this therapy as treatment for emotional difficulties with which the practitioner has had no prior experience. In other words, if you have not treated eating disorders prior to learning EvTFT, do not consider yourself capable of treating eating disorders because of your new knowledge of EvTFT. Proper professional ethics would recommend that a therapist obtain training and supervision before treating a new practice issue, or make an appropriate referral.

THE BDB GROUP[9] AND DEVELOPMENTS IN THE MODEL

In the process of using thought field therapy daily in our clinical practices we observed and listened to our patients as they experienced the process. We tried some variations with success and discovered methods that accomplished treatment goals more quickly and comfortably.[10]

We use the term *evolving* to signify this as a constantly developing method. The techniques of diagnoses and treatment have changed (for us) and will likely continue to change as we learn more about this form of psychotherapy. This book represents our procedures and thinking as of 2003 about what lies beneath the effectiveness of these methods. However, change is inevitable, and the evolving process of this form of psychotherapy will continue, especially through more clinical application and controlled studies.

Consider the following comparisons as an indication of where we stand in the evolution of this psychotherapy as of 2003. If you are new to thought field therapy, some of the terms and concepts will appear foreign, however they will quickly become familiar as you read through the chapters.

EvTFT has grown and now differs from thought field theory or TFT (i.e., Callahan Techniques™) in several important ways:

- EvTFT uses the touch-and-breathe (TAB) treatment method in lieu of tapping on meridian points. With TAB the patient need only lightly touch the acupoints and take one full respiration (in lieu of tapping acupoints 5 to 50 times) while he or she is attuned to the problem.
- EvTFT offers three energetically-related diagnostic methods involving two forms of *Contact Directed Diagnosis* and a *Thought Directed Diagnosis*. These interchangeable diagnostic methods allow for greater speed and versatility to adjust to therapist and patient characteristics. Thought field therapy basic has only one form of hands-on diagnosis.[11]
- EvTFT continues to use affirmation statements with the correction of psychological reversals (PR); affirmations are no longer part of Callahan's protocol.
- EvTFT enables the therapist to diagnose precise treatment sequences for psychological reversals that do not correct with the standard TFT basic methods.
- Diagnosis of specific treatment points in order to remedy belief related blocks (BRB) and unknown (unconscious) blocks to treatment are unique features of EvTFT.
- In EvTFT it is hypothesized that chi is a carrier frequency and that successful treatment also modifies the information-bearing signals flowing with, or carried by, the chi, which neutralizes or eliminates the energetic emotional source of the problem. In other words, EvTFT does more than just balance the flow of chi in the meridians; energetic information is also adjusted and results in *field-shifting*.
- EvTFT advances the hypothetical underpinnings of why and how this subtle energetic intervention works with the introduction of the emotional signaling mechanism and frequency resonance coherence.

- EvTFT expands clinical treatment to incorporate the diagnosis and treatment of positive emotions (elaters) that sustain self-sabotaging behavior.
- In EvTFT the future performance imagery index (FPII) was developed to evaluate and enhance successful performance outside the treatment setting.
- In EvTFT many protocols have been extended and elaborated, and intentionally developed when there were none. All protocol changes were made with traditional methods in mind so that learning and use would be compatible and user-friendly.

In the clinical practice of EvTFT we emphasize integration of these methods with those of traditional psychotherapy and close adherence to the ethical guidelines published by the American Psychological Association. We wish to stress that we do not promote the use of EvTFT as a stand-alone therapy or as a panacea or cure for psychotherapy patients.

Chapter 2

THE PARADIGM CHALLENGE

Always we must be disturbed by the Truth.
—Dogen Zenji

In this chapter we shall examine traditional definitions of thought and emotion, which have tended to be more descriptive than process oriented. We suggest that when process is considered in traditional psychotherapies, such as cognitive behavioral therapy or rational emotive therapy, it requires a series of steps that are organized on a perceptual level that frequently depends on the practitioner correctly labeling what the patient is experiencing. Seasoned practitioners make good guesses, but the paradigm from which they operate is more reflective of their experience than the protocols of their paradigms.

We propose that it is possible to examine these problems on a meta level by hypothesizing a working model for thought and subsequently *thought change* as some transformation of energy that is operative at the interface of mind and body. Just as heat, magnetism, electricity, and light are forms of energy and energy transmission that can be transformed into one another, we suggest that thoughts and emotions are transformations of energy that are designed for human communication and the human condition. Emotion may be the transformation of energy resonating in the soma. Thought may be the transformation of psychic energy existing outside the body that is stepped up or stepped down through the brain as some type of transformer or synthesizing processor (Tiller, 1997; Tiller, Dibble, & Kohane, 2001).

We begin the discussion of this hypothesis by describing how the Evolving Thought Field Therapy (EvTFT) model of psychotherapy naturally flows from Western philosophical and scientific traditions and

11

is easily linked to traditional methods of psychotherapy. We propose that the realm we are examining is one with which psychotherapists are already familiar; they only need to consider the process by way of a paradigm shift. There are many difficulties in the current practice and theory of psychotherapy; these problems call for a paradigm shift, and we shall explain how difficult it is to make such a shift by giving examples of the obstacles faced when attempts have been made to do so in other areas of science. We will also revisit some of the Western discoveries that may have led to the present idea of energy psychotherapy had the timing been different or the person who represented the idea been more persuasive. We will review and describe the role of thoughts, emotions, and energy influences on physical and psychological functioning and treatment. To do this, we must first turn our attention to the concept of *paradigm*.

WHAT IS A PARADIGM?

In the 1960s the scientific community took the word *paradigm*, a fifteenth-century word that meant "an example or pattern," and expanded its use to refer to a theoretical framework. *Paradigm shift* became the term used to describe the movement in or out of the paradigm.[1]

Changing any seated paradigm proceeds slowly despite growing evidence that supports change. Although healthy skepticism creates the opportunity for debate, dialogue, and evaluation, sometimes the changes are not supported because of politics, with the incumbent paradigm unwilling to relinquish power even for the greater good.

Because these difficulties seem characteristic of all discoveries that require an interpretation of an anomaly in observation or conceptualization, it is important to note that the problem may rest inside the very nature of being human. Thomas Kuhn describes a 1949 experiment by Bruner and Postman in which subjects were asked to identify, following short and controlled exposure, a series of playing cards. Many of the cards were normal, but some were unusual, so there might be a red 6 of spades or a black 4 of hearts. The normal cards were identified correctly, but the cards with anomalies were also categorized as normal without hesitation. When challenged about what they had seen, most subjects could realize the mistake in perception, but a few could not make the requisite adjustment of categories to fit the anomalies (Kuhn 1996). Kuhn concludes that this built in blindness to the unexpected may account for the resistance of a few men throughout history to accept new discoveries after they had been clearly supported by significant experimentation. To this point, Kuhn suggests that, "the man who continues to resist after his whole profession has been converted has ipso facto ceased to be a scientist" (Kuhn 1996, p. 159).

Whether for healthy or unhealthy reasons, when the seated paradigm becomes insecure because of the emergence of an innovative idea in its pre-paradigm period, there may arise frequent and deep debates over legitimate methods, problems, and standards of solution. Human nature is predictable in these developments, and students who stand outside the favored paradigm have less difficulty understanding the tenets of a newly proposed system because they are less invested psychologically (or politically) in the old system.

Taking into consideration zeitgeist and human nature, Kuhn wrote, "normal science means research firmly based upon one or more past scientific achievements, achievements that some particular scientific community acknowledges for a time as supplying the foundation for its further practice" (1996, p. 11). The key words in the statement are "for a time." Kuhn pointed out that normal science is not a single monolithic and unified enterprise that must stand or fall with any one of its paradigms. "Instead, it seems a rather ramshackle structure with little coherence among its various parts, with scientific education providing direct modeling and abstracted rules to newcomers" (1996, p. 46).

Despite the inconsistencies, the mature science is explained to the new student or the casual reader as if the path of study has been smooth and consistent, each step building from the past in a straight and upward direction. The key words here are "as if," because most textbook histories cannot recount the complexities of an entire process.[2] Complicated facts that cannot be integrated in the present time of the study may later prove revealing when future investigators either rediscover the same phenomena or investigate the historical work from their original sources. Friedrich Nietzsche commented that the value of antiquity lies in the fact that its writings are the only ones modern people still read with exactness. Perhaps this helps explain why old ideas that may have been unacceptable in the first days they are offered are rediscovered and sanctified years later.

In psychotherapy, we constantly experience such rediscoveries. One interesting rediscovery that will be important to our EvTFT discussion is the interest in the old and new brain. When Bender was studying undergraduate psychology in the early 1960s, it was thought that the cortex being developed as an "add on" to the old brain was a non-adaptive mutation. This mutation allowed humans to develop extraordinary technological capabilities even though humans remain constrained by primitive capacity of judgment. This belief about human structure and nature is limiting and suggests that humans are doomed to, for example, construct weapons of mass destruction and commit genocide[3] against other humans whose belief systems are different.[4]

Koestler (1967) wrote that one possible source for such problems lies in the lack of coordination between the phylogenetically old brain and the newer cortex. It appears that human intellectual functions are carried out in the newest and most highly developed part of the brain, whereas, human affective behavior continues to be dominated by the more primitive system. He went on to say that the distinction between "knowing" and "feeling," the difference between thoughts and emotions, dates back to the ancient Greeks, and we continually rediscover the distinction in psychotherapy. Koestler quoted Neurologist Paul MacLean: "Man finds himself in the predicament that nature has endowed him essentially with three brains. . . . Speaking allegorically . . . when the psychiatrist bids the patients to lie on the couch, he is asking him to stretch out alongside a horse and a crocodile" (1967, p. 277).

Each part of the brain holds some of the information, but the older structure has no language to put feelings into words and the connections among the parts are far from adequate. All people are familiar with the phenomenon of knowing with one's gut, and frequently patients may hold an irrational belief dominated by the influence of what may come to be understood as the memories of the inarticulate old brain. Koestler wonders why evolution superimposed a new brain structure over the old, rather than the old evolving as a whole into a newer structure. But be that as it may, one may also wonder why the connections among the brain parts are so limited.[5] Although we admit to the difference, only the newer psychotherapies have attempted to access the distinction and create a union for moving therapy toward exploring the possibilities of improving brain function.

The question of whether or not the human brain is capable of communicating from one level of evolutionary development to the next is intriguing. Advances in technology and the recognition of post-traumatic stress as a psychological disorder have led to a rekindling of interest in the ability of the old brain to communicate with the new brain and vice versa. Koestler quotes Judson Herrick, who argued that the history of civilization is a record of slow but dramatic enrichment of human life interspersed with episodes of wanton destruction, which leads to speculation as to the reasons. "Let the biologists go as far as they can and let us go as far as we can. Some day the two will meet" (1967, p. 267). It is clear to us that this meeting may be taking place in the work we do in EvTFT.

Why a Paradigm Shift in Psychotherapy?

We begin by asking, "why the need for a paradigm shift in psychotherapy?" Kuhn writes that scientific revolutions typically start with a growing sense of crisis, often restricted to a narrow subdivision of the scientific community, that an existing paradigm has ceased to provide necessary solutions to a growing problem.[6] Such a narrow subdivision in the psychotherapy community has arisen in clinical psychology countless times. Unfortunately, most of the solutions have provided systems that may be viewed in parallel rather than on meta levels.

We recognize that psychotherapy faces inherent difficulties in decisions about treatment since treatments need be contingent on whether humankind is essentially an evolutionary freak of nature that is destined for evil or an evolutionary wonder whose full capabilities have yet to be developed. Correlated to this philosophical issue are the important biological questions of Is the brain plastic or once formed unchangeable? and Could physically noninvasive techniques actually change and/or advance a person's thinking, behavior, or physical brain? Many of the questions remain unanswerable within the present models, and a paradigm shift is required to begin the search for clues. In addition to these formidable philosophical and biological problems, there are various pragmatic issues.

First, managed-care insurance has placed financial limitations on the number of sessions the patient may attend, and, as practitioners, we are constantly being pushed to find methods that speed up the therapeutic process. Second, increasingly busy schedules have placed further limitations on the amount of time the patient can spend in sessions. Third, as we in our particular culture and society become more consumer sophisticated and are able to read the proliferation of self-help material, the psychotherapist finds the patient has often already tried a variety of basic therapeutic methods and requires some newer strategies. Fourth, patients have become more and more interested in increasing their quality of life, rather than settling for merely existing. Fifth, and perhaps most important, as psychotherapists become more seasoned, they begin to experience more and more the frustrations that result when they are unable to help patients. In these instances, the psychotherapist may experience burnout.

The common element of these issues is the need for psychotherapy to develop methods for increased speed and enhanced efficacy. Unfortunately, the dogma that accompanies psychotherapy reduces the opportunities to tackle these goals.

Dogma Concerning Ways Psychotherapy
Does Not Work

Psychotherapy research tends to support the hypothesis that psychotherapy is efficacious; we know it works, but the research work, has brought us no closer to knowing *how* it works. How does cognitive behavior therapy work? How does Gestalt Therapy work? How does psychoanalytic therapy work? What are the mechanisms of action? Although, we do not know how psychotherapy works, psychology abounds with what does not work.

We generally think speed does not work. One of the dogmas is that psychotherapy is slow and takes time. There are varied allowances regarding how much time is required, with those involved with cognitive behavioral constructs willing to accept shorter time constraints than those who are psychodynamically oriented. Nevertheless, for most models it is not unreasonable to hear the pejorative "flight into health" and to question the legitimacy of treatment when a patient recovers too quickly from a psychological problem. Although we have examples from pharmacotherapy and electroconvulsive therapy that there are possibilities for rapid action within the system, we are reluctant to accept speed as part of the psychotherapeutic model in regard to any noninvasive treatments.

Another dogma surrounding psychotherapy is that the results have to be lasting. We tend as a community to always ask whether results are permanent, but in the world of medicine, what else is expected to last forever? The effects of aspirin do not. Would you not use aspirin for a headache because you know that in a week or a month you may have another headache?

Dogma three is that the placebo results are discountable since the patient is responding to variables outside those intended. For example, someone seeking help for a problem will find some relief from any treatment simply because seeking help in and of itself is healing. Therefore, any novel treatment may be successful simply because it is novel and not because of the unique merits of the therapy. Rather than thinking that something about novelty helps with treatment, we throw out the baby with the bath water and tend to ignore what may be a valuable clue to how psychotherapy works.

Dogma four is perhaps the most deleterious for the promotion of new psychotherapeutic models; that is, research in mind must be conceived and developed as if parameters of mind were equivalent to any other biological study. In addition to equivalence, we must ask which aspects of traditional psychotherapy and how it works need to be conceptualized anew. As we sit in our offices talking, instructing, desensitizing, and motivating our patients, how can we rethink the process of psychological change and redefine the mechanism that effects the change? We can discuss analysis, desensitization, and other process words, but we need a unifying hypothesis, one that addresses how the work in a psychotherapy session translates to work outside the session. We suggest that EvTFT can provide this unifying hypothesis.

DEVELOPING THE WESTERN STORY OF THOUGHT FIELD THERAPY

The following is offered as the theoretical underpinnings for the study of thoughts, emotions, and language as energetic substances that operate in fields and can be acted on in a fashion similar to other energetic substances. As explained earlier, the reader is introduced to these concepts to provide the necessary links to the hypotheses we propose in subsequent chapters. First, we will look at the Western concepts of force and fields as developed in physics and then at the somewhat parallel ideas that developed in medicine and biology.[7]

The Concept of Lines of Force

We start with the ingenious chemist and physicist Michael Faraday because it is from his work that we gain support for the notion of energetic processes. Faraday wrote in the first half of the nineteenth century that the various forms under which the forces of matter are made manifest have one common origin and are directly related and mutually dependent and convertible one into another. He believed in the ultimate unity of electricity, magnetism, and gravity and wrote, "A few years ago . . . magnetism was to us an occult power, affecting only a few bodies; now it is found to influence all bodies, and to possess the most intimate relations with electricity, heat, chemical action, light, crystallization, and through it, with the forces concerned in cohesion . . . [comes] the hope of bringing it into a bond of union with gravity itself" (Gillispie, 1960, p. 451).

At first, Faraday treated the lines of force describing the relationship of force as representational; however, at some point he began to think of them as actually existent as lines of force in the physical condition of space.[8] Furthermore, crucial to theory building for EvTFT, Faraday's discussions on the magnetic properties of crystallization abolished the boundary between matter and space for atoms in nonliving mediums and prepared the way for such discussion in reference to living organisms.[9]

There are those who argue that Faraday's intuitive abilities might have been restricted had he had a more formal education in mathematics. Whether this is the case is purely speculation; we do not know what Faraday would have done differently if he had been more educated. These are the problems of any historical evaluation because the story can never be run again under controlled circumstances. It is certainly correct to observe that no one today could enter the field of physics without a modicum of knowledge in mathematics. This is probably one of the biggest problems facing those involved in the behavioral sciences. Most in the field are not as capable in the applications of mathematics as are physicists and astronomers.[10] When we try to apply what has been gleaned from these fields to what we know about human nature, we become clumsy and easy game for any colleague who has a literary bent.[11] Nonetheless, there is sufficient basis for an educated person to see extensions of the work of Faraday and the research and thought studies of later astronomers and physicists to the thought field therapy model.

The Concept of Field

James Clerk Maxwell mathematized Faraday's discoveries and gave physics the word *field* in the early 1860s. Maxwell is quoted, "In speaking of the energy of the field, however, I wish to be understood literally. All energy is the same. . . . The only question is, 'Where does it reside?'" (Gillispie, 1960, p. 466). Maxwell went on to say, "On the old theories, it resides in the electrified bodies, conducting circuits, and magnets, in the form of an unknown quality called potential energy. . . . On our theory it resides in the electromagnetic field, in the space surrounding the electrified and magnetic bodies, as well as in those bodies themselves" (Gillispie, 1960, p. 476).

Maxwell proposed that the phenomena of fields does not occur as a result of direct action at a distance but may be imagined differently. The analogy he suggested was to understand the conducting space as an elastic membrane rather than a porous membrane. The hypothesized material does not flow through pores, but the pressure is transmitted from one side of the membrane to the other. He further described that each polarized molecule stayed where it was but the charge of each molecule was displaced such that one side became positive and the other negative. Thus there was no "flow," only the linear displacement of charge. Accordingly, Maxwell stated that "We cannot help regarding the phenomena as those of an elastic body yielding to a pressure and recovering its form when the pressure is removed" (quoted in Gillispie, 1960, p. 472).

It is clear that Maxwell's mechanical images were for the purposes of illustration and conceptualization, and they did not suppose that such a body exists.[12] For those who are interested in defining where the possibilities for the energy system lie for thought field therapy, this leaves the door open for the conceptualization of the space in which communication of ideas and emotions may function. This space may be the perfect place for mind-body interface.[13]

Application to Living Nature

Despite the start that Faraday gave to the concept that energy was a force to be reckoned with in living organisms, in the mid-nineteenth century Julius Robert von Mayer, a physician and medical physicist, remarked that applied mathematics had assumed the leading role in all but one of the sciences during the previous century. Only biological studies had failed to profit from the discoveries and methods of mathematics, and von Mayer urged that force be raised to a status equivalent to that of matter when dealing with life. Thus, force, whether heat, chemical bonds, electricity, magnetism, gravity, and perhaps others yet unperceived, were objects of science equal to kinds, pieces, and locations of matter (Gillispie, 1960).

Western Science of Medicine and Energy

Why didn't concepts of energy become part of biological and psychological thinking? What was it that kept energy from entering into the theory building for human biology and psychology? It was not because no one in Western science tried to use concepts of energy to describe and treat the bases of human actions and interactions; attempts were made on several occasions. Sometimes, however, the zeitgeist allows for more openness to the search; sometimes it is a particular person whose strength steers the course of the search. For biology and psychology, there was never a significant breakthrough, despite the many attempts to incorporate concepts of energy into these sciences. In Western medicine, Hippocrates started to forge a path of scientific study that was intricately tied to humanitarian and spiritual considerations. In the fifth century BCE, he wrote an oath for physicians that detailed the responsibilities of the physician and the rights of the patient under the physician's care. Some two hundred years later, Erasistratus, following in that tradition, set down strong foundations for methods of careful observation and the possibilities of the human body for self-healing. Unfortunately, Galen, in the third century CE, repudiated the work of Erasistratus by falsifying the results of his own studies, and for over twelve hundred years, Galen's studies misrepresenting the structure of the human body prevailed (Becker, 1990).

Philippus Paracelsus, born in Switzerland one year after Christopher Columbus's first voyage to the New World, was a contemporary of Nicolaus Copernicus, Martin Luther, Leonardo daVinci, and a host of other figures associated with the shattering of medieval thought and the birth of the modern world. In fact, Paracelsus played no less a part in this change than did these others. During his lifetime some called him the Luther of Medicine, and the scientific debates of the late sixteenth century were said to have centered more frequently on the innovations of Paracelsus than on the heliocentric astronomy of Copernicus. Paracelsus detested Galen for his fraudulent and duplicitous legacy, sharply criticized cherished beliefs derived from Galen's writings, and revived the tenet that the body could heal itself. Unfortunately, Paracelsus was unpleasant and quarrelsome, a bit of a mystic, and died young, so his name is less known to history than those who followed. He left his drawings and studies to Andreas Vesalius, the French surgeon, who ultimately published them when corroborated by his own experiments. It is Vesalius who is credited with dispelling the dogma of Galen (Becker, 1990).

Around the late sixteenth century and the turn of the seventeenth century, physicians like William Gilbert became interested in the forces of medicine, electricity, and magnets. As knowledge of the correct mechanics of the physical system of the body grew, there developed a controversy between *mechanists*, who viewed life as units of complex machines, and *vitalists*, who attributed life to an unknown force of some kind. As the argument heated, vitalists began to think that the source of vitalism might be electicity (Becker, 1990).

By the late 1700s, another remarkable physician, Luigi Galvani, stepped into this controversy. A thoroughly humanistic physician in the Hippocratic tradition, Galvani was also caught up in the fervor of the scientific experimentation of the time. He sought proof of the electrical nature of the life force and believed he had found it when he observed muscles contracting when connected to the spinal cord with metallic wires. Galvani termed this phenomenon *animal electricity*, postulating that this electricity was produced by the living body itself, but he neglected the alternative explanation that the effect could simply be attributed to the different metals from which the two wires were composed (Becker, 1990).

Alessandro Volta, a physicist and colleague of Galvani's, showed that the electricity in Galvani's study was produced by the junction between the two dissimilar metals, thus ostensibly refuting Galvani's conclusion. Galvani could have defended his position, but he did not do so publicly, and once again the understanding of the enormous energetic self-healing potential of human beings was given short shrift. Today, we know that there were two important discoveries in these events: Volta had developed an early revision of the storage battery and the possibility of continuous generation of large amounts of electricity; whereas, Galvani had actually found *direct current*, or continuously flowing electricity. Galvani had shown "animal electricity" as it flowed from injured tissue. Becker (1990) stated that Galvani, like Paracelsus, was far ahead of his time. Had Galvani defended himself more vigorously against Volta's attacks and continued his observations, the path of science might have been very different.[14]

The difference lies in how we think of medicine. If the flow Galvani uncovered had been explored further at the time, energy, polarity, and the body's ability to self-heal would perhaps have been acknowledged much earlier in medicine. By the time the electrical current found in any injured tissue was accepted as fact, it was relegated to the back burner of science. It is this *current of injury* and the polarity changes that occur during healing that offer possibilities for energetic mechanisms of action in psychology (Becker, 1990). It is probably of significance that it was during this time that the physician Franz Anton Mesmer encountered opposition when he became involved with the use of magnetism in the treatment of psychological disturbances. The tenet that energy in any form could be significant in human healing found no support in the zeitgeist of the time.

Some fifty years after Galvani's experiments, Emil DuBois-Reymond discovered that the passage of the nerve impulse could be detected electrically. The vitalists celebrated the fact that electricity had again been designated as the life force, acting through the brain and nerves. But this happy state did not last long. Within a year, Hermann Helmholtz had concluded that while the passage of the nerve impulse could be measured electrically, it was much too slow to actually represent the passage of a mass of electrical particles (Becker, 1990). In the late 1800s, Julius Bernstein proposed an alternate chemical explanation for the nerve impulse. "He believed that the ions (charged atoms of sodium, potassium, or chloride) inside the nerve cell differed from the outside tissue fluid, and that this difference resulted in the nerve-cell membrane's being electrically charged, or 'polarized.' In Bernstein's view, the nerve impulse was a breakdown in this polarization that traveled down the nerve fiber, accompanied by the movement of these ions across the membrane" (Becker, 1990, p. 22). It is unfortunate that the Bernstein hypothesis became limiting and the result was the dogmatic view that this was the only type of electrical activity permitted by the body.

Despite the opening of possibilities, it seemed as if each time energy concepts entered into the human behavior equation, they were stymied. By the beginning of the twentieth century, Wilhelm Ostwald, the founder of physical chemistry and the 1909 Nobel laureate for chemistry, suggested that mechanics impoverished science by refusing any handle to psychology. Ostwald objected to any theory that failed to appreciate the reality that energy does act, and whatever its transformations in an event, they were the event. He concluded that it was absurd to conceive of energy changes as mere extensions of mechanics. Energy changes were "real" and needed to be considered when dealing with the human condition (Gillespie, 1960).

"In 1941, Dr. Albert Szent-Gyorgyi proposed that the new method of electrical conduction, semiconduction, played a role in living cells. . . . Semiconductivity is a property of specific materials that have a crystal-like structure—that is, their atoms are arranged in a regular, latticelike fashion" (Becker, 1990, p. 39). Currents in semiconductors are always very small and only small voltages are necessary to make a current flow. Furthermore, such currents can be amplified by certain conditions available in living organisms.

When viewed in terms of energy transformations that are limited to polarized cell membranes as suggested by Bernstein, we cannot account for the speed of thought nor can we begin to develop a psychological theory that can include speed. When viewed as a linkup of the thinking and developments from Faraday to Szent-Gyorgyi, we can develop an attractive and theoretically possible hypothesis that the human body contains some informational system that uses both bones and cells as semiconductants and meridians as transducers.

A UNIFYING THEORY ABOUT
THE PROCESS OF PSYCHOTHERAPY

Unfortunately, the psychotherapy community is split on whether an informational system that deals with semiconductors and transducers has application to psychology and, if it does, how to research the possibilities. The problem is one of perspective, with some psychologists exclusively involved in academics, some solely in clinical practice, and only a few involved in aspects of both. Some of the problems that arise from this research versus applied perspectives are as follows. First, studying humans in groups for short periods may result in variables that are completely different from those obtained from studying individuals over long periods. Second, one cannot rerun a study with the same subjects because they are never the *same* subjects. Third, for the most part, psychologists who are heavily invested in research are usually lightly educated in physics and mathematics (other than statistics). This translates into staying within a model of thinking that cannot be outside the box of what is traditionally allowed in the study of psychology. We are fortunate that some researchers from the hard sciences, such as Ostwald, have come to understand psychology seasoned within their own profession and to infuse the discipline of psychotherapy with insights from their respective specialties.

Sometimes, we are fortunate to have additional insights from those who come from other clinical specialties. Bender and Diepold remember many years ago surgeon Bernie Siegal telling his audience of psychologists that he had noticed a profound difference in the survival length and quality of life in oncology patients who became engaged in their treatment after he talked to them with respect. He told us how he had written to a journal of surgery about his findings and they had written back that this was not surgery, but psychiatry. He then wrote to a journal of psychiatry about this discovery that he had made as a surgeon, and the editors replied that it was something they already knew.

Aristotle wrote some 2,300 years ago in his *On the Heavens*, "It is not once nor twice but times without number that the same ideas make their appearance in the world." Why does psychotherapy work? What had Siegel discovered again for the first time?

The Pen is Mightier Than The Sword

Siegel had discovered the power of communication and caring and their effect on motivation and quality of life. He had discovered the power of words, which was akin to a psychotherapist writing a surgery journal about the power of knives for cutting. The tools psychotherapists utilize are *words*. No matter the tradition, there is nothing but words. Once directions are included in any psychotherapeutic model, words become the organizing factor. What is not clear is why words work. Instructions on how to use words in psychotherapy differ according to the school of therapy, but the mechanism of action is not taught and is basically unknown. Besides the words we use within the process of psychotherapy, we describe on a meta level the function of words. We use terms like *communication*, *motivation*, and *desensitization*, but we do not know what about our words actually communicate, motivate, or desensitize.

Two important words representing two vast concepts used in psychotherapy are *thoughts* and *emotions*. Again, we find the abstractions intriguing but despite volumes written on the topics, we are at a loss for mechanisms of action. Research has concentrated on efficacy of one model versus another, but not on mechanisms of action, largely because we do not need mechanisms of action to use words, thoughts, and emotions in our present psychotherapeutic paradigms. Fortunately, the developing availability of sophisticated scientific instruments to peer within the brain is beginning to stir some scientists to attempt research to locate the processes of words, thoughts, and emotions. Nevertheless, such research is still dependent on the hypotheses generated by the seated paradigm.

Research of Thought and Emotion as Limited by Language

Convinced that our old paradigms are inadequate and no amount of extension and manipulation can put them right, we suggest that our wonderful psychotherapeutic tool of language could be enhanced by the addition of the EvTFT model. Although EvTFT calls for a paradigm shift, we believe that the shift does not move us away from the treasure of language and words but towards the mechanism of action underlying these phenomena and the potential for enhancement of these tools. The new paradigms of EvTFT and other innovative psychotherapies have advantages over the seated paradigms in this regard. In EvTFT we find not only hypothetical constructs about the ability of psychotherapy to make actual physical changes through noninvasive strategies, but we are also given the protocols, the means, for the psychotherapeutic session in which the needed communication mechanisms among the physical aspects of the brain are facilitated.

Our new paradigm is extraordinarily different in its presentation and offers a radical departure from some aspects of the old thinking, and yet it has a strong familiarity when reviewed with some historical perspective. We suggest that the new paradigm represents a rediscovered and reformulated former thinking at a time when the intellectual climate has advanced.[15]

In order to reformulate research possibilities, we start with the question of what happens with communication? Alfred Korzybski (1980) wrote that language is both expanding and containing. No language can be purely observational since it will always contain the subjective percept, yet it is language that has allowed humans to learn from one generation to the next without having personally undergone the experience. The major difficulty with passing the experience along with language is that interpretation and perspective of the experience are predicated on a paradigm and thereby limited by the form of the paradigm. By way of simple example, in Chapter 3 of this book we relate the difficulties in translating words like chi from Chinese to western languages since western culture does not have a word that matches chi. The reason the word may be missing from Western languages is that Western culture may lack the perspective in which the concept makes sense.

Along with language, we need to deal with the additional problem that psychologists, as members of the group they wish to study, are limited by their own human perceptual processes, and must move outside the limiting factors of these processes to form new paradigms of human perception.[16] The extent of the difficulty is underlined when we consider that research studies have shown that two subjects with the same retinal impressions can see different things, and two subjects with different retinal impressions can see the same thing. How do we get beyond this and other issues that are based on human nature?[17]

Can the experimenter step outside his or her subjective self? The answer is probably not. Scientists do not deal in all possible laboratory manipulations. Instead, they select those relevant to the experimenter's particular worldview and the zeitgeist of the time. Which bring us full cycle to the premise that scientists with different paradigms engage in different concrete laboratory manipulations, and those differences can result in findings that may be similar or different (Kuhn, 1996). Our paradigm is an attempt to take a metaposition regarding this loop. In our EvTFT paradigm we hypothesize that we move beyond circular reasoning when we are able to go beyond the descriptive level of language to the energetic level of language.

NEW TECHNICAL ADVANCES AND THE MIND

The significance of technological advances, such as the computer, magnetic resonance imaging (MRI), and the hologram, to our thought field therapy story can not be overstated because they lend theoretical constructs to the extension of a theory of mind that go well beyond the mere mechanics of brain. Not only do we gain new metaphors, but we also gain new methods to actually observe the phenomena.

In *On the Biology of Learning* (1969), a book of essays edited by Karl Pribram, we get some flavor of the excitement created in the minds of influential scientists dealing with the topic in the late 1960s.[18] In his contribution, "The Four R's of Remembering," Pribram writes about the hologram and how the hologram could account for Karl Lashley's finding that failure from as much as 80 percent of the sensory input mechanism of the brain would not impair pattern perception. Pribram explained that since any small part of the hologram contained all the information necessary to reconstruct the whole, such explanation could satisfy the condition in which there was no longer an isomorphic anatomical correlation. In another essay, entitled "Consciousness, Memory, and Man's Conditional Reflexes," surgeon Wilder Penfield (Pribram, 1969) repeated what he had articulated in many other writings, that when all is known of the functioning of the brain, we will not know all there is to know about the mind:

> The revelations of biological evolution and the history of the planets serve the purposes of science. But there is another school and a far more ancient scholarship, which have to do with social evolution and the history of moral and religious thinking. . . . Spiritual and moral truths that are no less important to man than the discoveries of science. . . . To say that such . . . are hidden in a man's genes, chromosomes, and nucleoprotein molecules explains nothing. It points merely to one of the approaches science may well make to the problem. . . . Physicians must make a double approach to the problem of man, for there is no thoroughfare of cause and effect between the brain and the mind of man, and there will be none until a new bridge is built. (p. 158)

Penfield continued, "we must bear in mind 'the possibility,' to use the words of Sir Henry Dale, 'that man's mind may never be able to achieve for itself an understanding of its own relation to the function of brain'" (p. 159).

ENERGY PSYCHOLOGY ROOTS IN WESTERN PSYCHOLOGY

The "new bridge" of which Penfield spoke may, in our opinion, be the interface between mind and body. To help define this interface, we draw first on the work of William McDougall. McDougall was a psychologist at Harvard who in the 1920s designed experiments to evaluate the likelihood that animals can transmit learned behavior to their young. He hypothesized that if he could find evidence, it would bolster Jean Baptiste de Lamarck's theories of evolution concerning the inheritance of acquired characteristics. If McDougall did not find evidence of such a transmission of learning, it could be viewed as evidence of Charles Darwin's theories of natural selection evolution. McDougall used standard white lab rats and trained them in a water maze. The rats were put into a tank of water from which they could escape only by swimming to a gangway and climbing up it. There were two such exits, one on either side of the tank. One exit was illuminated because it has been noted that rats will instinctively move toward light. If they chose this one they received an electric shock as they left the water. The other exit was dimly lit and shock free. The next time the rats were put into the tank, the gangway that was previously illuminated was now in dim light, while the other exit was lit up and electric shocks were given there. The rats had to learn that it was painful to leave by the illuminated exit but safe to take the other one.

The first generation of rats required an average of 165 trials before learning to take the dim exit. Subsequent generations learned more and more quickly, until by the 30th generation the rats averaged only 20 trials before learning the task. McDougall showed that this striking improvement was not due to genetic selection for more intelligent rats, because even if he selected the least intelligent rats in each generation as parents of the next, there was still a progressive increase in the rate of learning. He interpreted these results in terms of Lamarckian inheritance, that is, in terms of the modification of the rats' genes.

In 1954 in Melbourne, Australia, W.E. Agar and his colleagues found in a related study that the first generation of rats they tested in the water activity designed by McDougall were quicker to learn than rats in McDougall's original study. They tested 50 successive generations of rats over 20 years, and, like McDougall, found a progressive increase in the rate of learning in subsequent generations. But, unlike McDougall, Agar also tested control rats that were not descended from previously trained parents. Interestingly, these control rats also showed similar improvements. The investigators very reasonably concluded that the progressive increase was not due to Lamarckian inheritance; if it had been, the effects should have appeared only in the progeny of the trained rats. The effect has never been satisfactorily explained except when we consider the possibility of morphic resonance as an alternative hypothesis to Darwin or Lamarck (Sheldrake, 1995).

What is *morphic resonance*? Like Penfield and others, biologist Rupert Sheldrake contends that genetic material alone can never explain the memory involved in the development of an organism, especially the complicated development of human beings. Sheldrake proposes that such information may be contained outside the organism in fields analogous to known fields of physics that are capable of ordering physical changes, even though they themselves cannot be observed directly.

The theory of morphic resonance predicts that as animals of a given species learn a new pattern of behavior, other similar animals will subsequently learn the same thing more readily all over the world. The greater the number of animals or humans who learn a particular behavior, the easier it becomes for present and future generations to learn. The closer we are in time and space to the field, the greater the likelihood of resonance with the field and back-and-forth sharing of field to organism and organism to field.

If we allow for the possibility that information can be stored in fields, we could hypothesize that these fields (and hence thoughts) are not necessarily contained within the brain. The metaphor for such a model would be radio waves or television waves. If someone naïve to the workings of a radio found one and took it apart, it would cease playing. If this same person reassembled the pieces and found that the radio worked again, he or she might conclude that the sounds were stored within the device. In reality, the radio is a necessary, but not exclusive, source of the sounds. The sounds are transitionally contained in the radio, but their source is outside its physical parameters. Following this analogy, we may hypothesize that the relationship between brain and thoughts is similar, and would seemingly support the notion that the mind exceeds the boundaries of the physical brain (Sheldrake, 1988).

With these constructs as a basis for the interface of mind and brain, morphic resonance could be used to explain phobias that are unrelated to any trauma and are carried generationally, as well as other psychological symptoms that do not seem directly related to the patient's personal experience. We could posit intergenerational transmission of information locked up and resonating in the DNA molecules, and locked up and resonating in outside fields.

EVOLVING THOUGHT
FIELD THERAPY

Statements about what can or cannot be done in the physical world are really about science, not about nature. The tendencies toward simplification are limiting factors of Western science rather than a description of nature.[19] A description of the speed of light is set only by the limits of the instruments that measure this speed. "No one may say that nothing travels faster than light—It is only that we cannot be informed of it more rapidly. Information about measurements may be transmitted only by signals, light signals in the fastest case, and there is no significant statement in physics except about measurements. There is no measurement without an instrument, or ultimately without a physicist" (Gillispie, 1960, p. 517). Einstein wrote at the end of his autobiographical reflections, "Physics is an attempt to grasp reality as it is thought independently of its being observed" (Gillespie, 1960, p. 519). And who or what can grasp reality without observing?

Returning to the wisdom of Penfield (Pribram, 1969) that emerged for him only after years of familiarity with the responses of the brain during brain surgery, we read:

> Until the day ... we understand the nature of the mind, we can say only that each man uses his mind to condition, and to program his brain. The spirit, then, is really father to the brain. And our thoughts, we may be sure, will go on breeding other thoughts, through the brains of other men. (p. 167)

So the stage is set in Western science for a theory of mind that would stretch the limits of physics and biology and would allow a psychology in which thoughts are in fields and travel in speeds yet to be measured. Chapter 3 will continue this discussion by presenting some added studies from which EvTFT theory builds.

Chapter 3

THE ACUPUNCTURE MERIDIAN SYSTEM AND EvTFT

> Now, let me tell you about my appendectomy in Peking.
>
> —James Reston

Evolving Thought Field Therapy (EvTFT) is a meridian-based psychotherapy that utilizes the acupuncture meridian system (AMS) as the primary vehicle for diagnoses and treatment of psychological problems. This chapter gives a brief overview of traditional Chinese medicine (TCM) and the AMS as it is relevant to the practice of EvTFT. This chapter also includes a review of Western research on the AMS and evidence of its credibility. The vital concept of chi is introduced, followed by a description of the 12 major meridians and two collector meridians (vessels) used in EvTFT. This chapter serves as a beginning guide for practitioners who wish to develop an understanding of the AMS and the alarm and treatment points used in our approach. We provide information about associated positive and negative emotions that reportedly pertain to these meridians and offer this speculation as a guide for beginning EvTFT therapists. The concept of *therapy localization*, which originates in applied kinesiology, and the application of stimulating neurolymphatic reflexes as used in EvTFT are also explored.

TRADITIONAL CHINESE MEDICINE

Traditional Chinese medicine and acupuncture came to the attention of the Western world in 1971 when the journalist James Reston, who accompanied Henry Kissinger on his historic trip to China, had an emergency appendectomy in which acupuncture was used for anesthesia. Until that time, there was relatively little integration of Eastern and Western medicine, but Reston's personal report, amplified by Kissinger's press briefings, excited the American public, which immediately became interested in the phenomena associated with acupuncture. Over the following decades physicians, psychotherapist, chiropractors, and others who practice the healing arts began to explore and utilize some aspects of TCM. People of Chinese descent living in the United States, however, had been using these methods since arriving here over a hundred years ago. Suddenly, practitioners of TCM found themselves being consulted by a larger segment of the population and being asked to start schools as TCM became more accepted in Western culture.

To undertake a complete discussion of TCM and the meridian system would be beyond the scope and purpose of this text. However, the practitioner of EvTFT would benefit from a basic understanding of the philosophy and roots of TCM and acupuncture. A problem arises in conveying this information when one considers that the practices of Chinese culture have evolved on a completely different path from their Western counterparts. Thousands of years ago, the physicians of China formed from their culture, from their language, from their politics, and from their philosophy of life a tradition of medicine that was reflective of their worldview. The foundations of this practice were detailed in *The Yellow Emperor's Classic of Medicine*, which was compiled between 475 and 221 BCE and which predated modern Western medicine by nearly two millennia. When this and other important Eastern works were translated, the essence of the conceptualization of many words and ideas was lost. In writing this book, we have begun to appreciate the difficulty of defining Chinese practices to the Western mind: The difficulty of understanding another completely different set of linguistic rules is underscored when you look no further than the English language and the difficulties one generation faces when trying to understand the meaning of a younger generation's idiomatic expressions. It is with this in mind that we cautiously proceed in our explanations.

Traditional Chinese medicine, with some methods probably developed as early as the Stone Age, is built on a system of beliefs and practice that are alien to Western thought and medicine. Whereas Western medicine concerns itself with the Newtonian universe and cause and effect, Chinese medicine attends to relationships and patterns using methods as diverse as observation, tongue diagnosis, five element analysis, pulse and alarm point diagnosis, and thermal examination. For the Chinese, illness occurs simultaneously on all levels of a person's being, including physical, mental, and energetic. The Chinese do not distinguish between these nor treat them separately, as would their Western counterparts, and they prefer to observe and include all symptoms as part of the diagnostic picture. To do this, the TCM practitioner must see the person as a microcosm within a universal macrocosm and believe that the principles that determine the flow of energy in the larger body also determine the flow of energy in the human energy system (Gerber, 1988). A major principle governing this flow is that of *yin* and *yang*. The practitioner of TCM seeks to maintain a balance of the opposing forces of yin and yang, believing that their imbalance leaves the patient susceptible to illness. The twin forces of blood[1] and chi serve to circulate this flow of energy.

Basic to meridian-based psychotherapies is the concept of chi, also spelled *ch'i* or *qi*, the "life force" that we believe we are accessing and utilizing when we employ EvTFT. Chi has its corollaries in at least 97 other cultures, where it is variously known as *prana* (India), *ki* (Japan), *yesod* (in Jewish tradition), the Holy Spirit (in Christian tradition), and by myriad names in indigenous cultures around the world. Despite over 5,000 years of tradition describing the ideas and the existence of chi, and despite the libraries of books devoted to the topic, there is little scientific documentation of this life force. There are many definitions and descriptions of chi that include the phrases "life force," "that which influences," and more popularly in Western medicine, a form of "energy." Ted Kapchuk, author of *The Web That Has No Weaver* (1983), stated that "Chinese thought does not distinguish between matter and energy, but perhaps we can think of ch'i as matter on the verge of becoming energy, or energy at the point of materializing" (p. 35). Acupuncturist and neurobiologist Lonny Jarrett (1999) furthered this position in stating that chi supports the manifestation of both energy and matter:

> I understand qi as the quality of the Dao that supports the emergence of any functional relationship at a specific moment in time. Because a relationship is not a thing, the precise nature of qi can never be named with a word that denotes a measurable thing. I believe qi has no material substance, and that we are at peril when we assert that any thing measurable "is" qi. Rather, all "things" that exist depend on qi for their existence and function and may not be said to be qi.
>
> Qi, then, is that aspect of the Dao which supports the existence of the material plane, yet will ever elude our attempts to measure or precisely define it. (p. 302)

Jarrett's (1999) explanation of the Chinese character representing chi hints at the complexity of the Chinese worldview, their culture, their language, their philosophy, and thus the profound roots of the concept of *chi*.

> The top element of the character *qi* is radical 84, denoting "breath." The lower aspect is the character *mi*, denoting "rice," the most essential form of sustenance for the Chinese people throughout history. Together they depict vapor rising from boiling rice. This image evokes the sense of a fine essence emerging from and inherent to each thing that nourishes and sustains life. (p. 302)

There are many forms and subsets of those forms in the infinitely complex life influence called chi. While it is believed that there are multiple forms of chi, it is also believed that one form evolves from another, each having a specific purpose. Manfred Porkert, author of *The Theoretical Foundations of Chinese Medicine* (1974), offered nine variations of meaning for the term chi and described a minimum of 32 forms of chi. Regardless of its form, chi is always a specific type of energy (and information), with a determined direction, utility, quality, or purpose. With regard to function and purpose, Woollerton and McLean (1986) wrote,

> It is the function of acupuncture to maintain the health and efficiency of the cells by controlling the variable energy. Acupuncture achieves this by influencing the body's fourth circulatory system, which carries a form of electrical energy which the Chinese comprehend as ch'i . . . This fourth system appears to have three functions. Firstly, it forms a link between man and the environment of electromagnetic energy in which he lives. Secondly, it controls the internal distribution of energy from its supply to its consumption. The third function is the supply of information to and from the cells. Thus the acupuncture points have the capacity for exchanging information between the surface of the skin, and the related organs, and ultimately with the nuclei of the cells. (p. 8)

Three forms or sources of chi must unite to sustain human life (Woollerton & McLean, 1986). (1) *Yuan chi*, the catalyst-like form of *hsein-t'ien chi* (ancestral chi from the sperm and ovum), is transmitted from parent to child and carries inherited characteristics. This chi form circulates from the kidneys and regulates the transmutation of one form of chi to another form. (2) *Ku chi* is derived from the essential energy of food, and travels to the spleen and then to the lungs. (3) *Ta chi* (or *kong chi*) is the energy of the air that is taken into the lungs where it combines with *ku chi.* This combined chi energy is now called *tsung chi.* However, with the influence again of *yuan chi*, the *tsung chi* transmutes into *chen chi*, the basic nourishing energy. Some amount of *chen chi*, is transformed into *ching chi*, which is reported to be the available energy that circulates in the meridians. On yet a broader scale, there is *shen*, which is reported in ancient texts to be a more abstract concept than chi. While chi can be conceptualized as "energy in action" or "energy with a purpose," *shen* is thought to be a more speculative form of pure or guiding energy that defies direct perception. As Woollerton and McLean wrote, "In effect, the Shen functions can not be directly known or controlled. They constitute the spiritual aspects of mankind, which determine his deeds, and his attitudes to others" (1979, p. 21). This concept of *shen* in EvTFT is discussed again in Chapter 15 from a model-building perspective.

Clearly there are many different types of chi, each of which has different and equally important functions. There are myriad volumes devoted to this subject but for our purposes, chi shall be considered the force or energy that supports and influences life and all of its manifestations. It is this life-essential influence that we believe we engage when we diagnose and treat our patients in meridian-based psychotherapies.

OVERVIEW OF THE ACUPUNCTURE MERIDIAN SYSTEM

The acupuncture meridian system (AMS) is a complex network that, among other things, circulates the subtle energy of the chi influence throughout the body, much like blood and breath is carried through the circulatory and respiratory systems. "The complete meridian system, by which we mean all the pathways of energy between the surface of the body, and the organs, muscles and all other parts of the body, is uncharted. By the levels of contemporary understanding it is too complex to comprehend." (Woollerton & Mclean, 1986, p. 35). The AMS contains the acupuncture meridian points and is described by Jarrett as "internal rivers of the macrocosm, each acupuncture point along a meridian representing and harmonizing a specific aspect of the individual's inner kingdom" (1999, p. 341). These microscopic points are hypothesized to serve as a conduit between the physical body and the various internal, external, and inherited sources of chi.

Twelve networks known as *main* or *major* meridians are associated with the organs of the body; they are paired and run along identical bilateral paths both on the skin surface and deep into the body's organ system. In addition to the main meridians there are several other groups of pathways, including the eight *extraordinary* meridians. This group of extraordinary meridians includes the governing (*Dumo*) and conception (*Jenmo*) vessels, which are used in EvTFT. These two vessels are unilateral, have their own set of acupoints, and run along the front and back midlines of the body.

There are many guesses about how the meridians were discovered, but all are unauthenticated. One is that they were intuited or "seen" by people with the power to detect subtle energies; another, is that doctors on the battlefields noticed that soldiers wounded by a spear or an arrow in certain places would recover easily from their wounds. As early as 400 CE, a book titled *A Classic of Acupuncture and Moxibustion* was written on the topic of acupoint treatments. It described the points, including their locations, their names, and the protocols for using them in treatment. The book continues to be used by modern acupuncturists.

Research Describing the Acupuncture Meridian System

During the 1960s Korean scientist Kim Bong Han reported discoveries that imply the presence of a meridian system in dogs and rabbits. Han described the meridians as a vast network of microtubules that pass through and around vein and artery walls and body organs. According to Han, the microtubules circulate DNA, RNA, and the many neuropeptides and other biochemical messengers that engulf the brain (Lambrou & Pratt, 2000).

There is general agreement that the meridian system has electromagnetic characteristics. Studies have shown that acupuncture points have predictable electric characteristics, including a surrounding field. The pioneering work of German physician Reinhold Voll revealed that acupuncture points show a dramatic decrease in electrical resistance on the skin compared to non-acupuncture points on the body. In addition, Voll and his colleagues found that each acupoint seemed to have a standard measurement for individuals in good health and notable changes when health deteriorated (Voll, 1975). Robert O. Becker (1990), an orthopedic surgeon, reasoned from his extensive research that electrical currents flow along the meridians and that acupoints function as amplifiers boosting the electrical signals as they move across the body. It appears that the current generated by the meridian system is carried by the perineural cells (Becker & Sheldon, 1985). Through his research and observations Becker posited that the acupuncture meridian system was electric, with acupoints serving as transformers similar to electric lines.

Using a sophisticated measuring device of his creation, the apparatus for meridian identification (AMI), Hiroshi Motoyama obtains measurements of electrical conductivity throughout the meridian system. From readings resulting from application of calibrated low-voltage impulses directed into acupoints near the ends of the toes and fingers, Motoyama uses the data to infer whether the flow of chi is continual or distorted (Lambrou & Pratt, 2000). Physicist Zang-Hee Cho of the University of California at Irvine has used magnetic resonance imaging (MRI) to measure blood flow changes in the brain resulting from acupuncture. In a study published in the *Proceedings of the National Academy of Sciences* (1998), Cho described how the MRI was able to detect alteration of blood flow in the brain from an acupuncture treatment on the small toe, which has no known nerve, blood, or other brain influence (Lambrou & Pratt, 2000). It appears that scientific technology is beginning to verify physical mechanisms of change resulting from the ancient practice of acupuncture.

The 12 Main Meridians

There are an estimated 71 important meridian paths in the body (Woollerton & McLean, 1986), but meridian-based psychotherapy focuses on the 12 main bilateral meridians and the two vessels. The 12 main meridians used in EvTFT are those associated with the major organs, which are as follows:

Bladder: The meridian starts at the inside orbit of the eye socket at the bridge of the nose and travels over the top of the head, down the back in two paths on either side of the spine, down the back of the leg, ending on the side of the little toe and connecting 67 points. This is the most extensive meridian in the body and the only one that bifurcates (down the back).

Gall bladder: The meridian connects 44 acupuncture points beginning at the outside edge of the orbit of the eye socket near the temple, moving back and forth across the head, zigzagging down the side of the body, and ending at the fourth toe.

Stomach: The meridian connects 45 points beginning at the center of the lower eye socket, moving around the face, continuing down the front of the body and leg, and terminating at the end of the second toe.

Kidney: The meridian connects 27 points beginning on the sole of the foot in the middle of the ball, then goes up to the arch and around the inside ankle. It then proceeds up the inside of the leg, across the front of the torso, and terminates where the collarbone, first rib, and sternum meet.

Spleen/pancreas: The meridian connects 21 acupuncture points. It starts at the big toe, goes up the inside of the leg to the front of the torso and to the shoulder, and then continues down to its termination point about four inches under the armpit.

Liver: The meridian joins 14 acupuncture points. It begins on the inside of the big toe and traverses up the inside of the leg, crosses the hip, and moves outward to the side of the waist, where it reverses direction and moves up the ribcage and terminates at the eighth rib.

Lung: The meridian joins 11 acupuncture points and begins on the chest at the highest point of the pectoral muscle group, rises to the shoulder, and then traverses down the arm, ending on the thumb on the lower corner of the nail bed on the radial (inner) side.

Large intestine: The meridian, which joins 20 points, begins at the lower corner of the nail bed on the radial (inner) side on the index finger, goes across the ulnar side of the hand, and winds its way up the outside edge of the arm, across the shoulder, up one side of the neck, to the face, where it ends at the cheek.

Circulation/sex: The meridian connects nine points beginning at the nipple, extending up around the armpit and then moving down the middle inside of the arm to end at the lower corner on the nail bed on the radial (inner side) of the middle finger.

Small intestine: The meridian links 19 points and begins at the outside end of the little finger, runs up the side of the hand to the back of the arm, moves across the back of the shoulder and up the jaw to the cheekbone, and then terminates just in front of the ear.

Heart: The meridian connects nine points, beginning at the armpit, traveling down the inside edge of the arm, across the palm, ending at the lower corner of the nail bed on the radial (inner) side of the little finger.

Triple heater: The triple heater meridian is also known by the names triple warmer and thyroid meridian. Connecting 23 acupoints, it begins at the end of the ring finger, goes up the back of the hand and arm and up the shoulder and side of the neck, moves around the outside of the ear, and ends at the outside corner of the eyebrow.

Each meridian is described as having either predominate yin or yang flow of chi influence as a way of describing the aspects of the one-force, yin/yang. Worsley (1993) detailed six of the main meridians as predominately yin (heart, kidney, circulation/sex, liver, lung, spleen) and six as predominately yang (small intestine, bladder, triple heater, gall bladder, large intestine, stomach). Because every meridian is neither completely yin nor yang, it becomes inconsistent to think of yin/yang energy as purely electrical energy with a definite positive and negative, despite having electrical properties. In this regard, Woollerton and McLean offered an interesting perspective when they wrote, "Our own supposition is that Yang is analogous to high frequency and Yin to a lower frequency. We may then draw a simple scale from zero (no life) to Yin/Yang, on which 'more Yin' means a lower frequency, and 'more Yang' means a higher frequency" (1979, p. 28). This notion of frequency range and meridian activity is incorporated into our concept of frequency resonance coherence, which is presented in Chapter 15.

The Two Vessels

In addition to the 12 main meridians, there are two vessels that are believed to regulate these meridians. The Governing Vessel and the Central or Conception Vessel are described as chi reservoirs that collect and distribute chi throughout the meridians. Unlike the 12 main bilateral meridians, these vessels have only one primary pathway (either up the back or up the front of the body).

Governing vessel: The governing vessel connects 27 acupuncture points and regulates the yang meridians. It begins at the tailbone or coccyx, travels straight up the spine over the head, and ends at the center point between the upper lip and the nose, just above the two central incisors.

Conception vessel: The conception vessel connects 24 points and regulates the yin meridians. It begins at the perineum (between the genitals and the anus) and extends up the center front of the body, ending at the depression between the lower lip and chin.

The Alarm Points

Alarm points are one of the diagnostic indicators used by practitioners of TCM, applied kinesiology, and its hybrids, including EvTFT. Each of the 12 main meridians and two vessels have an associated alarm point that can be used as an indicator that a particular meridian is involved in some way with the problem being diagnosed. It is called an *alarm point* simply because testing it can alert the therapist or doctor to dysfunction in that specific meridian and its corresponding physical and psychological references. Most of the alarm points are located on or near the organ with which they are associated; however, the lung, liver, and gall bladder alarm points are located on their respective meridians (Walther, 1988).

For instance, the kidney alarm point is located directly on the kidney on the lower back just below the rib cage. Six of the meridians have bilateral alarm points. These are the gall bladder, kidney, lung, liver, spleen, and large intestine. Six of the meridians have only one alarm point and are located along the conception vessel, down the front midline of the body. These are circulation/sex, heart, stomach, triple heater, small intestine, and bladder. The alarm points for the two vessels are located on the midline of the face, in the same location as their treatment points as used in EvTFT.

Alarm Point Locations

The Chinese developed a measurement system that takes into account the size variations in human anatomy and that can accurately pinpoint the location of various points in the body, including the alarm points. The Chinese standard used is the width of a person's thumb, a unit known as a *tsun*. The location of several of the alarm points for the 12 main meridians can be found using the thumb, or *tsun*, measurement. The diagnostic process of EvTFT involves extensive use of the alarm points; therefore, clinicians are strongly advised to memorize their locations in order to facilitate the procedure.

The alarm points for the 12 meridians and two vessels are located as follows (see Figure 3.1):

- The *bladder* alarm point is located one *tsun* width above the center of the pubic bone or six finger-widths down from the navel.
- The *gall bladder* alarm point(s) is found at the bottom of either side of the front of the rib cage in line with the nipple.
- The *stomach* alarm point is located halfway between the bottom of the sternum and the navel.
- The *kidney* alarm point(s) can be found at the tip of the twelfth rib on either side of the lower back.
- The *spleen/pancreas* alarm point(s) is also bilateral and is located on the side of the body at the bottom of the eleventh rib. In our training we refer to this as the *teapot spot* because it is located where we bend to the side in the children's song, "I'm a little teapot."
- The *liver* alarm point(s) is located in the same place as its treatment point on the upper edge of the eighth rib, directly below the nipple. This is a spot some people find to be somewhat tender to the touch.
- The *lung* alarm point(s) is found in the depression at the outer side of pectoral area. If you hold your arm directly in front of you and swing it lightly back and forth, you can easily feel the depression between the shoulder and the end of the collarbone.

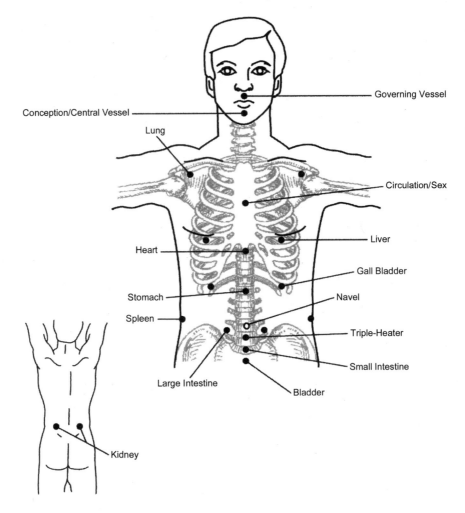

Figure 3.1 Alarm points for the twelve meridians and two vessels

- The *large intestine* alarm point(s) is one *tsun* down and one *tsun* to either side of the navel.
- The *circulation/sex* alarm point is found just below the center of the sternum.
- The *small intestine* alarm point can be found four *tsun* below the navel.
- The *heart* alarm point is found just below the bottom of the sternum.
- The *triple heater* alarm point is two *tsun* directly below the navel.
- The *governing vessel* alarm point is located in the same place as its treatment point, at the center point between the upper lip and the nose.

- The *conception vessel* alarm point is located in the same place as its treatment point, in the center point recess between the lower lip and the chin. Note that this is above, not on, the chin.

Therapy Localization

George J. Goodheart, Jr. originally observed that if a patient touched an area of dysfunction, a previously weak muscle became strong when reevaluated via muscle testing (Walther, 1988). Goodheart called his procedure *therapy localization*, a term that was used to identify the location of a problem, but not the nature of the problem. As initially described by Goodheart and later by Roger Callahan, therapy localization provides the basis for EvTFT alarm point assessment. In EvTFT, therapy localization is used with the alarm points of the 12 meridians and two vessels to determine which are relatively dysfunctional while the patient is attuned to a particular issue or problem. (Six of the meridians have bilateral alarm points and either one can be used in the therapy localization process.) An example of this method is as follows: The therapist first asks the patient to touch a specified alarm point on his or her body.[2] Next, the therapist asks the patient to think about the problem, and then the therapist simultaneously tests the response of the patient's indicator muscle. (The art of muscle testing is explored extensively in Chapter 4.) If the muscle tests strong while the patient is attuned to the problem, then that meridian is currently involved in the problem and in need of treatment. If the muscle tests weak while the patient is attuned to the problem, then that particular meridian is not involved in the problem at that moment.

It is important to emphasize Walther's caution that therapy localization tells us that *something* is wrong, but not necessarily *what* is wrong. We do not know precisely how the meridian or vessel is involved, or whether it is, in the parlance of acupuncture, undercharged, overcharged, damp, or any one or a combination of possible forms of deficiency or dysfunction. We can only determine through this therapy localizing method that this meridian or vessel is somehow involved at this moment with the targeted problem, and that treatment is indicated.

EVOLVING THOUGHT FIELD THERAPY TREATMENT POINTS

When an alarm point positively indicates meridian involvement while the patient is attuned to his or her problem, our protocol is to immediately treat that meridian at the prescribed location on that meridian. The AMS treatment points used in EvTFT are located almost exclusively at either the beginning or ending points of the meridians.[3] Only the triple heater and small intestine meridians are exceptions. For the vast majority of psychological issues, the patient can treat either or both sides of the bilateral meridian with equal effect. Exceptions are noted in Chapter 12.

The treatment points used with EvTFT are illustrated in Figure 3.2.

- *Bladder (BL-1):* The EvTFT treatment point(s) for the bladder meridian is the first point in the bladder meridian, which is located at the inside edge of the eye socket against the bridge of the nose. (The Chinese refer to the first bladder point as "bright eyes.")[4]

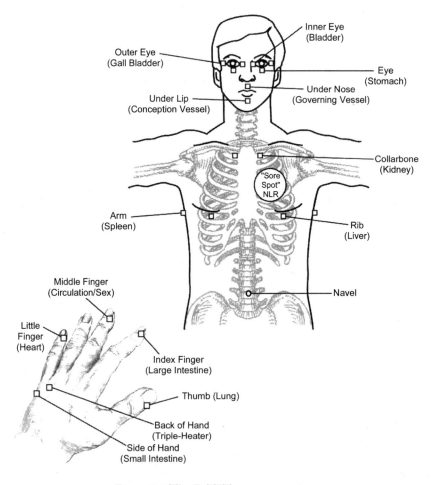

Figure 3.2 The EvTFT treatment points

- *Gall bladder (GB-1):* In EvTFT, the treatment point(s) for the gall bladder meridian is located at the outside edge of the orbit of the eye socket near the temple, the first point of the meridian.
- *Stomach (ST-1):* The treatment point(s) for the stomach meridian is located on the center of the lower eye socket (inferior border of the orbit), directly below the pupil when you are looking straight ahead. If you rub that spot lightly, you will feel a tiny notch where the treatment point is located.
- *Kidney (K-27):* The treatment point(s) for the kidney meridian is located in the hollow between the collarbone and the first rib, near the sternum. It lies approximately one inch down and one inch over from the sternal notch, located at the base of the throat. An alternate method of locating this point is to put your fingers under your collarbone at its points nearest your shoulders and to run your fingers along the bottom of the collarbone until you reach an indentation below and to the side of the sternal notch.
- *Spleen/pancreas (SP-21):* The treatment point(s) for the spleen meridian is located about four inches below the armpit in the sixth intercostal space.
- *Liver (LV-14):* The treatment point(s) for the liver meridian is located on the upper edge of the eighth rib, directly below the nipple. Some people find this spot to be somewhat tender to the touch.
- *Lung (LU-11):* The treatment point(s) for the lung meridian is located at the lower corner of the thumb-nail bed on the radial side.
- *Large intestine (LI-1):* The treatment point(s) for the large intestine meridian is located at the lower corner of the index fingernail bed on the radial side.
- *Circulation/sex (CX-9):* The treatment point(s) for the circulation/sex meridian is located at the lower corner of the middle fingernail bed on the radial side. This meridian, which deals with the blood circulatory system and the sex organs, is also known as the *pericardium* meridian.
- *Small intestine (SI-3):* The treatment point(s) for the small intestine meridian is located on the outer edge of the hand (karate chop side) at the topmost large crease created when a fist is made.
- *Heart (HT-9):* The treatment point(s) for the heart meridian is located on the lower corner of the little fingernail bed on the radial side.
- *Triple heater (TH-3):* The treatment point(s) for this meridian is located on the back (dorsal surface) of the hand at a spot that would constitute the third point of an equilateral triangle whose base is the space between the knuckles of the little finger and the ring finger.
- *Governing vessel (GV-27):* The treatment point for the governing vessel can be found at the center point between the upper lip and the nose.

- *Conception vessel (CV-24):* The treatment point for the conception vessel is found in the center of the face in the depression between the lower lip and the chin.

Neurolymphatic Reflex

In addition to 12 bilateral meridian treatment points and two unilateral vessel points, there is one additional treatment place, the neurolymphatic reflex (NLR) area or "sore spot," as some call it. Frank Chapman, who associated them with poor lymphatic circulation, first described the neurolymphatic reflexes in the 1930s. Goodheart experimented with these spots and found that when palpated, individual reflexes strengthened in what he found to be related muscles. Applied kinesiologists use the NLR areas, which are associated with specific glands, organs, and health conditions, to improve muscle functioning. There is also conjecture that stimulating the NLR area helps to flush body toxins that could be contributing to the observed deficiency in muscle response. The NLR area is the only non-meridian related site used in EvTFT treatment.

The NLR is bilateral, but the mechanism of action seems strongest on the left side above the heart. On the left side, it can be found over the left breast, several inches below the clavicle and in line with the nipple (see Figure 3.2). In explaining this to patients, have them put their hand across their chest over their heart, and then keeping their hand in place, fold the fingers into a fist. If they then rub the area beneath their fist with their fingers, they will find an area that is often sore. This particular spot is tender for most people.

In a model that uses the acupuncture meridian system as its base, the NLR area seems an anomaly. It is one of the many areas that need further exploration regarding its effectiveness.

Meridian Alarm and Treatment Point Charts

To assist the clinician with learning the alarm and treatment point locations used with EvTFT, Figure 3.3 and Table 3.1 are provided as guides for easy reference. Learning this information is like learning the alphabet; after you have memorized it, it becomes second nature to identify and use this information. Figure 3.3 provides both alarm and treatment point locations in visual form on a single human diagram. Table 3.1 addresses the same information, but in written, descriptive form.

Meridian Treatment Points and Related Emotions

The literature on traditional Chinese medicine cites seven emotions that can affect the organs: joy, anger, sadness, grief, pensiveness, fear, and fright (Kapchuk, 1983), but it does not necessarily correlate these emotions with any one particular organ. The relationship emotions have with the body is an important but frequently abused construct in Western psychology. We have struggled with how to present this apparent relationship without losing what we believe to be the essence of the EvTFT model for diagnosis and treatment. Other energy psychology methods have treated emotions as if there were specific, one-to-one correlations between the emotion and a meridian. However, being mindful of the Chinese philosophy of emotions as described above, we do not want to sanction these direct correlations. For example, what one person may describe as anger may not be the same anger experienced by another person. Perception of the event that triggers the word or feeling "anger" may be quite different from person to person and therefore resonate differently in some, which would suggest variable meridian involvement or activity. Yet the thinking about meridian-emotion correlations can be useful, and we do not want to discard a useful and practical tool. We believe that providing a meridian-emotion guide will provide a bridge for the beginning EvTFT clinician who has been schooled in emotion oriented psychotherapy.

The teachings of the founder of general semantics, Alfred Korzybski (1980),[5] provide an essential link between Western and Eastern psychology when correlating emotions and meridians. Korzybski wrote that the map is not the territory, and the map is not all of the territory. That is, the word you may have attributed to the emotion may not be the emotion per se, and it certainly is possible that it may not be all of the emotion. For example, on seeing the patient scowl, a therapist may infer that the patient is angry. However, this is only conjecture on the part of the therapist since no one can say what should represent or inspire a particular emotion. Upon asking the patient what he or she is feeling, the patient might reply that he or she is disgruntled, irritated, unsettled, or any of a myriad of emotions not inferred by the therapist.

When working with meridians, we can only speculate in the most general of ways what the patient might be feeling. If you sense what you (the therapist) have learned to call *anger* from your patient, and get a meridian that is associated with grief, it may mean that you misread the associated emotion, or that another emotion was more prominent, or both, or none. Our point is that language can be confining and we may be limited by our selection of words for emotions. We wish to emphasize that there is no isomorphic "emotional" word corresponding to a meridian because of all the variables.

The meridian-emotion correlations provided in Table 3.1 are culled from TCM literature, including Kaptchuk (1983), Diamond (1985), and Whisenant (1994). The list is composed solely of negative emotions, which have been the primary targets of thought field therapies and most psychotherapy in general. No doubt meridian activity is also part and parcel of pleasant emotions; however, there have been no treatments in thought field therapy utilizing positive emotions prior to the work on elaters in the EvTFT model, which is discussed in Chapter 11.

As depicted in Table 3.2, the meridian-emotion correlations are summarized below.

- *Bladder (BL-1):* The bladder meridian relates to a constellation of emotional states involving fear, frustration, and hyper-vigilance, which are frequently connected to trauma. The use of BL-1 is of interest because, in acupuncture, it is believed to control the pituitary gland.[6]
- *Gall bladder (GB-1):* The emotions most frequently associated with this meridian include rage, excess anger, fury, wrath, and powerlessness. The issue of powerlessness in the gall bladder relates to loss of power or power being blocked, rather than never having had power. For instance, gall bladder meridian dysfunction may become evident when a person is in a traffic jam: One has the power to drive but is blocked by other cars, construction, and so on. Power has been temporarily lost. The gall bladder meridian is sometimes associated with emotional exhaustion, and it can influence the decision making process. There are implications that anger and rash decisions are a result of a disharmonious gall bladder (Kaptchuk, 1983). A person with an undercharged gall bladder meridian may feel that his or her power is being drained or blocked.
- *Stomach (ST-1):* The emotions of disgust, bitterness, fear, and anxiety are most commonly associated with the stomach meridian. This may be the meridian most sensitive to emotional disturbances. How many times when we are upset do we have a knot or butterflies in our stomach. In both Western and Eastern medicine, stomach ulcers have traditionally been associated with anxiety and stress. The stomach meridian dysfunction is usually found in the anorexic picture and can be associated with psychosis (Whisenent, 1994).
- *Kidney (K-27):* In addition to being associated with neurological disorganization, the kidney meridian appears to be connected to fear and

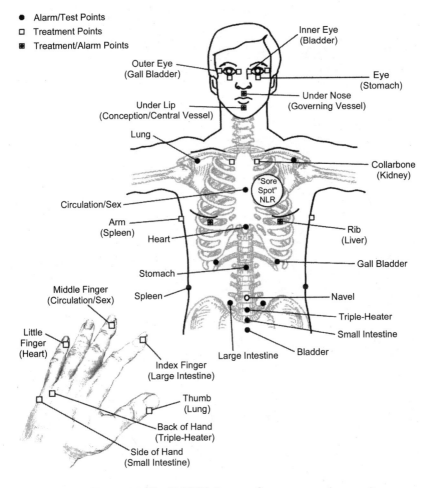

- ● Alarm/Test Points
- ☐ Treatment Points
- ▦ Treatment/Alarm Points

Inner Eye (Bladder)

Outer Eye (Gall Bladder)

Eye (Stomach)

Under Nose (Governing Vessel)

Under Lip (Conception/Central Vessel)

Lung

Collarbone (Kidney)

"Sore Spot" NLR

Circulation/Sex

Arm (Spleen)

Heart

Rib (Liver)

Gall Bladder

Stomach

Middle Finger (Circulation/Sex)

Spleen

Navel

Triple-Heater

Little Finger (Heart)

Small Intestine

Large Intestine

Bladder

Index Finger (Large Intestine)

Thumb (Lung)

Back of Hand (Triple-Heater)

Side of Hand (Small Intestine)

Figure 3.3 The EvTFT alarm and treatment points

fright, indecision, cowardice or lack of courage, lack of sexual interest, and lack of self assurance.

- *Spleen/pancreas (SP-21):* Worry, anxiety about the future, and pervasive anxiety are the emotions that dominate the spleen meridian. Not surprisingly, the spleen meridian figures prominently in the peak performance protocol discussed in Chapter 12.
- *Liver (LV-14):* Throughout Western and Eastern cultures, the liver has been associated with anger. This anger tends to be excessive, pervasive, and is generally directed at all things, not one specific target. It can involve denied gratification and can figure prominently in the addiction picture.

Table 3.1
Meridians: Alarm & Treatment Points

MERIDIAN	ALARM POINT LOCATION	TREATMENT POINT LOCATION
Bladder	One *tsun* above the center of pubic bone	Inside orbit of eye socket against bridge of nose (BL-1)
Gall Bladder	In line with the nipple, bottom of rib cage	Outside orbit of eye socket (GB-1)
Stomach	Halfway between the bottom of the sternum and the navel	With the eye looking straight ahead, directly below the pupil on the center of the lower eye socket (ST-1)
Governing Vessel	Under nose	Under nose (GV-27) at the center point between the upper lip and the nose
Conception Vessel	Under lip (in depression between lower lip & chin, NOT on chin)	Under lip (CV-24) at the depression between the lower lip and chin
Kidney	Tip of the 12th rib on the lower back	Collarbone point (K-27) in the hollow between the first rib and collarbone near the sternum
Spleen/Pancreas	On either side of torso where we bend, at bottom of 11th rib	Four inches under armpit (SP-21)
Liver	Upper edge of 8th rib, directly below nipple	Same place on rib (LV-14)
Small Intestine	Four *tsun* directly below navel	Outer edge of hand at crease from palm when fist is made (SI-3)
Triple Heater	Two *tsun* directly below the navel	Back of hand. 3rd Point of equilateral triangle between knuckle of little finger & ring finger (TH-3)
Lung	Outer side of pectoral area in space between shoulder and collarbone	The lower corner of the thumb-nail bed on the radial side (LU-11)
Large Intestine	One *tsun* down and one *tsun* to either side of the navel	Lower corner of the index fingernail bed on the radial side (LI-1)
Circulation/Sex	Just below center of sternum	Lower corner of the middle fingernail bed on the radial side (CX-9)
Heart	Just below bottom of sternum	Lower corner of the little fingernail bed on the radial side (HT-9)
Neurolymphatic Reflex (NLR) Area or the "Sore Spot"	This is *not* a meridian or alarm point	Upper left chest, about where you would put hand over the heart

Table 3.2

Meridians, Related Negative Emotions, and Psychological States

MERIDIAN	DIAMOND[1] CORRELATIONS	WHISENANT[2] CORRELATIONS	KAPTCHUK[3] CORRELATIONS
Bladder	Frustration, impatience, restlessness	Hypervigilence, Hyper arousal, Fear	
Gall Bladder	Rage, fury, wrath	Rage, power is blocked; control	Anger, indecision, timidity
Stomach	Disappointment, disgust, greed, emptiness, deprivation, bitterness	Phobia, schizophrenic process, anorexia, deprivation	
Governing Vessel	Embarrassment	Inferiority, powerless; money issues	
Conception Vessel	Shame	Negative sense of self; issues of self worth	
Kidney	Sexual Indecision	Fear	Fear, fright
Spleen	Future Anxiety	Fear, recklessness, morbid introspection	
Liver	Unhappiness	Anger (generalized); anger, unexpressed, irritability; depression; suspicious	Anger
Small Intestine	Sadness, sorrow	Over responsible, obsessive, compulsive, overwhelmed	
Triple Heater	Depression, despair, grief, hopelessness, despondency, loneliness,	Depression, mania, mood disorders	
Lung	Disdain, scorn, contempt, intolerance, prejudice, arrogance	Grief, sadness, poor self-concept	Sadness, grief
Large Intestine	Guilt	Clings to dysfunctional relationships; toxic interactions, commitment issues	
Circulation/Sex	Jealousy, sexual tension, regret	Impulse control, addiction, hysteria	
Heart	Anger	Control	

[1] Diamond (1985).
[2] Whisenant (1994).
[3] Kaptchuk (1983).

- *Lung (LU-11):* The hallmark emotions for this meridian are sadness and grief. It is interesting to note that in Western tradition lung cancer used to be called the "disease of the hopeless." (For example, physicians will sometimes tell stories of older patients who have recently lost a spouse succumbing to lung cancer within a very short time of their loved one's death.) The lung meridian is also associated with prejudice, intolerance, and disdain.

- *Large intestine (LI-1):* The emotion most strongly linked to this meridian is guilt. It can also be part of the clinical picture with people who are caught in dysfunctional relationships and those who have problems with attachment.

- *Circulation/sex (CX-9):* Many emotions and behaviors are related to this meridian, including those involving impulse control, addictive behavior, regret, remorse, jealousy, stubbornness, sexual tension or repressed sexual feeling, hysteria, and fear of punishment. This meridian can also be prominent in allergic reactions.

- *Small intestine (SI-3):* The main emotion associated with this meridian is vulnerability, including fear of injury or abandonment. It also is linked to obsessive thoughts, compulsive and perfectionist behavior, as well as overly responsible behavior.

- *Heart (HT-9):* This is the third meridian whose dominant negative emotion is anger. But whereas the gall bladder's anger is rageful and the liver's anger is pervasive, the anger of the heart meridian tends to be specifically directed at a particular person or target. The heart can also be associated with vengeance and control issues.

- *Triple heater (TH-3):* The associated emotions of this meridian are depression, sadness, hopelessness, grief, and despair. The triple heater has also been linked to pain control. From a clinical perspective, much "older emotional stuff" is frequently associated with this meridian.

- *Governing vessel (GV-27):* Emotional states connected with this vessel are frequently those involving embarrassment, willpower, inferiority, and lack of power. As distinct from the gall bladder, this lack of power concerns never having had adequate power or the ability to manipulate one's environment satisfactorily. Interestingly, money and employment issues tend to be evident with this meridian.

- *Conception vessel (CV-24):* The conception vessel seems to be associated with emotions about one's sense of self. This encompasses shame and feelings of being undeserving or not good enough. It is frequently associated with people who have been abused and with children of alcoholics. Often negative or defective core beliefs begin with an imbalance in the conception vessel.

Chapter 4

ACCESSING AND USING THE HUMAN PSYCHO-SOMA SYSTEM

The body never lies; however, we must ask
the right questions in the right way.
—George J. Goodheart, Jr.

This chapter outlines the history and basis of muscle testing (kinesiology), and explains how it is used with the acupuncture meridian system in Evolving Thought Field Therapy (EvTFT). The concept and procedures of therapy localization are also described, several forms of manual muscle testing are delineated, and research in the field is cited. Appropriate patient preparation and the issue of touching patients in order to muscle-test are addressed. The therapist's physical proximity in muscle testing is also discussed. When manual muscle testing reveals that the patient's energy system is not functioning optimally (e.g., neurologic disorganization), corrective treatments are offered.

THE INFLUENCE OF APPLIED KINESIOLOGY

Applied kinesiology (AK) is a subspecialty of chiropractic that developed from the work of George J. Goodheart, Jr. Muscle testing or kinesiology was originally developed by physical therapists as a means of diagnosing neuromuscular and musculoskeletal disorders. Pioneered in the 1930s by Robert W. Lovett, kinesiology was later advanced by the work of Florence Peterson Kendall and Henry Otis Kendall (Kendall & Kendall, 1949). In the early- to mid-1960s Goodheart incorporated a unique method of manual muscle testing developed by Kendall and Kendall that permitted evaluation of muscle and bodily function by comparing relative strength and weakness of an indicator muscle (Walther, 1988). Goodheart called his healing art *applied kinesiology*. Goodheart developed the system of AK by combining the muscle-testing response, the acupuncture meridian system, and his studies of the work of English medical and acupuncture researcher Felix Mann (Walther, 1988; Gallo, 1998). In his seminal text *Applied Kinesiology: Synopsis* (1988), David Walther details the mechanics and intricacies of this discipline and explains how Goodheart's central thesis—that the body is self-correcting and self-maintaining—is utilized in AK.

Goodheart correlated muscle responses as sensitive indicators of the body's neurological, lymphatic, respiratory, vascular, and energetic functioning, which included the mental and emotional realms (Gallo, 1998). He noticed that if patients touched certain areas on their body, or if their eyes were turned in a particular direction, that a change in muscle-test response often occurred. Goodheart also clinically experimented with the interconnection of organs, glands, and muscles with the acupuncture meridians, and he discovered the effectiveness of applied pressure and tapping on acupuncture points for treating physical disorders. What is relevant for the field of psychotherapy is that he observed that emotional problems were discernable by muscle-testing and could be corrected through nutritional and structural interventions (Walther, 1988).

Goodheart discovered that a patient's muscle would remain strong when thinking about something pleasant or factual, and it would weaken when thinking about something unpleasant or false. Goodheart deduced from this that thoughts and emotions were connected in some way to the acupuncture meridian system and were reflected in the body's muscular response.

Implications for EvTFT

For our purposes the meridian system is considered an energetic highway. We hypothesize that when the body energy is working properly, the energetic integrity is maintained as indicated by a strong muscle response when we think about events or facts that are pleasant and true. The energetic system is compromised when we think about unpleasant events or false information as indicated by a weak muscle response. Caution is necessary, however, when interpreting muscle-testing responses because there are various factors that can affect the results. Diamond (1988) expressed concern that some testers are not adept at the required skills and others are unaware of their own unconscious desires to obtain what may be misleading or preconceived results.

The idea that a muscle will go weak when a person hears or thinks of something unpleasant is not new. Many are familiar with the words, "sit down, I have some bad news for you." This is said in advance because the predicted response will be a weakening and perhaps a collapse of the muscles of support. We somehow know that our muscle system can weaken under physical or emotional stress. EvTFT and its predecessors use the phenomena of muscle strengths and weaknesses as an executive basis of the model. Frequency resonance coherence, a possible explanation of this phenomena, is explored in Chapter 15.

MANUAL MUSCLE TESTING

In EvTFT, muscle-testing is the method of exerting a small amount of physical force against a resisting muscle or muscle group in order to make a diagnostic determination. We are not seeking to evaluate the absolute power of the muscle, but rather the relational aspect of the muscle response with the thoughts and feelings of the individual. The therapist can then determine if the thought field has a stabilizing or weakening effect on the individual and use the muscle responses to guide treatment.

Developing the art and skill of manual muscle testing takes practice and experience. Learning how much pressure to apply to the patient's muscle, learning which muscle to test so as not to inadvertently cause discomfort to patients with existing injuries, and neutralizing tester bias are important skills to master.

The Validation of Muscle Testing

In the literature of applied kinesiology and physical therapy there are several studies as of 2003 that validate the effectiveness and efficacy of manual muscle testing. Notable among these was research done by Monti, Sinnott, Marchese, Kunkel, and Greeson (1999) in Philadelphia in which it was found that significant differences in muscle strength occurred when subjects were making congruent versus incongruent self-referential statements.

Not only has the validity of muscle testing itself been studied, the question of whether or not muscle testing by humans is as effective as muscle testing by machine has also been addressed. Despite attempts to mechanize muscle testing, Walther contends that the single best muscle-testing "instrument" is a well-trained human tester. He cites the double-blind studies of Constable and Hanicke (1987), which found a 78%

agreement between examiners testing the same subjects. Similarly, a 1981 study by Jacobs found an 81.9 % agreement between two testers (Walther, 1988).

This method of assessing information via manual muscle testing has been both heralded and criticized. Diamond wrote, "Indicator muscle testing is a major means whereby the process of life-energy analysis is carried out. It is an incredible research tool affording us instant access to the depths of the unconscious" (1988, p. 11). Diamond also views muscle-testing as "a test of the integrity of the acupuncture system" (p. 12). Psychiatrist David R. Hawkins described muscle testing as a source of "unlimited information about any subject, past or present" (1995, p. 10), a statement with paradigm shifting implications. Critics, however, are skeptical about the likelihood of tester manipulation and challenge the validity of muscle-testing responses. However, the aforementioned study by Monti et al. found, under tightly controlled procedures for tester and subject, that a significant difference did occur in muscle-test responses.

There are many other therapeutic techniques, which are not necessarily linked to thought field therapies, that make use of kinesiology methods. Among these are Touch for Health (Thie, 1979), behavioral kinesiology (Diamond, 1979), the neuro-emotional technique (Walker, 1990), Nambudripad allergy elimination technique (Nambudripad, 1993), and Brain Gym (Dennison, 1994); all of these methods use manual muscle testing as part of their protocol. The muscle-testing procedures are also used for a variety of other healing purposes, from diagnosing allergies and energy toxins to discovering nutritional deficiencies and prescribing medications and vitamins using Versendaal and Versendaal-Hoezee's contact reflex analysis (1993).

Explaining Muscle Testing to Patients

When explaining muscle-testing to the patient, we suggest that the therapist give some introductory information about EvTFT, along with a description of muscle testing. The explanations can be simple or detailed, depending on the level of comfort and sophistication of the patient. In some instances patients may have had prior experience with muscle testing by health care practitioners experienced in the various forms of applied kinesiology, especially chiropractic. Therapists might want to explain that muscle testing began as a form of diagnosis in physical therapy and that it evolved into the use of the muscle system as a form of biofeedback to guide the diagnostic process. We find most patients to be interested, curious, and open to an experience that they ultimately find validating. After experiencing muscle testing in the therapist's office, some patients might suggest the use of muscle testing to solve many of their other therapy issues. For example, in the course of one talk therapy session, Britt was discussing with a client which of many problems they should address that day. After a few moments, and with some slight exasperation at Britt's indecision, the patient said, "Why don't you just muscle-test me so we can get on with it!"

Touching Patients When Muscle-Testing

A primary consideration when using muscle testing is that therapists touch their patients briefly in a limited way. Muscle testing must be done in a professional and respectful manner with the full knowledge, permission, and understanding of the patient. Patients must be clearly informed about what is going to happen in the muscle-testing session, and their permission to proceed must be obtained.

A second consideration concerns the differences among various psychotherapeutic disciplines regarding patient contact. Physicians, psychiatrists, psychiatric nurses, chiropractors, and other health-care professionals include touching as a viable component to facilitate diagnosis and treatment. Accordingly, muscle testing is easily integrated within the framework of these disciplines. Psychotherapists who come from social work traditions are also comfortable with the minimal touching required in the EvTFT protocol. However, some psychologists at workshop trainings have inquired about the use of touch as part of psychotherapy. They wondered if touching for diagnosis would be a violation of ethical principles or the code of conduct. Based on our reading of the American Psychological Association's (APA) Ethical Principles of Psychologists and Code of Conduct, there would be no violation. The APA ethics code prohibits touch of an inappropriate sexual nature, which is clearly different from the touching required for muscle testing. In addition, it is neither necessary nor recommended that a therapist touch the acupuncture alarm or treatment points on the patient's body during the diagnosis and treatment procedures.

Muscle testing involves touching the patient either just above the wrist or at the fingers when employing a diagnostic procedure in EvTFT. We initially ask our patients, "Is it okay if I touch your wrist (or hand)?" and "Is it all right if I stand (or sit) this close to you?" These questions are asked at the beginning of each treatment session until the patient comfortably states that asking is no longer necessary. Some practitioners may want to obtain a written release before proceeding, especially if they follow the tradition of obtaining releases when practicing other methods of psychotherapy.

A core concern when initiating any form of psychotherapy is the safety of the patient. It is paramount that the patient feels safe when participating in EvTFT, and it is the therapist's duty to ensure that the patient feels safe and is safe. The therapist may know that EvTFT will do no harm, but the patient may be skeptical. Remember, these EvTFT methods are likely to be different from the patient's previous psychotherapy experiences. Accordingly, the therapist needs to consider the following questions:

1. Is there a history of trauma involving emotional, physical, and/or sexual abuse?
2. Are there serious transference or counter transference issues that are immediately evident?
3. Are there gender issues that could interfere with the minimal required touching? These issues may stem from questions 1 and 2.
4. Are there religious prohibitions to touching?
5. Is the patient uncomfortable having the therapist stand or sit close to him or her?
6. Are there physical problems that would preclude muscle-testing a particular muscle group?

If the answer is *yes* to any one of these questions, it would be prudent for the therapist to describe and discuss in more detail the muscle-testing component with the patient. Sometimes it takes a few sessions before a more fragile patient will allow a therapist to come into close physical proximity. It is better to be overly cautious with these patients than to move too quickly. It should be noted that once engaged in treatment, we have found such patients extremely amenable to muscle testing; more importantly, they are helped by the therapy. Trust in the therapist and the EvTFT methods must be earned. The therapist should be patient and gentle with this sensitive population.

The Mental Stance of the Therapist

Muscle testing is an elegant means of communicating both internally and interpersonally. Donna Eden noted in *Energy Medicine* that muscle testing "reinforces the link between your brain and subtle energies in your body, establishing new levels of internal communication. New areas of self-awareness begin to unfold" (1998, pp. 48–49). She elaborated by saying that muscle testing is comparable to "launching a communication in which your awareness is working in tandem with subtle energies" (p. 49).

We wish to state that muscle testing is not only an intrasubjective event, but also, an intersubjective one. It is clear to us that when Sigmund Freud wrote about transference and counter transference, he had become aware of the connections that can occur between human beings. However, Freud may have been unaware that humans cannot avoid an energetic connection, despite the noblest of efforts. Although we suggest that the therapist do everything possible to remain objective and neutral when muscle-testing a patient, we have come to think that such neutrality may never be possible. The therapist can, however, free himself or herself of preconceptions and expectations about the outcome of the muscle tests. This is important because such preconceptions and expectations can undermine neutrality in the degree of force the therapist uses when pushing on a muscle. The therapist should learn to exert a similar force on the muscle for both aspects of any response. The therapist can also influence the patient by way of subtle energy transfer without varying the pressure exerted on a muscle, and this influence is more difficult to control. The patient may read the therapist's intention or belief and respond accordingly, despite the therapist's efforts towards neutrality.[1]

Another more obvious objective is to intentionally avoid eye contact during muscle testing because much can be communicated with the eyes, certainly enough to influence the test. We recommend that therapists look just far enough away to keep the patient's face in their peripheral field of vision. We hypothesize that the therapist serves as a conduit, allowing the exchange of energetic information to assist in the diagnosis and treatment process.

To help foster a more objective stance, the therapist should clear his or her mind before conducting the muscle tests. There are many ways this mind clearing can be accomplished. Some involve taking a deep or cleansing breath, focusing on the still point (e.g., the place between the inhale and exhale), gazing at a focal point nearby, and reminding oneself to keep the mind open to the truth. Each therapist will find his or her own manner of maximizing the desired mental stance while muscle-testing.

Selecting and Qualifying the Indicator Muscle

In order to begin manual muscle testing one has to choose an appropriate muscle to test. Applied kinesiologists call this selecting an *indicator muscle* (IM). Although therapists have a choice of several different muscle groups in EvTFT, the most common muscle that is tested for the assessment of emotional problems in meridian-based psychotherapies is the deltoid (shoulder) muscle of an outstretched arm (Diamond, 1979; Durlacher, 1994; Gallo, 2000). Muscle testing the pectoral (chest) muscle, or pulling apart tightly held fingers (e.g., the thumb and any one of the fingers, may be used when testing of the deltoid muscle is not feasible (e.g., because of a neck or shoulder injury).

After selecting the indicator muscle (based on patient input and clinical judgment), the therapist then ascertains whether it is an appropriate muscle to use by performing the following procedure:

Muscle Testing in the Clear

After obtaining patient permission, ask the patient if he or she has any physical problems that would prohibit you from lightly pushing on the patient's arm to test the muscle response. Next, inquire which arm the patient feels most comfortable using; simply asking, "which arm do you prefer?" allows the patient to self-select. In order to isolate the deltoid muscle, have the patient extend the arm out straight and to the side, palm down, on a plane level with the shoulders, parallel to the floor, and perpendicular to the body (see Figure 4.1). The patient's other arm should hang free at his or her side. The same is also true for the tester.

As you are clearing your mind, you should ask the patient to do the same so that you can get the most accurate muscle response. Next, place

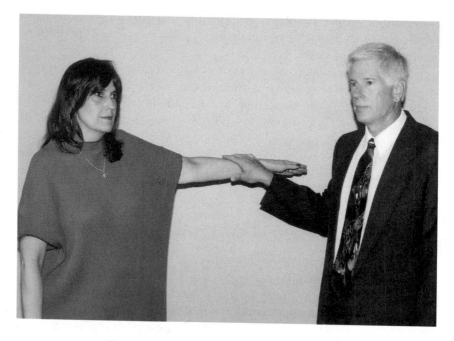

Figure 4.1 Muscle-testing in the clear (deltoid)

your hand just above the patient's wrist—remember to place pressure above the wrist on the forearm side—on the extended arm and ask the patient to, "hold" or "hold strong" (see Figure 4.2). If further clarification is needed you might remind the patient to "hold strong to keep your arm from being pushed down." Using a firm but gentle touch, press down for one to two seconds on the arm, exerting about 7 to 10 pounds of pressure. (To ascertain what is 7 to 10 pounds of pressure, press down on a bathroom scale placed at shoulder height.) In doing this, you will discover what "strong" feels like for the patient and thus establish a baseline for the indicator muscle. Generally, with a strong response, you will notice that the muscle seems to be in a locked position with no discernable weakness. The purpose is to get a feel for the muscle response while the patient is free of intentional thoughts and feelings. In applied kinesiology, this is known as testing in the clear.

Amount of Pressure or How Hard to Push

The amount of pressure needed to manual muscle-test can vary a great deal depending upon variables like size, strength, age, gender, and health of the patient and the therapist. Although the procedure of

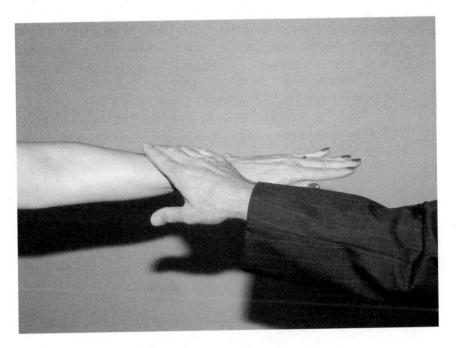

Figure 4.2 Hand placement above wrist

muscle-testing the deltoid is most often done with both parties standing, it can also be done with both parties seated. Testing a 16-year-old athletic boy is very different from testing a 75-year-old woman. Be careful to use only the amount of pressure needed to test the patient's muscle. All pressure should be applied in a smooth, continuous motion. There is never a need to force a muscle to give way. In this way you will also avoid hurting or unnecessarily fatiguing the muscle.

On occasion you may find that some clients try with all their might to resist when you are testing them. For these clients, you may want to remind them that this is not a wrestling contest or test of strength. State that muscle testing is a team effort and show the client the difference between being strong "with a fight" and simply being strong. Tell the patient that you simply need to determine relative strength for these testing conditions, rather than absolute strength.

Calibrating the Indicator Muscle

To further calibrate the response of the patient's indicator muscle and to get a feel for the patient's response style, the therapist can ask the patient to "hold" or "hold strong" while making a series of statements that require a *yes* or *no* response. Any true/false statement will suffice, but we routinely use the following:

1. Ask the patient to state his or her correct name using the following format: "Say, 'my name is . . . ,' and tell me your name." After the patient states his or her name, say, "hold" or "hold strong," and test the muscle response. The muscle should hold strong. Then say, "Tell me a name that is not your own [and not the therapist's]." After the patient states a phony name, say, "hold" or "hold strong," and test the muscle response. The muscle should test weak.
2. Following the same format, have the patient say, "two plus two equals four." Then say, "hold" or "hold strong," and test the muscle response. The muscle should test strong. Now have the patient say, "two plus two equals seven." Say, "hold" or "hold strong," and test the muscle response. The muscle should now test weak.
3. The same format is followed by having the patient now say, "Today is (say the correct day of the week)." Say, "hold" or "hold strong," and test the muscle response. The muscle should test strong. Then have the patient say, "Today is [say an incorrect day of the week]." Say, "hold" or "hold strong," and test the muscle response. The muscle should test weak.

When the patient makes a true statement, the muscle should remain strong. When a false statement is made, the muscle should weaken. As strength varies for each patient, so do manifestations of weak and strong muscle responses. Accordingly, weakness can mean anything from a person's arm dropping dramatically down to the side to a slight weakness signaled by a momentary lessening of resistance. Some patients are easy to manually muscle-test because the weakness is obvious, whereas others require greater sensitivity on the part of the therapist to discern muscle response changes.

It takes a great deal of practice to learn how to detect and adjust to the nuances of muscle testing and to become proficient at this skill. Therapists should be patient and open to what patients may teach them about their response style. In the beginning, we suggest that therapists practice muscle testing as much as possible with friends, family members, or colleagues to increase their ability. To further develop skills and confidence in the technique, therapists can also test "in the blind"; that is, ask practice partners a question to which the therapist does not know the answer (e.g., what is your mother's birth name?) and muscle-test their reply. For example, the practice partner could say, " My mother's name is Rosemary" and then "My mother's name is Gloria." The therapist tries to ascertain, via muscle testing, which answer is correct. This can also help the therapist clear his or her mind of expectations since the therapist has no idea of the outcome. Often a skeptical patient who alleges that the therapist pushed harder the second time, will respond positively to being tested "in the blind."

Muscle-Testing Children and Adolescents

When dealing with a child, it is always necessary to discuss the muscle-testing procedure with the parent or guardian and to obtain permission to proceed before introducing EvTFT. Demonstrating the process to the parent can help them understand the mechanics and put them at ease. Some therapists will illustrate the method by doing a small piece of work with the parent; for instance, helping them with their anxiety about the child's circumstance or disturbance. Depending upon the comfort level of the parent and child, the therapist's style, and the case circumstances, it might be advisable to have the parent remain in the room while conducting this portion of the treatment.

Children and adolescents are usually open to and intrigued by the EvTFT process, especially muscle testing. They tend to find it exciting, fun, and different from the other forms of therapy they have experienced, though sometimes they need an extended introductory phase so that they can play with the process. Many times children ask to muscle-test the therapist or their parents to see if it really works. Most often they are trusting and accepting of the results and do not require theoretical explanations.

However, children frequently need special instructions. The therapist should teach the child how to hold his or her arm (or fingers) and show the child what "hold" or "hold strong" means. Often, children, especially boys, will try to be extremely strong when tested, as if they were in a wrestling match. Like some adults they need to be shown the difference between "be strong" and "be strong with a fight."

Using Muscles Other Than the Deltoid

When it is not possible to use the deltoid muscle, or if the therapist or patient prefers to use another muscle, the therapist can consider using the following as the indicator muscle in the testing procedure. The therapist will get equal results using any of these alternative muscles.

The Pectoralis

This muscle group is located between the breast and the collarbone. One way to isolate the pectoralis for muscle testing is to have the patient extend his or her arm straight out in front, holding it at shoulder level and perpendicular to the body with the thumb pointed downwards and palm facing outwards (see Figure 4.3). Take a position in front of and slightly to the side of the extended arm. Place your fingers just above the patient's wrist near the topside of the forearm. Clear your mind and ask the patient to clear his or her mind. Then ask the patient to "hold" or "hold strong" while you push against the patient's arm to the outside. Use about seven to ten pounds of pressure for one to two seconds. This will begin to establish your baseline strong response. Now proceed with the set of yes/no or true/false statements to get a feel for the difference between strong and weak responses.

Another way to use the pectoralis is to invite the patient to extend a straight arm forward with palm facing down. Position yourself in front of the patient and place your hand over top of the patient's extended arm with the palm of your hand on his or her forearm just above the wrist, as shown in Figure 4.4. Proceed to calibrate the indicator muscle as previously described.

Using the Fingers

Finger testing may be ideal for many patients and therapists where size or strength differences are of concern. This finger-testing alternative

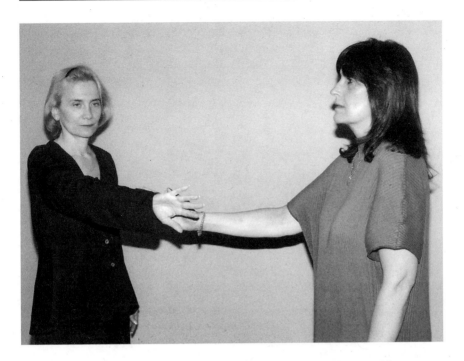

Figure 4.3 Muscle-testing the pectoralis (pushing to the outside)

allows both parties to remain seated; it is physically easy for patients who have neck and shoulder problems that preclude their arms from being tested, and it can be less tiring for some patients. Sometimes the tester may be physically weak or small in comparison to some patients, so finger testing provides an excellent substitute and yields the same results as the other indicator muscles.

To test the finger muscles, have the patient touch his or her thumb to the index finger, forming the OK sign as shown in Figure 4.5. Using your thumb and index finger, lightly grasp the patient's fingers by placing your thumb over the nail of his or her thumb and your index finger under the pad of the patient's thumb. Grasp the patient's index finger in the same way, using your other hand (see Figures 4.6 and 4.7). Clear your mind and ask the patient to clear his or her mind. Then ask the patient to "hold" or "hold strong" while you attempt to pull apart the fingers. This will begin to establish your baseline strong response. Now proceed with the set of yes/no or true/false statements to get a feel for the difference between strong and weak responses. Proceed to calibrate the indicator muscle as previously described.

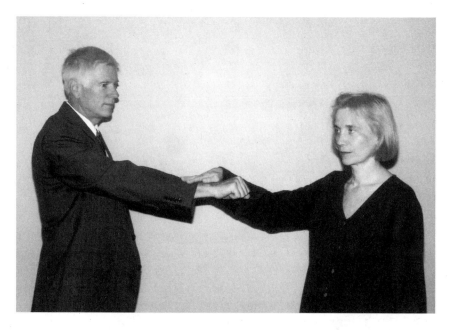

Figure 4.4 Muscle-testing the pectoralis (pushing down)

When the thumb and forefinger are too strong to permit the therapist to pull the fingers apart, try testing the thumb paired with the middle or ring finger. You may also test the thumb and the little finger to further reduce the strength factor.

Troubleshooting Variations in Muscle Response

In the EvTFT protocol, when a patient demonstrates a weak muscle response to a true statement and a strong muscle response to a false statement, or the patient muscle-tests the same to both statements (i.e., either strong/strong or weak/weak), corrective action is warranted. The following are first line methods of corrections. The discussion relevant to these corrections is continued in Chapter 6.

Weak/Weak Response

Here the patient is unable to maintain a strong muscle response and shows a weak response to both positive and negative statements. When this happens in the beginning of treatment, have the patient drink two to eight ounces of water. Often these patients are dehydrated, which adversely affects their ability to hold a strong muscle. This small amount

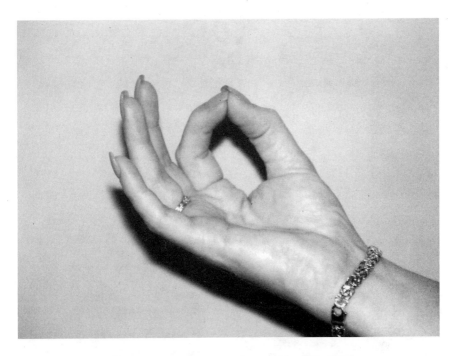

Figure 4.5 Muscle-testing fingers (the OK sign)

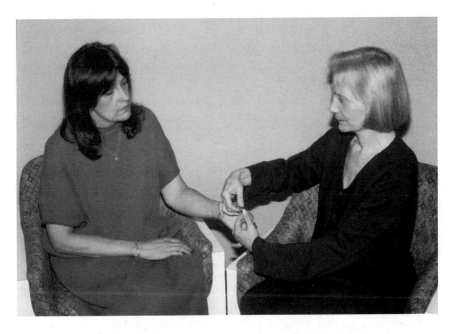

Figure 4.6 Muscle-testing patient using fingers

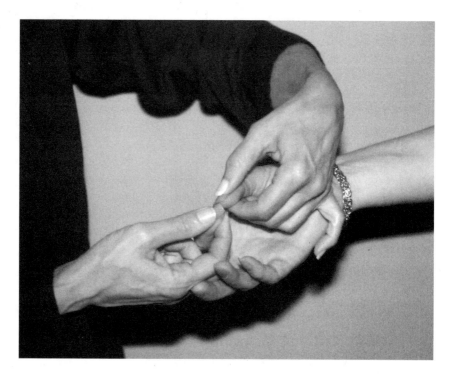

Figure 4.7 Muscle-testing fingers (close up)

of water usually restores strength, and thus the ability to demonstrate a differentiated (strong/weak) muscle response. Testing for hydration is described on page 68.

There are, however, reasons other then dehydration for a weak/weak muscle response. For example, during treatment and after an extended time engaging in muscle testing diagnosis, the patient's muscle may become fatigued because of the frequent muscle tests. At these times it is prudent to ask if the patient's indicator muscle (e.g., arm) is tired. This is more often the case than not. When a patient confirms the tiredness, switch to the other arm or another muscle group. In Chapter 6 we discuss other methods of working with a weak/weak response that may arise during the course of treatment.

Strong/Strong Response

Here the patient shows a strong muscle response to both positive and negative statements. Sometimes this happens because the therapist is a novice with muscle testing and unsure how much pressure to use on the muscle. However, if you are experienced with muscle testing you may need to explore other options. First, you could shift to a different indicator muscle to see if you can get a differentiated response with that muscle. This strong/strong response can result from a number of conditions (e.g., therapist or environmental influences,[2] food or clothing); however, in order to obtain the diagnoses, this response pattern needs to be cleared or corrected. We suggest doing one (or more if needed) of the several energy correction methods described later in this chapter.

When the energy correction methods fail to "unlock" the muscle to obtain the working polarized response, the therapist must endeavor to discover another possible cause. The strong/strong muscle response is interesting in that it can result from the unintentional influence of the therapist. Callahan and Callahan (1996) conjectured that such a muscle response results from the therapist being *psychologically reversed*. We have observed that it may also stem from the therapist sharing an issue (usually unresolved) with the patient, about which the therapist may be reversed. It is strongly recommended that the therapist treat himself or herself for the possibility of reversal when demonstrating the energy corrections to the patient. These concepts will be detailed in Chapter 6.

A strong/strong response may also be indicative of an environmental influence. For example, Diepold observed that a student athlete demonstrated a strong/strong muscle response that was uncorrectable with the various energy correction methods. This was highly unusual because the young man had a history of polarized muscle responses over a several month period. In asking him if anything was different, it turned out he was wearing a new unlaundered wrestling tournament shirt that his coach had just given him. Since he had another shirt with him, he was asked to change shirts. Now, surprisingly, he demonstrated the working polarized muscle response. When he put the new shirt back on, he once again demonstrated the strong/strong "locked" muscle response. Moreover, when he merely held the new shirt in his hand at his side he could not be muscle-tested. After the shirt was washed several times the suspected interfering properties disappeared, and he was able to wear it and demonstrate working polarized muscle responses.

Reversed Muscle Test Response

Here the patient muscle-tests weak to a true statement and strong to a false statement. This response pattern suggests that there is an issue with body polarity that warrants correction before proceeding. The subject of polarity and the reversed muscle-test response is described fully in Chapter 6.

Hydration Testing

Water, which makes up about 70 percent of the human body, is needed for virtually every biological process, chemical reaction, and mechanical action that takes place in the body. Thus, it is important that the patient be adequately hydrated in order for their muscles to function appropriately for muscle testing. If a subject is showing a weak/weak response to testing in the clear, then inadequate hydration is usually the issue. The following two hydration testing methods are adapted from Touch for Health (Thie, 1973): (1) Muscle-test indicator muscle while the patient tugs lightly on his or her hair; (2) Muscle-test indicator muscle while the patient presses gently on the tip of his or her nose. The second method is preferred for abused patients, who may have had their hair pulled during the abuse; this method will avoid triggering them. When the indicator muscle is weak, have the person drink two to eight ounces of water.

NEUROLOGIC DISORGANIZATION/SWITCHING

The condition of *neurologic disorganization* (ND), as used in applied kinesiology, "appears to result from afferent receptors sending conflicting information for interpretation by the central nervous system" (Walther, 1988, p. 147). When a therapist is using manual muscle testing, "it is necessary that the nervous system be organized to provide correct information . . . disorganization may also result in failure to find dysfunction or may indicate problems that are not actually present" (p. 148). Walther further wrote that "the most common cause of neurologic disorganization is dysfunction of the cranial sacral primary respiratory mechanism" (p. 150), which comes from the structural side of the triad of health. ND may also result from imbalances generated on the chemical/nutritional side or the mental side. Robert Blaich (1988) speculated that the phenomenon of ND occurs naturally in a transformation process whenever the body adjusts to new limits of higher performance after being pushed beyond the usual comfort zone. In this regard, diagnosis and treatment of ND is critical to attainment of higher levels of functioning.

The concept of ND, also called *switching*, becomes important in EvTFT when the therapist begins to get nonpolarized muscle responses from the patient. At a more subtle level, it may also become evident when the therapist notices a pattern of single point drops in the subjective units of distress (SUD) level, or no drop at all, while using EvTFT methods. It is important to remember that when ND is active, diagnostic information may become misleading, and treatment results may be compromised.

There are many behavioral indicators that ND might be influencing the patient. Here are several easily recognized signs that suggest ND:

1. Gait irregularities, as evidenced by an unbalanced and/or truncated arm swing (e.g., one arm swinging considerably more or less than the other, or a lack of a swing in either or both arms while walking).
2. Experience of physical awkwardness or clumsiness at the extreme end, and coordination inconsistency where timing and performance abilities are off at the lesser end.
3. A pattern of transposing letters or numbers, and even words.
4. A pattern of reversing two intended actions (e.g., putting an empty glass in the refrigerator and the milk carton in the sink).
5. A pattern of falling asleep while reading, regardless of the fatigue level of the person.
6. A left/right confusion whereby the patient states or points in one direction but means the other (e.g., directing someone to go left when he or she mean, right).
7. Patient history of learning difficulties involving aphasia, delayed speech, stuttering, below-level reading performance, poor quality handwriting, frequent spelling errors, and others such difficulties are also suggestive of ND according to the work of Delacato (Blaich, 1988).

The primary test for the presence of ND, as used in thought field therapy, was originally described by Callahan (e.g., 1998). This evaluation method requires the patient to touch (therapy localize) the collarbone treatment points (K-27) in a sequential and alternating pattern while being muscle-tested. The therapist muscle-tests the patient eight times using eight different hand or finger positions representing changes in body polarity and cross lateralization. When the patient demonstrates neurologic organization, the indicator muscle should remain strong through all the tests. However, a single weak muscle response is suggestive of ND, and corrective treatment is recommended. The testing steps to evaluate ND are as follows:

1. Have patient touch (therapy localize) the *right* collarbone point (K-27) with the palmar side of the fingers of his or her *right* hand while you are muscle-testing an indicator muscle on his or her left side.
2. Have patient touch the *left* collarbone point (K-27) with the palmar

side of the fingers of the *right* hand while you are muscle-testing an indicator muscle on his or her left side.

3. Have patient touch the *right* collarbone point (K-27) with the knuckles of his or her *right* hand while you are muscle-testing an indicator muscle on his or her left side.

4. Have patient touch the *left* collarbone point (K-27) with the knuckles of the *right* hand while you are muscle-testing an indicator muscle on his or her left side.

5. Now reverse the procedure. Use the left hand to therapy localize and the right arm to muscle-test. Follow the same pattern as described in steps 1 through 4. See Figures 4.8 and 4.9 for examples of hand placements.

If the indicator muscle weakens at any of these test points then some degree of ND is evident. However, the therapist may go through all the test points to observe the complete pattern presented by the patient. When indicated, we recommend treatment using the brief energy correction, the simplified collarbone breathing treatment, or the neurologic organizer treatment, depending on the place in treatment or patient pat-

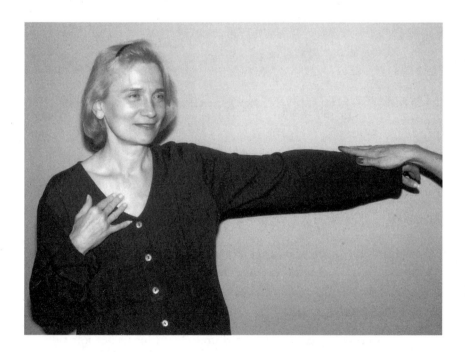

Figure 4.8 Muscle-testing for neurologic disorganization (fingers)

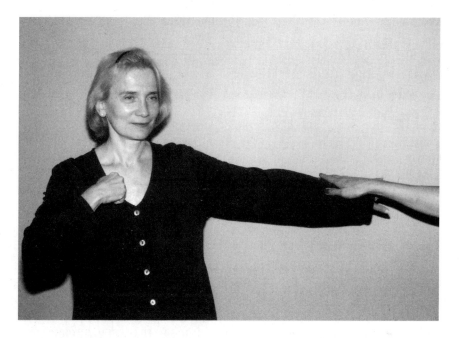

Figure 4.9 Muscle-testing for neurologic disorganization (knuckles)

terns as described in the following section. Upon completion of any treatment for ND, all test points that initially tested weak should be retested. The correction and restoration of neurologic organization are thought to be successful when the indicator muscle responds strong when therapy localization testing is repeated.

Treatments for Neurologic Disorganization

The simplified collarbone breathing (SCB) treatment, the neurologic organizer treatment (NOTx), and the brief energy correction (BEC) were developed by The BDB Group as alternative procedures in response to patient resistance and noncompliance with Callahan's original collarbone breathing treatment. These procedures take less time and are simpler to perform and easier to remember. They are also more user-friendly and appear to be as effective as Callahan's original method. The three alternative methods all use the touch-and-breathe (TAB) treatment approach. SCB and NOTx incorporate two additional phases of respiration that are commonly used in applied kinesiology interventions. The BEC, which is the briefest of the three, is derived from the basic unswitching procedures used in applied kinesiology (Walther, 1988).

SCB and NOTx can be used prior to the start of the EvTFT protocol, as well as during treatment if the need arises. These neurologic organizers may also be effective treatments on their own for a variety of symptoms with some patients.[3] In keeping with the findings of Blaich (1988), we have integrated these neurologic organizing treatments into our workshops as a teaching aid to facilitate the learning of a great deal of information in a short amount of time. More specifically, the BDB Group workshops impart a great deal of information, which can be overwhelming to participants because of the paradigm shift. Thus, we have attendees repeatedly practice neurologic organizing techniques in order to assist their efficient assimilation of information. Participants often report that they think more clearly about the material being presented, and feel more refreshed, less anxious, and more ready to learn. As mentioned previously, we base our use of neurologic organizing techniques in our workshops on a 1988 study by Robert Blaich titled "Applied Kinesiology and Human Performance," in which participants were "pushed to perform past their comfort zone" (p. 8). Blaich found that using a treatment for ND that included therapy localizing to the collarbone points, the eight phases of respiration, and Callahan's correction for psychological reversal increased the average rate of reading two and a half times over base rates. Blaich (1988) further commented that

> Since a high percentage of the participants developed or redeveloped ND by being forced to read beyond their comfort zone, but then were able to read 25% faster with just being unswitched, it could be speculated that being pushed beyond one's comfort zone creates or recreates ND which, if corrected allows the people to expand their comfort zone and obtain and maintain a new level of performance. (p. 11)

Neurologic organizing treatments have a broad range of application. Britt uses SCB and NOTx to treat patients who experience continual, inappropriate sexual arousal. Diepold strongly recommends the use of these approaches with athletes before and after practice, games, matches, and races to help the athlete obtain higher levels of performance. These treatments also appear to help academic activities when performed prior to starting homework, writing a report, reading, or studying, and when there is a type of "brain lock" typified by blockage in creativity or the inability to find the right words for what the person wants to write. Treatments can be useful in all performing arts as well.

Simplified Collarbone Breathing
Treatment (SCB)

The collarbone treatment points are located approximately one inch down and one inch over from the sternal notch, in the hollow between the collarbone and the top rib, near the sternum. When doing SCB, the patient is instructed to continuously touch the collarbone points while performing the following breathing sequence:

The Breathing Sequence

1. Breathe normally, one full respiration.
2. Take a full breath in and hold for two seconds.
3. Gently force more breath in and hold for two seconds.
4. Let breath out about halfway and hold for two seconds.
5. Let breath all the way out and hold for two seconds.
6. Gently force more breath out and hold for two seconds.
7. Take a half breath in and hold for two seconds.

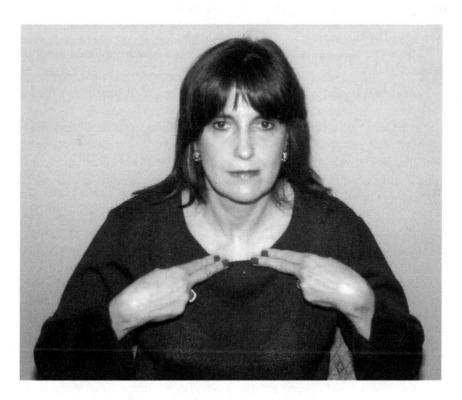

Figure 4.10 SCB—using the collarbone (K-27) treatment points

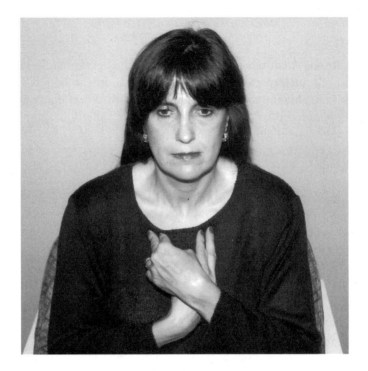

Figure 4.11 SCB—using the collarbone (K-27) treatment points (cross-over)

8.　Breathe normally.

*The Touching Positions and the Placement of Finger
and Knuckles*

Fingertips are on the palmar side of the hand and knuckles are on the dorsal side of the hand. Palmar and dorsal sides of the hand have a different polarity, which is discussed in Chapter 6.

1.　Place fingertips (usually the tips of the index and middle fingers) of the right hand on the right collarbone point (K-27) and fingertips of the left hand on the left collarbone point, as shown in Figure 4.10. Do respiration sequence as previously described.
2.　Place knuckles of the right hand on the right collarbone point (K-27) and knuckles of the left hand on the left collarbone point. Repeat the respiration sequence.
3.　Cross your hands at the wrists and place the fingertips of the right hand on the left collarbone point (K-27) and the fingertips of the left hand on the right collarbone point, as shown in Figure 4.11. Repeat the respiration sequence.

4. Keep hands crossed and place the knuckles of the right hand on the left collarbone point (K-27) and the knuckles of the left hand on the right collarbone point. Repeat the respiration sequence.

The Collarbone Breathing Exercise: Historical Note

Callahan's collarbone breathing exercise (Callahan & Trubo, 2001) uses five breathing positions; he does not use the forcing of more breath in and out, as well as the final normal breathing components. The BDB Group, however, chooses to maintain these components in keeping with procedures originating in applied kinesiology (e.g., Walther, 1988; Blaich, 1988). We, like the practitioners of applied kinesiology, have found the effects from the two forced breath positions advantageous, and in fact find their use beneficial in working with all populations and

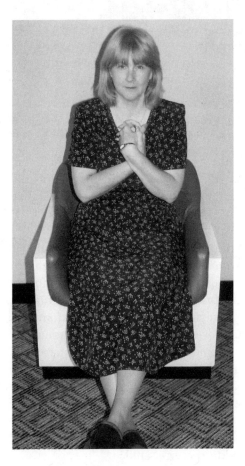

Figure 4.12 The neurologic organizer treatment (NOTx) position

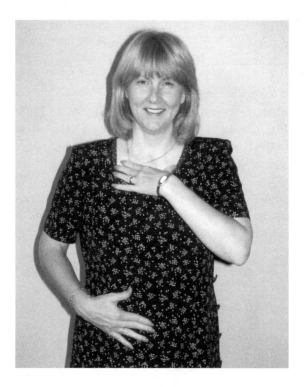

Figure 4.13 The brief energy correction (BEC; position 1)

consistent with some practices of yoga, music, and voice training. Callahan's exercise also differs from ours in that he instructs the patient to continually tap on the gamut spot (back of the hand at TH-3).

The Neurologic Organizer Treatment (NOTx)

This neurologic organizing treatment was developed by The BDB Group and is an amalgam of the collarbone breathing exercise and the over energy correction.[4] It clears ND and is easy for clients to learn and perform. It is a treatment that is routinely prescribed for use in anxiety reduction before studying, any practice or performance activity, and as needed to maintain overall neurologic organization and while doing the EvTFT protocol. Some users have dubbed the exercise "square knot breathing" because of the left-right opposed positions of the ankles and wrists, which is analogous to tying a square knot (left over right, then right over left; see Figure 4.12).

A. Ankle and wrist positions
　　1. Place *left* ankle *over right* ankle.
　　2. Put hands out straight, back to back.

3. Place *right* wrist *over left* hand.
4. Interlock fingers, fold hands in, and rest knuckles high on the chest in the area of the collarbone points (K-27).

B. Breathing pattern
   1. Take three normal respirations.
   2. Place tongue tip on the roof of mouth and take one full respiration.
   3. Place tongue tip on the floor of mouth and take one full respiration.
   4. Relax tongue and do the following:
      a. Take a full breath in and hold for two seconds.
      b. Force more breath in and hold.
      c. Let breath about half way out and hold.
      d. Let breath all the way out and hold.
      e. Force more breath out and hold.
      f. Take a half breath in and hold.
      g. Breathe normally.

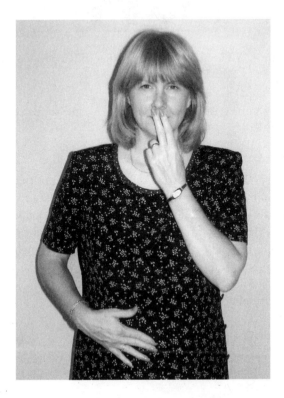

Figure 4.14 The brief energy correction (BEC; position 2)

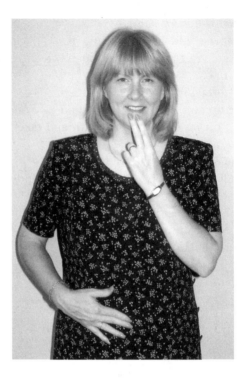

Figure 4.15 The brief energy correction (BEC; position 3)

Reverse ankle and wrist positions in step A, and repeat entire breathing pattern in B.

The Brief Energy Correction

The brief energy correction (BEC) is another procedure that can be used as a treatment for neurologic dosorganization (ND), and is ideal when polarity problems are noticed early in treatment. It consists of a sequence of steps that derive from applied kinesiology and the Basic Unswitching Procedure (Gallo, 1998) and the use of the touch-and-breathe method. Although a treatment for ND, we primarily use the BEC for treatment of nonpolarized and reversed muscle responses in the hand over head polarity check, as discussed in Chapter 6.

A. Place fingertips of one hand on the navel.
B. With the other hand do the following:
   1. Touch both collarbone points (K-27) and take one full respiration (see Figure 4.13).

2. Touch under the nose (GV-26) and take one full respiration (see Figure 4.14).

3. Touch under the lip (CV-24) and take one full respiration (see Figure 4.15).

4. With the palm of the hand, touch the base of the spine and take one full respiration (see Figure 4.16).

C. Now place the opposite hand on the navel.

D. With the other hand, repeat the same four steps in B above.

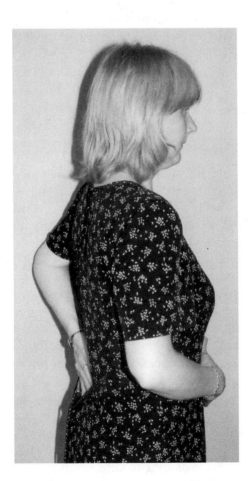

Figure 4.16 The brief energy correction (BEC; position 4)

Chapter 5

THE TOUCH-AND-BREATHE
TREATMENT TECHNIQUE

And the Lord God formed man of the dust of
the ground, and breathed into his nostrils the
breath of life; and man became a living being.
                                        —Genesis 2:7

This chapter details the discovery and use of touch-and-breathe (TAB),[1] the procedure used in lieu of tapping in all Evolving Thought Field Therapy (EvTFT) treatments. A historical overview of tapping and TAB are described from both Western and Eastern traditions. The argument is made that clinical observations indicate that TAB is more user-friendly, as well as more congruent with current information and research about the human bioenergy system.

Roger Callahan (1985) introduced the method of using fingers to tap designated acupoints (e.g., 5 to 50 times) for the treatment of negative emotions, as well as for dealing with blocks to successful treatment (psychological reversal). He reasoned that tapping transmitted external kinetic energy that is transduced and integrated into the body's energy system,[2] which then has a direct influence on the perturbations in the specific thought field being addressed. However, there is no empirical evidence from experimental studies to support that it is specifically the tapping that facilitates the rapid emotional resolve. While other means of stimulating acupoints are available (e.g., rubbing, pressure holding, cold lasers, and even imagining tapping on an acupoint), Diepold (2000) reported that the TAB approach used with EvTFT is more congruent with the growing body of information about the human body's subtle energy system. Thus far, TAB has been shown to be equally, if not more, effective and user-friendly than tapping. Perhaps the practice of "tapping" into the body's energy system has been taken too literally. Let's first examine where the tapping concept originated.

80

RATIONALE FOR TAPPING

The practice of using the fingertips to tap as percussion tools on acupuncture points for the treatment of psychological problems was a choice of Callahan in his Callahan Techniques™ over 20 years ago. Callahan's decision to adopt tapping was influenced by his study of applied kinesiology (AK) with Walther and Blaich, and the work of Goodheart. In *Applied Kinesiology: Synopsis*, Walther described a meridian treatment approach in AK called the *entry or exit point*, which involves stimulating the entry or exit acupoints of the meridians located on the fingers and toes. Walther wrote that "stimulation of these points helps transmit energy from one meridian to the next, if there is a blockage in the continuity" (1988, p. 210). The use of entry or exit points, coupled with the AK beginning-and-ending technique, which involves tapping the beginning or ending acupoints of meridians that begin or end on the head, appears to have served as the foundation for Callahan's choices of which meridian points to tap. Nearly all the treatment points in the Callahan Techniques™ are on, or close to, the beginning or ending points of the involved meridians.

In *Five-Minute Phobia Cure*, Callahan wrote: "Rhythmic tapping at a specific point on a meridian will improve the condition of the associated vital organ. This, they[3] say, occurs because the 'energy flow' within that meridian is freed to move again" (1985, p. 32).

Callahan also presented additional statements in support of tapping. For example, in *The Rapid Treatment of Panic, Agoraphobia, and Anxiety* (1990) he stated:

> The tapping provides an external source of energy which, when done correctly, at the right spot, with the mind tuned to the problem being treated, balances the energy in a particular energy system in the body which is suffering from a deficiency or imbalance. We hypothesize that the energy from tapping is transduced into the system into usable energy as needed. (p. 7)

Callahan (1992) later commented on his practical and theoretical ideas related to tapping.

> The points we tap are related to the ancient meridians of acupuncture. Tapping the PROPER point when the person is thinking of the problem is quite effective. . . . It appears to me that these points are transducers of energy; where the physical energy of tapping can be transduced into the appropriate (probably electromagnetic) energy of

the body so that the person with a problem can be put into proper balance by a knowledgeable person. (p. 11)

Although Gallo wrote about other treatment methods like rubbing, pressure holding, imagined tapping, and use of cold lasers on acupoints as "effective at times" (1999, p. 150), no other method of stimulation has captured the attention of psychotherapists. Despite the fact that there is no evidence to support tapping in preference to other methods, tapping on the meridian treatment points continues to be the most widely used treatment approach employed with meridian-based psychotherapies. As a result, thought field therapy and many of the meridian-based psychotherapies are sometimes called *tapping therapies*.

Although the authors have tapped our way to psychotherapeutic success hundreds of times, we did encounter resistance to tapping in both our patients and ourselves. This did not reflect on the efficacy or non-efficacy of treatment, but more on the delivery of treatment. Like good clinicians we observed our patients and began to notice patterns of resistance to the treatment. More importantly, we began to notice certain behaviors during treatment delivery that caused us to speculate about treatment options in the context of patient needs and preferences, and in accordance with the increasing information about subtle energy fields.

These observations and theoretical musings formed the basis of the paper Diepold presented in 1998 in which he offered an alternative to tapping, *touch-and-breathe* (TAB; Diepold, 1998). There was a great deal of excitement when Diepold presented TAB because for many therapists, it was the answer to many of the problems encountered with tapping.[4]

THE ORIGIN OF THE TAB APPROACH

Watching and listening to patients while they tapped proved highly interesting and informative, and Diepold observed that if patients were not reminded of the number of taps to use, they would often tap as many times as matched a full respiration before inquiring or looking for guidance. Noting the respiration and posture of patients, Diepold shared his observations and believed that he noticed an important behavior when other therapists reported that a full breath or sigh (from the patient) often accompanied the tapping procedures. These discussions led to the sharing of other information that validated that the level of discomfort about tapping that patients admitted to their therapists was more extensive than was acknowledged in any of the written literature.

Patients were occasionally heard to make statements such as: This looks stupid. I feel silly. I can't do this in public. It hurts if I do tapping too much. Tapping distracts me. I couldn't remember how many times I was told to tap. How hard do I tap? Accordingly, compliance with "homework" as follow-up self-care between sessions also suffered because of concerns like those voiced above. One other important problem that had not been addressed was revealed when some therapists related that this method was completely out of the question for some of their patients who were victims of abuse and refused to tap on themselves because they related the tapping to abuse.

In response, Diepold began to question the mechanisms and importance of tapping as the delivery of stimulation for treatment. His observations and theoretical explorations ultimately led to his development of the TAB approach to treatment. To Diepold's amazement, every patient to whom he introduced TAB preferred the TAB approach to the tapping. Users of TAB also reported more profound, comfortable, focused, and relaxing effects with this treatment approach. TAB has been presented to and utilized by hundreds of therapists since 1998. Anecdotal reports have supported the initial findings that patients respond positively and treatment is successful. Although it is impossible to know if treatment is more successful than tapping, it is reasonable to assume that patient compliance is important to treatment success, and TAB produces more patient compliance than tapping does in a variety of circumstances. Since 1998 we have exclusively employed TAB with patients and in our workshops while working within the thought field therapy protocols.

MECHANISMS FOR TAPPING: THE PIEZOELECTRIC EFFECT

Goodheart wrote that prolonged tapping for nearly two minutes or more on the first tonification point of an involved meridian provided the "proper stimulus" to relieve pain. He reasoned in regard to the process of tapping that "a steadier type of stimulation would cause adaptation; the fibers being stimulated are large fibers which adapt to constant stimulation. If your tapping is adequate stimulation, the muscle will now test strong" (quoted in Walther, 1988, p. 263). While describing Goodheart's utilization of the Melzack and Wall gate control theory of pain in AK, Walther wrote, "The most productive tapping is when there is a bony backup to the tonification point. If possible, direct the tapping to obtain a bony backup" (p. 263). For that reason it is speculated that tapping may cause a piezoelectric effect due to bone stimulation at the acupuncture points. The piezoelectric effect occurs when tiny amounts of generated electrical current result from stimulating the crystallized calcium in the bone and thus impact the meridian system (Gallo, 1998). Walther (1988), however, wrote an interesting hypothesis about the failure of tapping to yield results, as in the failure to obtain pain reduction:

> Another factor that may cause less than adequate results with the Melzack-Wall technique is *tapping at an improper frequency* [italics added]. It is often necessary to reduce the tapping rate. Two to four Hz appear to be the most productive. (p. 263)

Several writers and practitioners (e.g., Callahan, 1995; Durlacher, 2000; Gallo, 1998, 2000; Lambrou & Pratt, 2000) have speculated that tapping creates a piezoelectric effect that puts a form of energy *into* the meridians, perhaps via the receptive antenna-like capability of the acupoints. In addition, they propose that adding the needed energy restores a balance to the flow of chi/energy in the meridians. Their assumption is that the added chi/energy from tapping eliminates the meridian deficiency, which is reflected in the change of indicator muscle response.

Walther (1988) reported that Goodheart observed "an antenna effect" regarding the acupoints that he believed could be easily demonstrated. Durlacher (2000) described a paper presented in 1974 at a meeting of the International College of Applied Kinesiology by Robert Pearlman, a chiropractor colleague in which such a demonstration was presented. Pearlman reported on the electromagnetic aspects of acupuncture energy and the antenna properties of stainless steel acupuncture needles. He observed that when the insertion of an acupuncture needle corrected a meridian disruption as measured by manual muscle testing, placing a leaded ceramic cup over the acupuncture needle negated the previously observed results. He concluded that the lead blocked the meridian from receiving (via the needle in the acupoint) the required subtle energy needed to effect a correction.

If we take this as the model, one could say that TAB is similar to what happens when a person touches the antennae of a television set that is not cable-connected. When static interference distorts the sound or the picture received through the antenna, often just touching and holding the antenna, without moving the position, is enough to clear the problem. In this example, touch enables the body to function as an energetic extension of the physical antenna and to refine the television's reception. However, as soon as you release your hand from the antenna the static problem recurs until you adjust the antennae and locate the optimal position for reception. In keeping with the television metaphor, the TAB method

1. extends and maximizes the bioenergetic contact at the acupoints by touch,
2. uses the body's natural function of breath to facilitate the flow of subtle energetic influences (chi), which
3. facilitates the combined antenna/transmitter capacity of the acupoints.

This combination of sustained touching and breathing, while attuned to the target thought field, enables the acupoints to receive and transmit chi influence and hypothetically establish a homeostatic condition called *frequency resonance coherence*, which will be described in Chapter 15. Most important, however, is that this gentle breath-assisted touch serves to focus intention in a mindful and effortless fashion.

THE ANCIENT SYSTEM OF ANMA AND THE MUDRAS

The TAB approach with meridian-based psychotherapy (EvTFT) may have similar mechanisms of action as the ancient system of *anma* and the mudras. Diepold had no knowledge of mudras prior to his participation in the First Energy Psychology Conference in Europe[5] in Furigen, Switzerland, in July 2001. There, in a conversation about TAB, Donna Eden[6] commented that TAB was similar to mudras. Diepold had never heard the term *mudra* before, but he made a point to learn about them. Two months later, Graham Anderson, a colleague from Australia who had read about TAB on the Internet sent Diepold an e-mail inquiring if he was familiar with *The Book of Life* (1979) by Roshi Jiyu-Kennett and Daizui MacPhillamy (personal communication, September 27, 2001). This book is about mudras.

The use of mudras has an ancient origin and relates to the harmonization of mind and body via the cleansing of karma. According to MacPhillamy (Jiyu-Kennett & MacPhillamy, 1979), the art of *anma* can be traced through tradition to the period of the legendary Chinese Yellow Emperor more than 4,500 years ago as described in a document known as the *Nei Ching*. The oldest account in existence of this ancient art was written by Wang Ping and dates to 762 CE. MacPhillamy states that acupuncture, moxibustion, shiatsu, and many other related arts stem from these ancient practices.

Buddhism encountered the *anma* arts upon its entrance to China during the first century CE. At that time *anma* was already fully integrated with the traditional Daoist cosmology regarding the interaction of yin and yang. While Buddhists did not necessarily accept the Daoist explanation for the success of *anma*, the *anma* arts were assimilated into Buddhist religious practices. Many years later Dogen Zenji (1200–1253) was credited with determining that the harmonization of mind and body was the core of Zen. Written accounts reportedly show that Hakuin Zenji (1686–1769) combined the use of self-*anma* with directed breathing and seated meditation. Modern Zen practices continue to show the influence of the *anma* arts.

Anma is defined as "the practice of touching points on the body for the purpose of enhancing well-being" (Jiyu-Kennet & MacPhillamy, 1979, p. 53). The particular points (or sequence of points) along the meridians of *anma* that are touched with fingertips of the left and right hands comprise the mudras. The use of mudras, for example, is considered less invasive and manipulative than acupuncture or massage, and more consistent with an emphasis on personal intention and self-enlightenment in terms of the problem being addressed. Although self-treatment is preferable, there are guidelines to respectfully assist another person if they are unable to treat themselves. Depending upon the mudra selected, specific hand placements and postural positions are recommended.

Selection of mudras appears similar to the selection of thought field therapy algorithms. (Algorithms will be presented in Chapter 13.) MacPhillamy (Jiyu-Kennett & MacPhillamy, 1979) wrote that choosing a mudra is based on information about the problem or tension, then selecting mudras that are found to be of potential value for that specific concern. There are many charts and tables that illustrate the purpose of treatment, with the corresponding left and right hand placement on the meridian points. The majority of mudras affect one of a pair of the bilateral *anma* meridians. Either a "left mudra" or a "right mudra" can be selected by intuition or by a conscious choice to do one or both.

TAB and Mudras

The TAB approach is a "a gentle, mindful, and natural treatment, used in lieu of tapping, to facilitate energy and/or chi influence along the acupuncture meridians" (Diepold, 2000, p. 112). Traditional acupuncture meridian theory, as discussed in Chapter 3, holds that chi is a form of bodily energy that is, in part, generated in internal organs and systems (Tsuei, 1996). Further, it is believed that chi enters the body from the outside through breathing and through the numerous acupuncture points. Chi, often called the life force, combines with breath to circulate throughout the body along complex pathways called *meridians* and *vessels*. In essence, *breath facilitates the flow of chi in its most natural state.* Imbalance of flow or distribution of chi throughout the body is considered by many acupuncturists to be the blueprint for physical and psychological problems. Such imbalances become evident at the acupuncture points through definite changes in electrical activity and possibly through felt tenderness when touching the treatment point.

At first glance mudras may appear similar to TAB, but they are also quite different. Use of mudras often combines a specific pattern of sequential meridian point contacts and meditation for 2 to 30 minutes for each step of the mudra. During the time of meditative contact the person holds the points gently "until the pulsations you feel in the tips of the fingers of both hands have become equal in speed, pattern, and strength. . . . When the pulsations are balanced in strength, speed, and pattern it *may* be time to move to the next step of the mudra; you . . . must decide this intuitively" (Jiyu-Kennett & MacPhillamy, 1979, p. 62). Mudra steps and procedures are considerably more involved than TAB, and they require more time and sensitivity to touch and sensation than one or several respirations. Meditation is essential for mudras to be maximally effective in reducing or eliminating the "tensions" in the meridians. While most likely a qualitatively different experience than Zen meditation, attunement to the thought field also involves intention and focused direction, which is essential for successful treatment outcome when using TAB.

MERIDIAN ACTIVITY AND THE TAB APPROACH

Not only is the TAB approach consistent with traditional and contemporary Chinese thinking about the flow of chi influence and the system of mudras, but TAB is consistent with emerging evidence suggesting the complexity of bioelectric currents throughout the body.

The research and theories of physicist William A. Tiller have shed more light on the interplay among mind, body, spirit, and subtle energies. We believe his work is particularly relevant to the applicability of TAB for use with meridian-based psychotherapies. Considering the complex array of electrical and electromagnetic circuitry in and around the body, Tiller theorized that "the body can be thought of as a type of transmitting/receiving antenna" (1997, p. 107). Tiller envisioned the autonomic nervous system (ANS) as a sophisticated signal carrier, wave-guide, and signal conductor that utilizes both the sympathetic and the parasympathetic branches in impacting the full range of body functions. He described the acupuncture points as a set of antenna elements that "provide an exquisitely rich array with capabilities exceeding the most advanced radar system available today. These sensitive points are coupled to the ANS via the fourteen known acupuncture meridians" (1997, p. 117).

It appears to us that the tapping treatment has focused solely on the generation and reception of energy at the acupoints. In our opinion, the prevailing approach has been remiss in not including the added possibil-ity that chi/energy may need to be released, transmitted, or exchanged in the meridians via the transmitter-like capacity of the acupoints, as Tiller intimates. This important aspect of acupoint functioning is also utilized in the TAB treatment approach.

Diepold (2002) hypothesized that meridian acupoints are "frequency modulators" and therefore they have the potential to regulate *both* the reception and transmission of chi influence. Whether a particular merid-ian receives or releases chi influence is determined by the synergistic relationship between and among the meridians as they resonate with the thought field. When we do a diagnostic procedure (therapy localize) we learn only that there is a problem (as evidenced by a weak indicator muscle response relative to a thought field) involving that meridian, or subset of meridians, but not the precise nature of the problem. The popular view is that meridian energy is blocked, thus the prescription to tap to infuse energy. We believe that the aberrant muscle response serves only to indicate that there is a disruption in chi influence in that meridian when attuned to the thought field. Such a disruption signifies either deficiency or over-abundance of chi influence related to the tested meridian. In conditions of profuse chi it is more reasonable to expect that acupoints would transmit or dissipate the excess chi as needed, which is what we believe is also facilitated with TAB. Adding more chi influence/energy to a meridian where there is already too much makes as much sense as adding more air to a balloon that is about to burst. Perhaps tapping does something other than, or in addition to, the trans-duction of energy into the meridians.

It can be hypothesized that inserted acupuncture needles may serve as actual antenna or transmitter extensions of the acupoints, which proj-ect into the biofields around the body. Over thousands of years Chinese acupuncturists learned that different conditions and different treatment locations respond better to different size needles. Acupuncture needles differ in thickness and length, which may relate to needle vibration fre-quency and how far the needle needs to extend into the surrounding layers of the biofield to obtain or release the subtle energies (e.g., chi influence). When we needle, TAB, or tap acupoints with our fingers, we stimulate ion flow at the physical level, "which reacts at the etheric[7] level to unclog the meridian flow channel" (Tiller, 1997, p. 121). Tiller stated that the unclogging results from a reaction involving the etheric level. We are of the opinion that the reaction at the etheric level incorporates the antenna/transmitter aspect of energy-information exchange and not merely the addition of more energy to facilitate the clearing.

When using TAB, we extend the antenna/transmitter capacity of the body in maintaining contact at acupoints with a direct-feed to the held acupoint. The intrinsic mechanisms of the acupoints, which are engaged via TAB, then modulate both the flow of subtle energies and the energetic information contained therein relative to the thought field. In contrast, tapping repeatedly *connects, then disconnects*, the direct but brief energetic contact with the acupoints. Thus, tapping potentially creates an inconsistent or disrupted energetic signal to the body. Perhaps the tapping treatment is more in line with chaos theory, where tiny disruptions in the prevailing pattern result in broader system changes. For example, chaos theory explores how tiny aberrations in initial conditions (i.e., adding to or disrupting the condition of chi influence in a meridian) can drastically change the long-term behavior and emotional response of a nonlinear, dynamic system (i.e., the human body and levels of consciousness). However, TAB may also be operating in accordance with chaos theory in a more subtle fashion.

In *Energy Medicine: The Scientific Basis* (2000), James L. Oschman provided a wealth of scientific data about the human body as a living, dynamic matrix of energy and information exchange. It appears that the crystalline mechanisms of our "living matrix" function as "coherent molecular antennas" that radiate and receive signals. The connective tissues of the body appear to be "a semiconducting communication network" that allows bioelectric signals to be received and transmitted to all areas of our body. In other words, when we touch our skin, especially acupoints, we contact a continuous interconnected matrix that communicates electric, magnetic, electromagnetic, vibratory and resonant interactions, which impact the regulatory biological, chemical, and molecular structures of our body.

Breath and the Piezoelectric Effect

Tapping on a bony structure is not the sole source of the piezoelectric effect in the human body. Nearly all of the tissues in the body are crystalline or liquid crystal and therefore generate electric fields (Oschman,

2000). When the tissues of the human body are moved, bent, stretched, or compressed, minute amounts of electric pulsation begin to flow. The resulting oscillations and their harmonics contain precise information relative to the forces acting upon the tissue. As previously discussed, the use of one complete respiration (one easy inhalation and exhalation), as used with TAB, is postulated to be the most natural vehicle of chi circulation. We additionally postulate that a complete breath also creates a piezoelectric effect via vibration and sound (sonic resonance). It is in this regard that Tiller (1997) wrote:

> An additional indirect mechanism exists for emissions from the body. Here, the primary stimulus comes from the sound spectrum (also called the phonon spectrum) of the body's cells, muscles and organs associated with their relative motion. The sonic resonances for a particular body part occur in a significantly lower frequency range (by a factor of ~1 million to ~10 million) than its EM [electromagnetic] resonances. This is so because the sound wave velocity through tissues is about 1 million times slower than the EM wave velocity. Because collagen, tissue and bone are all piezoelectric materials, the small stresses produced by the sound wave patterns generate associated electric field patterns and thus emit EM wave patterns. Thus movements of a particular body part give rise to two emitted EM wave pattern signatures. One signature occurs at a very high frequency due to direct ion movement while the other occurs at low to intermediate frequencies via electrically neutral mass movement coupled to the piezoelectric response mechanism. (pp. 106–107)

It appears that the natural motion and sound of the breathing process creates a powerful energetic influence involving the piezoelectric response mechanism. The radiation of this energy conceivably enhances the antenna/transmitter function of the body as it is directed to the specific acupuncture points by way of sustained touch. Perhaps this relationship explains why various types of breathing with movement have been such an integral aspect of many Eastern health practices (e.g., yoga, qigong) used to facilitate a balanced flow of chi.

Goodheart recognized a relationship between breathing and meridian activity. He specifically recommended that when there is difficulty therapy-localizing (diagnosing meridian involvement), the therapist should "have the patient quit breathing for ten seconds prior to testing; this slows down meridian activity" (quoted in Walther, 1988, p. 262). Diamond (1980) also connected respiration with the flow of chi and the impact on muscle-testing results. He concluded, "muscle weakness on kinesiological testing is no more than the inability of the incorrect respiration to supply enough breath, enough Chi, enough energy, to the meridian which has been weakened" (pp. 33–34). Diamond also pondered, "Perhaps the first manifestation of stress is an instantaneous freezing or fixation of the natural spontaneous respiration" (p. 30). By incorporating breath as an integral aspect of meridian-based treatment, we further impact the body at a fundamental level.

Breath and Intention

Tiller believes that "breath is a carrier of intention" (Tiller and Diepold, personal communication, September 27, 1999), which, in our opinion, adds an important dimension to treatment when using TAB. Tiller reached his conclusion as a byproduct of his many years of experimental research. For example, in 1972 Tiller observed and reported that variations in mental alertness caused significant changes in the electrical characteristics of the acupuncture skin points. We conjecture that such electrical changes possibly reflect the influence and impact of intentional thought attunement to the thought field. The result of several thousand experimental tests conducted or directed by Tiller from 1977 to 1979 revealed that mind direction or intentionality is evident and measurable, and this intentional thought energy is not indicative of a "classical electromagnetic energy" (1997, p. 10). Accordingly, Diepold (2000) hypothesized that treatment of therapy-localized acupuncture meridians will be more profound using TAB rather than tapping or pressure alone because of the combined enhancement of energetic contact, use of breath, and a more mindful experience of intention.

Advantages of Incorporating TAB into Meridian-Based Psychotherapies

The use of TAB now extends the successful use of thought field therapy to reluctant or sensitive populations, and in general allows meridian treatments to be more consumer-friendly. If the therapist is already familiar with another meridian-based psychotherapy approach that employs tapping as treatment, he or she will find that the TAB procedure is easily inserted in place of tapping. However, as previously mentioned, there is one small change in the treatment site for the bladder meridian; it is now restored to the bladder 1 (BL-1) acupoint (inner eye/medial canthus at the bridge of the nose) when using TAB. The bladder 1 acupoint is the preferred treatment point in the beginning-and-ending technique used in applied kinesiology with yang meridians. However,

Walther (1988) cautioned about the possibility of eye injury when tapping the bladder 1 acupoint. Accordingly, Callahan exercised the same caution and deferred to the bladder 2 treatment point at the inside edge of the eyebrow, which is unnecessary with TAB.

According to Woollerton and McLean (1979), the BL-1 treatment point as used in acupuncture is thought to control the pituitary gland. They further wrote,

> The hormones controlled by the pituitary gland include the growth hormone, ACTH, gonadotropic hormones, lactogenic hormones and thyrotropic hormones. The pituitary gland, through the hypothalamus, affects our emotions and the autonomic nervous system. ACTH, or adrenocorticotropic hormone, influences the adrenal glands, which produce epinephrine. This controls blood pressure, pulse, respiration and blood sugar content. It relaxes the bronchial muscles, and it is the trigger for the alarm reaction in an emergency, which releases the reserve of chi stored in the kidneys. (p. 66)

It is little wonder that we have noted a more profound treatment effect when using TAB at BL-1, compared to BL-2, when treating trauma-related issues.

The TAB approach also permits energy-psychotherapy treatments to become more versatile and user-friendly. The authors have observed in their individual practices and during professional workshops that almost all patients, when given the choice between tapping and TAB, prefer the TAB approach. The treatment effects of TAB, when used within the thought field therapy framework, are parallel to tapping. However, the subjective experience when using TAB is more focused and mindful compared to tapping, and it diminishes the criticism of distraction during treatment. Based on our own and colleagues' experiences, as well as the response from patients, we use and teach only TAB as our treatment method. In addition, patients have been more likely to comply with follow up self-care at home because TAB is more palatable and less conspicuous than tapping.

We strongly encourage empirical study to evaluate these hypotheses and methodologies. While anecdotal reports indicate that tapping and TAB are effective treatment approaches, research is needed to discern quantitative energetic differences between the two approaches, as well as qualitative differences experienced by individuals utilizing tapping and TAB. Empirical and clinical study is also encouraged regarding the potential effectiveness of *imagined-touch-and-breathe* (i-TAB), where the patient only imagines touching the treatment point while also taking one full respiration. Use of imagined-touch-and-breathe (i-TAB) may be applicable in treating individuals who are physically incapable of touching the acupoints or who are too self-conscious to do so publicly.

Using TAB in Lieu of Tapping

While TAB has been unique to EvTFT in its development and application, it is by no means exclusive to EvTFT in that TAB can be comfortably applied to all meridian acupoints. The TAB treatment approach is applicable with all meridian-based psychotherapies where the patient attunes a thought field and where a tapping method of meridian treatment had been used (e.g., Callahan Techniques™, Emotional Freedom Technique, Gallo's EDxTM).

Implementing TAB is quite easy. With TAB, the patient is invited to lightly touch the prescribed treatment sites along the acupuncture meridians with one to four fingers (depending on the treatment site) *and* to take one complete respiration at their own pace, preferably through the nose, while maintaining contact at each designated acupoint. That is it! No hard pressure, rubbing, or percussion is required to affect the info-energy exchange at the mind-body interface. Intentional deep breathing is neither warranted nor necessary; the patient takes one full respiration at his or her normal tempo. However, it has been observed that some patients will spontaneously take two or more respirations at a treatment point, which is entirely permissible. We suspect that these observations are indicative of the potential for idiosyncrasies and variability in the mind-body-energy interface as the patient experiences change.

Just as our breathing seems to adjust to our cognitive, behavioral, and emotional experiences, there are specific treatment interventions in EvTFT that allow for additional breaths and direct the use of at least three complete breaths (e.g., using the future performance imagery index). Additional breaths are also part of the pain management protocol (see Chapter 12) in which the patient is invited to "breathe through the area of discomfort" as they TAB on the specified meridian treatment point. Augmented breathing patterns, as spontaneously displayed by the patient, are also observed with some clinical conditions (e.g., dissociative identity disorder, acute anxiety disorders).

It should be noted that the TAB method does not replace the treatment of rubbing the neurolymphatic reflex area (NLR), also referred to as the sore spot. The NLR area, as described in Chapter 3, is the only non-meridian treatment site used in thought field therapy, EvTFT, and other meridian-based psychotherapies. The neurolymphatic reflex areas require actual muscle movement to function effectively, which is why this area is rubbed or massaged in a clockwise direction.

Chapter 6

SYSTEM DISRUPTIONS
AND TREATMENT BLOCKS

To think is to act on the plane of thought, and
if the thought is intense enough, it may produce an effect on the physical plane.

—Paracelsus

This chapter is a glimpse into what happens when psycho-energetic
activity in the mind-body interface is compromised. The terms *polarity compromise* and *block* are introduced to describe what has traditionally been called *resistance* in the psychological community. The measures
of polarity and methods of uncovering polarity dysfunction are discussed
as various forms of treatment blocks that hinder treatment effectiveness
and sustain self-defeating patterns. These phenomena are described
along with their respective procedures for diagnosis and treatment. We
also speculate as to their cause and nature.

It is interesting that psychotherapy works. The questions are *how* does
it work and, when an impasse is reached, *why* is it not effective. It is
easy to understand the patient who admits to no desire to change, but
it is difficult to grasp what prevents a patient who, with the best of
intentions and hard work in therapy, cannot move beyond the position
in which he or she is stuck. This inability of the patient to change self-
defeating thoughts and behaviors is one of the mysteries of psychology.
The literature typically describes this as *resistance* and attributes the
problem to some unconscious role of the patient. Resistance is a formida-
bly vast unmapped territory. To further complicate the matter, there is
no way to explain the territory because the language of resistance implies that the patient must resist interpretations in order to maintain the
gains obtained through the resistance itself. The explanations become
circular and may loop without any possible entrance point. One of the
most distinguishing characteristics of Evolving Thought Field Therapy

(EvTFT) is that, in this model, resistance has a map and can be diagnosed and treated.

MUSCLE TESTING AND POLARITY

In EvTFT, an interesting phenomena is utilized for diagnostic purposes. It has been noticed that when you put the palm of your hand over your head, a short distance above the scalp, and have any of your muscles tested for strength (see Figure 6.1), the muscle being tested will hold strong. If you position your hand palm skyward over your head the tested muscle will weaken (see Figure 6.2). This difference in muscle response is so consistent that at first it appears that the muscle response may be simply an anatomic circumstance in which the hand placement puts muscles in a position that locks or unlocks their holding abilities. We find that this hypothesis does not hold because there are times when the palm down results in a weak muscle response and palm up is strong. In EvTFT, the circumstances we have described are called *polarity measures*. When the patient has a weak muscle response with palm down over the scalp and a strong response with palm upward, the condition is

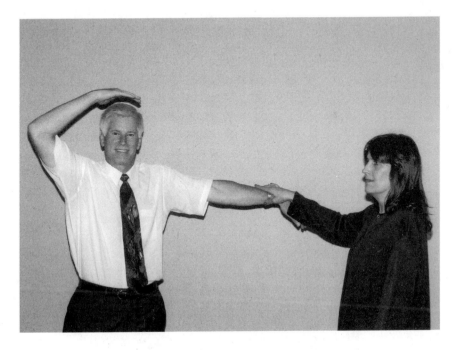

Figure 6.1 Hand over head polarity test (palm down)

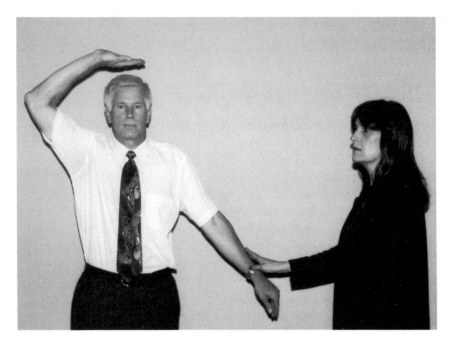

Figure 6.2 Hand over head polarity test (palm up)

called *polarity reversal*. When polarity measures obtain either weak/weak or strong/strong, the condition is labeled *nonpolarized*. Polarity reversal and nonpolarized responses are correctable, and they must be corrected as a first step in the EvTFT protocols because we cannot proceed in diagnosis until we get a strong muscle response for palm downward over the scalp and a weak muscle test for palm upward. To proceed without correction, can lead to misleading diagnostic information and impede treatment.[1]

Beyond describing the possible manifestations of the phenomena and correcting it, there is little in the literature on how and why this polarity reversal comes about and whether or how the correction would take place under other conditions. As eloquently demonstrated by muscle testing, it seems the body quickly responds by way of polarity measures when the patient is attuned to varying thoughts and feelings, or when in contact with certain environmental agents. In this regard we are intrigued by *Webster's* definition of polarity as: "a. the property or characteristic that produces unequal physical effects at different points in a body or system, as a magnet or storage battery, b. the positive or negative state in which a body reacts to a magnetic, electric, or other field" (1996, p. 1496). While some environmental agents (e.g., high tension electric lines) may be easy to recognize as field influencing, the observation that thoughts and emotions also affect body response at an energetic level lends credence to the concept and influence of thought operating in fields, which influence polarity.

We are extremely interested in the phenomena of polarity changing and muscle-testing and believe it has some extraordinary meaning in human psychological organization and thinking. In Chapter 2, we discussed how Western science offered evidence that energy could be a useful concept in psychology, not simply as metaphor, but also as concrete phenomena that could be manipulated within the EvTFT paradigm. From Michael Faraday to Albert Szent-Gyorgyi, from the concepts of vitalism to those of Robert Becker, we find constructs that help pull together the pieces of the complex puzzle.

Becker (1990) studied dedifferentiation of cells and current of injury. In his studies, it became clear that all rapidly growing tissue is found to be negative in polarity. Of interest to us is that changes in polarity signal differences in ability to physically regenerate. This being the case, we are drawn to the wisdom of Paracelsus. Is the paradigm of mind affecting the physical plane reflected in body polarity? Would the body in proper polarity, ready for whatever living requires, be analogous to a properly-tuned musical instrument, ready for whatever music is to be played?

Polarity Patterns That Block EvTFT Diagnosis and Treatment

The protocols of EvTFT involve interactions between the therapist and the patient. When working with the EvTFT model, one of the conditions that precludes an effective interaction between therapist and patient is the condition of polarity reversal, or nonpolarity, in either patient or therapist. Consider the use of cardiopulmonary resuscitation (CPR) as an analogy. In the CPR protocol, you check the airways before any attempt at resuscitation. If the airways are blocked, they must be unblocked. The system must be clear before any attempt to introduce air; otherwise, such efforts are futile. Similarly, a block in polarity must be cleared before introducing EvTFT diagnosis and treatment. As in CPR, corrections of blocks are part of the diagnosis and treatment procedure and not separate from them.

Polarity is involved on two levels as an indication of impasses in the EvTFT model. The first, as already described, relates to what might be characterized as a factor in the readiness of the total body to any interventions. The second is a description of the response we get when muscle testing during any phase of EvTFT from the beginning through to the final step.

Many interactions between the therapist and the patient in EvTFT are judged in terms of the muscle-test response. Unlike the palm up/palm down polarity test, in most cases the response is obtained through a linguistic statement made in parallel to a muscle test. A muscle is tested to assess relative strength or weakness when thinking about a problem, and the resulting muscle response guides the therapist's decision as to which steps to take next in the diagnostic and treatment process.

In EvTFT, we expect that under proper conditions of polarity the muscles will test strong when patients make positive statements and weak when they make negative statements. If a patient makes a negative statement and is strong when muscle-tested and is weak when tested for a positive statement, the condition is called a *polarity reversal* in reference to that particular thought. If a patient makes both a positive or negative statement and shows strong for both, or makes such statements and shows weak for both, the condition is labeled as *nonpolarized* in reference to that particular thought. The conditions of reversed polarity and nonpolarized responses require correction and are correctable in the EvTFT procedures. The next part of this chapter deals with the complexities of blocks, both polarized and nonpolarized, in the EvTFT model.

THE CONCEPT OF BLOCKS

The EvTFT model categorizes resistance to treatment as part of an overall class called *blocks*. As defined in Webster's, *blocks* "hinder the passage, progress or accomplishment by or as if by imposing an obstruction" (1996, p. 147). This dictionary also defines a block in medical practice as the "interruption of normal physiological functioning" (p. 147). The BDB Group broadens the definition of *block* to include the experiential component of a class of psycho-energetic disrupters that interferes with diagnosis and treatment in the EvTFT model. Accordingly, we offer the following definition of the term *blocks*: Blocks are both a physical and psychological manifestation of an individual's state of being, which, when present, may maintain self-defeating attitudes and behaviors, thus preventing positive change from either taking place or being maintained, and directly hindering the process and progress of treatment and personal growth. In our EvTFT model, there are several different types of blocks. The first one to be discussed is called *psychological reversal.*

Psychological Reversal in Perspective

John Diamond observed that patients would sometimes muscle-test in a reversed manner to statements dealing with morality. Diamond noted this phenomenon of testing weak to a morally appropriate statement and strong to the immoral inverse of the statement with both broad and specific issues (Diamond and Diepold, personal communication, January 13, 2001). When it occurred on broader issues of morality (e.g., love/hate, good/bad, right/wrong), Diamond called it a "reversal of the body morality" (1988, p. 15). He reported that when this condition was evident, healing could not occur because life-energy was not properly directed and utilized.

Roger Callahan observed the same phenomenon but termed it *psychological reversal* (PR), which he defined as "a state of the body and the mind that blocks the natural healing (energy) force within and prevents effective therapeutic intervention" (1991, p. 42). In PR, "the usual motivational state of the person" appears to be reversed, and "it appeared to turn the person against self-interest and toward self-defeat" (Callahan & Callahan, 1996, p. 15).

Callahan's PRs, like Diamond's reversals, appear to represent a literal reversal of body–energy polarity specific to a thought field. The reversal serves to block both natural healing processes and treatment efforts. Once these unconscious but physically manifest forms of self-sabotage are identified and treated, the stage is set for psychological (and physical) healing to progress with greater effectiveness.

Callahan (1996) specified four forms of PR: massive, specific, mini, and recurrent. Massive PRs reflect a global or systemic interference, whereas specific PRs have a more delineated context. Mini PRs become evident in mid-treatment, sometimes after other reversals have been treated and before complete resolution of the problem. Should a successfully treated problem recur, Callahan often evaluates for either a *recurrent* PR or evidence of an "energy toxin."

Additional delineations or levels of PR have also been described. For example, Callahan has described a level 2 or maxi PR, the term he used when efforts to maximize one's potential were reversed. Additionally, Durlacher (1994) and Gallo (1994, 2000) have explored the identification and correction of beliefs and "criteria-related reversals" that hinder successful treatment.

Evolving Nomenclature of Psychological Reversal

In rethinking the concept of PR, we have reclassified the terms to provide greater specificity and adherence to procedural aspects. For example, we changed Callahan's term from *massive psychological reversal* to *generalized psychological reversal* to more accurately reflect the effect and scope of this reversal. In a similar vein, we prefer the term *issue-specific* to *specific* because the phenomenon relates directly to the specific issue or problem being treated. We have also proposed the term *process-specific* in lieu of *mini* to clarify that this PR only occurs during the process of *completely* resolving the targeted issue.

Generalized Psychological Reversal

Generalized PR reflects general, global, or systemic interference to treatment. In this regard generalized PR may be considered a predominant or first-degree PR in the hierarchy because treatment cannot progress successfully when a patient exhibits this form of PR.

To test for the presence of a generalized PR, the therapist asks the patient to say, "I want to be happy," and then muscle-tests his or her indicator muscle. Normally, a person should maintain a strong indicator muscle when saying this. Then the therapist asks the patient to say, "I want to be unhappy" and muscle-tests again. Usually, the indicator muscle is weak when a patient makes this statement. However, if the opposite results are obtained (i.e., a *weak* muscle test to "I want to be happy" and a *strong* muscle test to "I want to be unhappy") then generalized PR is present and must be corrected before proceeding with further work.

Issue-Specific Psychological Reversal

Issue-specific PRs are more delineated in context and are limited to the particular issue or problem. An example might be a patient who is successful in most aspects of his or her life, but identifies a disconcerting fear of bees. To test for an issue-specific PR, the therapist asks the patient to say, "I want to be over this problem[2] (its cause and all that it means and does to me)" and then muscle-tests him or her. Following this, the therapist asks the patient to say, "I want to keep this problem (its cause and all that it means and does to me)." If the muscle test is *weak* to the first statement and *strong* to the second, then an issue-specific PR is present and must be corrected.

Process-Specific Psychological Reversal

Process-specific PRs are evident in mid-treatment and inhibit complete resolution of the problem. They occur during the course of an EvTFT session when the therapy appears to be progressing in a positive manner, but full relief has not yet been achieved. It could be considered a partial block in that the patient was able to precede in treatment for a period of time but the progress stalls, indicating that there is a block to completing the treatment. Generally, process-specific PR occurs when the reported Subjective Units of Distress (SUD; see Chapter 8 for a discussion of the Subjective Units of Distress Scale) level has dropped two or more points but is not down to a one or zero. It is at this point that the therapist must check for a process-specific PR.

To test for a process-specific PR, the therapist asks the patient to say, "I want to be *completely* over this problem (its cause and all that it means and does to me)" then muscle-tests the patient. The therapist then asks the patient to say, "I want to keep *some* of this problem (its cause and all that it means and does to me)." If the muscle-test is *weak* to the first statement and *strong* to the second, then a process-specific PR is present and must be corrected in order to proceed with the EvTFT diagnosis and treatment.

Recurrent Psychological Reversal

The recurrent PR is a less common form of psychological reversal that is found in cases where a successfully treated problem returns sometime after treatment is completed. If a patient reports in the following session that the problem returned several hours or days after the treatment, a recurrent PR may be suspected. Therefore at the end of a treatment session, it is usually helpful to check for this form of block even after the SUD or SUE (see Chapter 11) level has reached zero, as it can appear as a hidden impediment to maintaining successful resolution of the problem.

The recurrent PR is characterized by a weak muscle response to the statement, "I want to be over this problem once and for all," and a strong muscle response to, "I want this problem to keep coming back." A non-polarized muscle response to these statements also warrants treatment for correction.

TREATMENTS TO CORRECT PSYCHOLOGICAL REVERSALS

During the EvTFT diagnosis and treatment procedure, all PRs must be treated when they become evident. The corrections for the various types of PR have a clearing effect that reorient body polarity and permit the change process to continue. Failure to identify and correct a PR can literally block treatment from starting or stall the treatment partway through the process. When PRs are corrected, there may be a reduction in the patient's subjective level of disturbance, which they sometimes verbalize. While it is the exception and not the rule, correction of PRs may serve occasionally as treatments in themselves. After the correction of any PR, the therapist is then able to resume the EvTFT diagnosis and treatment protocol, following the appropriate next step in the procedure.

Considering the fluidity of energy, it is always recommended that both the therapist and the patient perform the corrective treatment. The rationale goes beyond modeling because it is a possible indication that either or both the therapist and the patient are energy disrupted when the patient muscle-tests strong for both ends of a polarity or PR test.

Part of the process of correcting PRs involves the patient repeating a self-affirming statement as he or she touches the appropriate treatment point. This repetition is part of Callahan's original protocols. We continue in that tradition despite the fact that over the past several years Callahan has gradually discontinued its use. Apparently, the purpose of this change in procedure was to demonstrate and emphasize the energetic underpinnings of the Callahan Techniques™ and to differentiate the treatment results from those of cognitive psychotherapy. However, we, Gallo (1998, 2000) and Durlacher (2000) have continued to advocate the use of affirmations in the treatments of psychological reversal. In our opinion, the use of language in correcting psychological reversals neither negates the energetic foundation of EvTFT nor makes it just another cognitive psychotherapy.

The use of language (affirmations) appears to facilitate attunement to a thought field by way of additional sensory (auditory) input. Language also connects related aspects of the thought field, via the patient's idiosyncratic meaning and associations, to the whole of his or her life experience. In this regard, affirmations may help resolve past, present, and future issues related to the thought field and thus affirmations have an added preventative quality.

The volumes of studies on the inextricable relationship between language and thought have contributed to our belief that this relationship is essential to the psychotherapeutic process. The originator of general semantics, Alfred Korzybski, in his book *Science and Sanity* (1980), contended that humans had progressed because of a flexible nervous system capable of symbolism. Language allowed humans to summarize their experiences and pass them along so others might learn from their mistakes. Although it seemed that language and communication were built in, Korzybski suggested that humans needed to be properly trained in the use of language to prevent misevaluation of nonverbal realities. He formulated his *law of non-identity*, also called the *law of individuality*, which states that no two persons, situations, or stages of processes are the same in all details. Korzybski noted that there are fewer words and ideas than unique situations, and this leads to confusion when dealing with more than one situation. As Korzybski indicates, language has constraints, and it is important that we allow that affirmations are metaphorically another avenue to access the interface of mind and body.

In EvTFT, affirmations usually begin with the words, "I deeply accept myself. . . . " In some ways this is reminiscent of the work of psychologist Carl Rogers, who believed that in order for people to effect change, they must first accept themselves as they are. Affirmations are an interesting and sometimes profound part of the treatment, and will be discussed further as we proceed. The wording of the affirmations to be used with EvTFT is only provided in suggested form in this book. In keeping with Korzybski's writings, the affirmations will be perceived as unique for each person's experience, so they can and should be modified in accordance with a patient's age, culture, and history.

There is a parenthetical phrase included in the affirmations: "its cause, and all that it means and does to me." The decision to add this phrase is left to the clinical discretion of the therapist. Sometimes it is sufficient and appropriate to simply have the patient say the affirmation without this phrase, while at other times, it is helpful and more specific to add "its cause" and either or both of the words "means and does." We add this because, at times, there is a deeper unconscious meaning to the problem, to which neither the patient nor the therapist has conscious access. This may be particularly relevant when treating an issue for which the cause is preverbal or no longer conscious. The additional statement can act as a signal to the psyche that it is now time for the meaning of a problem to shift in either emphasis or epistemology. Similarly, the notion of adding "does to me" can deepen the treatment effect by encompassing the spectrum of side effects attendant to the problem (e.g., states of fear, flashbacks, and bodily sensations).

In the corrections for blocks, we use circumscribed treatment points. These points will handle most situations that arise. After discussing the usual correction sites, we will detail in Chapter 12 how to diagnose and treat the blocks that do not correct at these locations.

Correction for Generalized Psychological Reversal

When a patient is found to show evidence of a generalized PR, the primary way to correct this is to have him or her rub the neurolymphatic reflex area ("sore spot") on the upper left side of the chest. As the patient rubs in a clockwise direction with a gentle but deep pressure, invite him or her to say (three times), "I deeply accept myself with all my problems and limitations." (An alternate correction statement for the generalized PR could be, " I deeply [and profoundly] accept myself with all the problems and limitations that contribute to my being unhappy.") It is very important to always verify the correction upon completion of the correction method. Verification requires having the patient repeat the statements "I want to be happy" and "I want to be unhappy" while retesting the indicator muscle. The patient should now test strong when making the first statement and weak when making the second.

The majority of generalized PRs are corrected in this manner. However, in a small percentage of cases, rubbing the neurolymphatic reflex spot will not correct the generalized PR. In this case, the patient should touch-and-breathe (see Chapter 5) on the small intestine treatment spot (SI-3), located on the (karate chop) side of the hand, while repeating this affirmation three times, "I deeply (and profoundly) accept myself with all my problems and limitations." The therapist should verify the correction, which should now be manifest. In the rare instance that a generalized PR remains, diagnose the required treatment site(s) as described in Chapter 12.

In the EvTFT model, affirmations are usually said three times. The historical basis for saying something three times is folklore that indicates "three's a charm" or "say something three times and it belongs to you." We can remember that in *The Wizard of Oz*, Dorothy clicks her heels three times and says, "there's no place like home. . . . " When people say things three times it increases the chance that they are understanding the words in a more profound way.

While correcting a generalized PR, we sometimes find that the affirmation "I deeply (and profoundly) accept myself with all my problems and limitations" may elicit a tearful response or other indications that the patient has difficulty with the meaning they attach to these words. Indeed, the patient is sometimes unable to say the words because they *are* generally reversed and, in truth, they do *not* accept themselves. When helping a patient to do this and other corrections, it is usually helpful for the therapist to mirror the treatment by doing it himself or herself and saying the words with the patient. Sometimes, if patients are unwilling to make this statement, we ask them if they could either say the words silently in their head or have the therapist say the words for them. The therapist can point out to the patient that the correction is similar to other medical treatments that produce momentary pain yet promise help in healing (e.g., receiving an injection of medication). Regardless, the patient has already heard the words spoken by the therapist

and responded in his or her personal way, which serves as an acknowledgement of the patient's understanding.

Correction for Issue-Specific Psychological Reversals

In order to correct an issue-specific PR, the therapist should have the
patient touch-and-breathe on the small intestine treatment spot on the
side of the hand (karate chop) while saying aloud three times, "I deeply
accept myself even though I have this problem (its cause and all that it
means and does to me)." The therapist should then verify the correction.
After correction, the therapist should get a *strong* muscle response to the
statement "I want to be over this problem (its cause and all that it means
and does to me)" and a *weak* muscle response to the statement "I want
to keep this problem (its cause and all that it means and does to me)."
The large majority of issue-specific PRs will be corrected in this manner.
If this correction fails, the therapist may have the patient gently but with
deep pressure rub the neurolymphatic reflex area on the upper left side
the chest in a clockwise direction while saying three times, "I deeply
(and profoundly) accept myself even though I have this problem (its
cause and all that it means and does to me)." The therapist should then
verify the correction. After correction, the patient should demonstrate a
strong muscle response to the statement "I want to be over this problem
(its cause and all that it means and does to me)" and a *weak* muscle
response to the statement "I want to keep this problem (its cause and
all that it means and does to me)."

Diagnostic evaluation of the issue-specific PR initiates the targeting
of treatment for the specified problematic thought field. If no issue-
specific PR is found, the therapist may proceed with the diagnosis of
alarm points for treatment. If an issue-specific PR is present, it is necessary to correct it immediately in order for treatment to be effective. If
the therapist forgets to check for an issue-specific PR, and the treatment
sequence does not reduce the SUD level, it is a good indication of the
presence of an issue-specific PR.

Correction for Process-Specific Psychological Reversals

Process-specific PRs can only be treated effectively at the point in the
EvTFT protocol where part of the problem is relieved, but other aspects
remain. The treatment of a *process-specific* PR consists of having the patient touch-and-breathe on the small intestine treatment site on the side

of the hand (SI-3) and say aloud three times, "I deeply (and profoundly) accept myself even though I *still* have *some* of this problem (its cause and all that it means and does to me)." The therapist should then verify the correction. The patient should now demonstrate a *strong* muscle response to "I want to be *completely* over this problem (its cause and all that it means and does to me) and a *weak* muscle response to "I want to keep *some* of this problem (its cause and all that it means and does to me)."

Correction for Recurrent Psychological Reversal

The recommended correction for a recurrent PR involves rubbing the NLR area and saying (three times), "I deeply accept myself, even though this problem has come back." Clinically, the recurrent PR is more frequent in cases involving addictions and obsessive-compulsive disorders, although it can occur in any thought field.

Verification of Corrections

Note that we have placed strong emphasis on verifying all corrections of PR. Verification involves repeating the evaluative statements or methods used before initiating the correction procedures. It is important to do so in order to be sure that the correction indeed took place because sometimes it does not take place on the first attempt. When correction of a PR or belief related block is not evident after the initial corrective treatment, the therapist must use an alternate treatment point and repeat the corrective treatment. (The majority of corrections are attained after the initial treatment; however, use of an alternative treatment site, or diagnosis of the needed acupoint[s], may be required in some cases.) We also believe that it is affirming, and sometimes relieving, for the patient to see and to experience that their mind and body are now in sync. As mentioned earlier, there are a small percentage of occasions when neither the primary nor the secondary attempts at correction are successful; we discuss the protocols for diagnosing PR in Chapter 12.

BELIEF RELATED BLOCKS

Durlacher (2000) and Gallo (1994, 2000) introduced *belief* and *criteria-related reversals* into their work to better assist patients whose core negative beliefs were sabotaging treatment. In thought field therapy, these reversals are often called *deep-level reversals* or PR2. These blocks concern patients' core beliefs about themselves and are akin to psychologist Jeffrey Young's schema-focused approach (Young, 1999). Belief related blocks (BRB) will sometimes translate linguistically, as can be readily seen in the long lists of possible limiting beliefs provided by Durlacher and Gallo. However, in EvTFT, expressive language is not the only means to determine and treat core beliefs that interfere with treatment. We will describe our nonverbal method of accessing and treating these challenges when we discuss unknown blocks later in this chapter.

BRBs sometimes manifest themselves differently from PRs in an EvTFT session. Although BRBs often present in a polarized but reversed manner, they may also present as nonpolarized responses during treatment. Accordingly, a therapist suspects a BRB when the patient demonstrates a strong/strong muscle response to belief related statements with two alternatives. BRBs seem to tap into the patient's core belief system relative to the thought field, and they have the power to block treatment. A BRB can occur at any point in the session and should be considered an important factor throughout the entire treatment process.

The therapist should be especially alerted to the possibility of a BRB in four instances:

- A BRB is usually present when a patient thinks about the targeted problem (thought field) and the indicator muscle response is strong despite a reported SUD level greater than zero. This condition can arise at any time before or during treatment, even though there is confirmation of proper body polarity when the patient is not attuned to the thought field. It is expected that when a patient is thinking about a problem, and reports a SUD level greater than zero, the muscle response ought to be weak for treatment to proceed. The strong muscle response suggests a block in the form of a BRB, which impedes further treatment if undetected or uncorrected.
- A BRB is usually evident at the end of treatment when there is a disparity between the patient's reported verbal SUD and his or her muscle-tested SUD level of zero. A common example is when a patient verbally reports a SUD level of one or more, but muscle testing indicates a SUD level of zero. The muscle-test response to the thought field will also be strong. It appears that though the body response is clear at that time, there are belief related issues that still interfere and could jeopardize the overall treatment if uncorrected.
- When the SUD level fails to drop after a treatment sequence is performed and there are no indications of a process-specific PR or neuro-

logic disorganization (e.g., there is proper body polarity when tested in the clear, the collarbone test is clear), then a BRB is suspected.

- The presence of either a strong/strong or weak/weak response to both alternatives of the test statements.

Three primary categories of BRBs have emerged over the years; these pertain to issues involving the patient's *future*, *safety*, and sense of *deservedness*. In keeping with the idea that language can be both expansive and limiting, we choose to see these categories as expansive in their meanings. For example, the word *future* is used to refer to issues of expectation, pessimism, despair, or hopelessness; *safety* expands to issues of vulnerability, risk, and trust; *deservedness* expands to issues regarding the basic sense of shame and one's birthright for forgiveness and healing. Many BRBs fall into these three categories, and they should be explored first when any of the four previously outlined conditions are present.

When trying to ascertain which one of these blocks is currently active, it is best to use clinical judgment and intuition about the patient and his or her issue. For instance, if the presenting problem is a phobia, it would be prudent to evaluate future and safety aspects. If self-esteem issues are being addressed, a good assumption would be to evaluate the possibility of a deservedness related belief. Often the patient directs us to the correct choice by verbalizing a fear such as, "I don't think I will ever be able to get over this problem." At this point, the therapist may want to check for a future BRB.

The Future Belief Related Block

The future BRB carries the idea that the future will not bring an end to the patient's problem. To test for a future BRB, the therapist asks the patient to say, "I *will* be over this problem (its cause and all that it means and does to me)" and then muscle-tests him or her. Immediately following this, the therapist asks the patient to say, "I will never be over this problem (its cause and all that it means and does to me)." (An alternative statement might be, "I will keep this problem [its cause and all that it means and does to me].) If the muscle response is weak to the first statement and strong to the second, or strong (or weak) to both statements, then a future BRB is present and must be corrected.

Our standard initial correction point for a future BRB is on the governing vessel at a point under the nose (GV-26). To treat, the patient is asked to touch-and-breathe under the nose, and say three times, "I deeply accept myself, even if I will never get over this problem (its cause and all that it means and does to me)." As always, the therapist must verify the correction. The patient should now have a strong muscle response to the first statement and a weak response to the second statement. In a small percentage of cases where the reversal or nonpolarized block does not correct at the governing vessel, the patient should touch-and-breathe on the small intestine side of the hand (SI-3) and repeat the same affirmation above. The therapist should then verify the correction.

The Safety Belief Related Block

Inherent in the safety BRB are issues of vulnerability, risk, trust, and safety, not only for oneself but also sometimes for others. For example, a man who presented with a fear of flying was found to have a BRB around the safety of others since he was fearful of what would happen to his children should he die in a plane crash. While the safety BRB is occasionally evident in the treatment of phobias and trauma-related experiences, there are no hard and fast rules. Clinical observation suggests that there is a great deal of variability regarding if and when safety issues manifest. The point, however, is for the therapist to be mindful of the potential role of such safety issues in the course of therapy.

To test for a safety BRB, the therapist asks the patient to say, "It is safe for me to be over this problem (its cause and all that it means and does to me)" or "It is safe for others for me to be over this problem (its cause and all that it means and does to me)," and muscle-tests the patient. Immediately following this, the therapist asks the patient to say, "It is not safe (unsafe) for me to be over this problem (its cause and all that it means and does to me)," or "It is not safe (unsafe) for others for me to be over this problem (its cause and all that it means and does to me)," and muscle-tests him or her. If the muscle response is weak to the first statement and strong to the second, or strong to both statements, then a safety BRB is present and must be corrected.

Our initial standard correction site for the safety BRB is on the governing vessel at a point under the nose (GV-26). To treat, the patient is asked to touch-and-breathe under the nose and says three times, "I deeply accept myself even if it is unsafe (not safe) for me to be over this problem (its cause and all that it means and does to me)." Or, when appropriate, the patient can say, "I deeply accept myself even if it is unsafe (not safe) for *others* (or a specific person can be named) for me to be over this problem (its cause and all that it means and does to me)." The therapist should then verify the correction. The patient should now have a strong muscle response to the first statement and a weak response to the second statement. In a small percentage of cases where this block or reversal does not correct with this procedure, the patient should touch-and-breathe on the small intestine side of the hand (SI-3) and repeat the same affirmation three times again. As before, the therapist should verify the correction.

The Deservedness Belief Related Block

The deservedness BRB carries a linguistic theme familiar to all therapists. This block is often evident with people who have negative core beliefs involving shame, a sense of worthlessness, or self-condemnation (with, for example, children of alcoholics and victims of abuse). To test for a deservedness BRB, the therapist should ask the patient to say, "I deserve to be over this problem (its cause and all that it means and does to me)" and then muscle-tests him or her. Immediately following this, the patient should say, "I deserve to keep this problem (its cause and all that it means and does to me)," and then the therapist muscle-tests him or her. If the muscle response is weak to the first statement and strong to the second, or strong (or weak) to both, then a deservedness BRB is present and must be corrected.

Our initial standard correction point for the deservedness (Gallo, 1994b) BRB is on the conception vessel at a point under the lip (CV-24). To treat, the patient should touch-and-breathe under the lip and say three times, "I deeply accept myself even if I deserve to keep this problem (its cause and all that it means and does to me)." The therapist should then verify the correction. The patient should now have a strong muscle response to the first statement and a weak response to the second statement. In a small percentage of cases where the block does not correct at this treatment site, the therapist should have the patient touch-and-breathe on the small intestine side of the hand (SI-3) and repeat the same affirmation again three times. As before, the therapist should verify the correction.

An interesting event sometimes happens when patients say the deservedness affirmation: They sometimes change the word *if* to *though*, as in "I deeply accept myself even *though* I deserve to keep this problem." Although we may or may not make a gentle correction when they say it the second time, they tend to persist using *though* because of the idiosyncratic relevance to them. This is certainly diagnostic information in the traditional sense and is one of the many ways a therapist can use EvTFT to enhance his or her understanding of the overall treatment picture.

The Process-Specific Belief Related Block

As with PRs, BRBs could also have process-specific blocks. The process-specific BRB is a far less common block than the others, but it does occur. Process-specific BRBs only become evident during the course of treatment, and after a prior BRB is corrected. Their presence is suspected when the SUD level fails to drop and the patient remains strong to the thought field. Although there is no hard or fast rule, a process-specific BRB usually occurs when the SUD levels are below three.

The test statements for diagnosing and the treatment point(s) for correcting process-specific BRBs are similar to those of the process-specific PR. For example, to test for a process-specific future BRB, the therapist asks the patient to say, "I will be *completely* over this problem (its cause and all that it means and does to me)" and then muscle-tests him or her. The therapist then asks the patient to say, "I will never be *completely* over this problem (its cause and all that it means and does to me)." (An alternative statement might be, "I will keep *some* of this problem [its cause and all that it means and does to me].") If the patient's muscle response is weak to the first statement, and strong to the latter, then a process-specific future BRB is present and needs to be corrected.

To correct this process-specific future BRB, the patient should touch-and-breathe on the small intestine treatment spot on the side of the hand (SI-3) and say three times, "I deeply accept myself even if I will never get *completely* over this problem (its cause and all that it means and does to me)." The therapist should then verify the correction. The initial correction site for all process-specific BRBs is the side of the hand.

Assessment and correction of safety and deservedness process-specific BRBs follow the same steps as above. The language of these test statements and the affirmations must reflect the process-specific form with the identified BRB.

Additional Belief Related Blocks

Although the safety, future, and deservedness BRBs are the most frequently occurring in our clinical experience, there are many other beliefs that can block successful treatment. We look for these other blocks when it is apparent that a BRB exists, but it is not represented by any of the three primary categories. For some patients, the language of the statements brings an added conscious dimension to their understanding of the problem. It is then that we have the option to collaborate with our patients, exploring other beliefs unique to the patient that may be blocking treatment. However, interfering core beliefs do not need to be verbalized for correction. Beliefs can be energetic and not linguistically formed (e.g., experienced at a preverbal level) and can be diagnosed and treated as an *unknown block*. Themes pertaining to responsibility, trust, abandonment, and defectiveness are among the many possibilities for additional BRBs. The corrections are similar to those used with the three primary BRBs and all begin with, "I deeply accept myself even if. . . ." Examples of some additional BRBs and their suggested correction points can be found in Appendix 2.

UNKNOWN BLOCKS

Unknown blocks manifest themselves in a manner that neither the patient nor the therapist can identify or define with a verbal belief statement that can be evaluated via muscle testing. It took us several years of clinical practice to realize that this category of blocks existed, partly because this was uncharted territory in the world of energy psychology and partly because these blocks are not common. When they do appear, it is often towards the end of a session when the SUD level is low and many times when the SUD level is between 0 and 1. However, there are no hard and fast rules and these unknown blocks can and do crop up anywhere in the EvTFT procedures. One option a therapist has after checking for and failing to confirm a future, safety, or deservedness BRB is to regard all other blocks as unknown rather than going through lengthy lists of possible BRBs.

The protocol for working with unknown blocks begins with asking the patient if they are aware of any blocks that may be obstructing the resolution of the problem. If the answer is *no*, the therapist invites the patient to "tune into whatever it is that is blocking you from completing this treatment, which you may or may not be aware of with words (consciously)" and then muscle-test him or her. Inviting a patient to attune to an unknown block may sound like an odd request; however, the patient seems to know at some level when something is blocking him or her and is able to inwardly focus on whatever it is, even when it is an unknown entity. When the muscle response is weak an unknown block is indicated.

When the therapist has ascertained that an unknown block is present, then he or she must test the patient for an issue-specific PR for the unknown block. To do this, the therapist asks the patient to say, "I want to be over this (unknown) block (its cause and all it means and does to me)," then muscle-tests him or her. Following this, the patient should say, "I want to keep this (unknown) block (its cause and all that it means and does to me)." If the muscle response is *weak* to the first statement and *strong* to the second, or strong to both, correction is needed.

Correction procedures are the same as for any issue-specific PR. To correct an issue-specific PR for an unknown block, the patient should touch-and-breathe on the small intestine treatment spot on the (karate chop) side of the hand (SI-3) while saying aloud three times, "I deeply accept myself even though I have this (unknown) block (its cause and all that it means and does to me)." As usual, the therapist should verify the correction. There should now be a strong muscle response to the statement about wanting to be over this unknown block, and a weak muscle response to wanting to keep the unknown block.

Most issue-specific PRs regarding an unknown block will be corrected in the above manner. If this correction fails, the therapist has the second option of having the patient gently but with deep pressure rub the neurolymphatic reflex (NLR) area on the upper left side the chest in a clockwise direction while repeating three times, "I deeply accept myself even though I have this (unknown) block (its cause and all that it means and does to me)." The therapist should verify the correction as described above.

There are instances when neither of these corrections is effective. In those cases, the specific treatment point(s) will need to be "diagnosed." The protocol for diagnosing treatment points for issue-specific PR and unknown blocks is found in Chapter 12.

Probable Causes of Psycho-Energetic Blocks

We do not know or understand what causes psycho-energetic blocks or disruption of information transfer or processing at the mind-body interface. We can only posit that, like metal filings in a magnetic field, muscle testing can make the field visible in a way that was previously not possible. We hypothesize that one source of production and resolution of psycho-energetic blocks comes from interaction with certain subtle energy fields. For example, we typically observe that patients with addictions become reversed when they come in contact physically with the addictive substance. Indeed, many times, thinking about the substance is sufficient to cause their energy system to be disrupted. Blocks in the form of PRs, BRBs, and unknown blocks can occur when patients come in contact with substances or subtle energies that are not necessarily addictive but are toxic to them, such as certain cleaning fluids or allergens. (See Chapter 12 on special protocols for additional discussion on the subject of energy toxins.) These contacts with toxic or negative subtle energies seem to shift a person's energy field in such a way that the person becomes reversed regarding the possibility of change. The toxic or negative energies may possibly even influence the person to pursue self-destructive behavior.

We also posit the intergenerational transmission of subtle energetic fields (e.g., Sheldrake, 1988), perhaps locked up in the DNA code, which may cause family members to be psychologically/polarity reversed over a particular issue. Examples of this are transmission of phobias, obsessive-compulsive behavior, or patterns of inexplicable behavior, such as members of a family having a high propensity for accidents.

Psychological/polarity reversal could also happen when an individual comes into contact with a person to whom he or she has a strong negative reaction, or a person with whom he or she is involved in an ongoing negative relationship. Expansion of this concept would lend support to psychoanalytic notions of transference and counter transference. We begin to postulate that one cannot *not* influence.[3]

It is extremely interesting to us that a person does not have to be in direct contact with any person or substance to evidence reversal; we consistently observe the occurrence of the psychological reversal phenomenon when a person merely thinks or tunes into a particular thought field. The causes may involve cognitive belief related issues or perhaps reach further into the depths of a thought field (see Chapter 15).

Chapter 7

DESCRIBING AND EXPANDING THE THEORY/MODEL

> We see that each human being ... participates in an inseparable way in society and in the planet as a whole. Such participation goes on to a greater collective mind, and perhaps ultimately to some yet more comprehensive mind in principle capable of going indefinitely beyond even the human species as a whole.
>
> —Bohm and Hiley

This chapter explains the terms and theoretical framework that originated in the Callahan Techniques™ pertaining to the concepts of thought fields, perturbations, active information, subsumption, and holons. In addition, this chapter introduces new concepts advanced by the authors, including elaters, harmonizers, and the emotional signaling mechanism, all of which serve to expand both the clinical application of EvTFT and the theoretical model.

THE LANGUAGE OF THOUGHT FIELD THERAPY

Many of the terms used in thought field therapy are taken from other specialties. This practice has precedent in the modern philosophy of science, which has repeatedly borrowed words from other traditions. For example, Rudolf Clausius, a mid-nineteenth century physicist, resurrected the word *entropy* from the Greeks; Clausius preferred to use words from ancient languages for the names of important scientific quantities because they could have the same meaning in all living tongues (Gillispie, 1960). The word *entropy* is reprised in information theory. As discussed in Chapter 2, the search for the words to describe an idea is one of the great difficulties of communication. Language, one of our chief means of communication, can only reflect the social and political zeitgeist of the speaker's time. It does not necessarily convey anything more than what is seen, experienced, and described by those living during that time. Nature, however, is not similarly limited (Gillispie, 1960).

This chapter defines some of the more esoteric terms Roger Callahan introduced to thought field therapy from physics, biology, and other sciences in an effort to build a meaningful vocabulary with which to understand his observations and interventions.[1] Although some critics think Callahan misapplied terminology and information, we believe that his approach constitutes a conceptual hurricane that takes us by storm over the traditional shores of psychodynamic and cognitive-behavioral psychotherapies. The hypothetical energetic substructures of disturbing emotions are now detectable and treatable via the mysterious acupuncture meridian system, which lies outside of the words and medication of traditional psychotherapies.

The Use of the Term *Fields* in *Thought Field Therapy*

Callahan hypothesized that thought fields are psycho-energetic entities that serve as causative agents influencing human behavior, emotions, and experience. Theorized to be more like an electromagnetic pattern in structure than either a chemical or cognitive pattern, a thought field can be conceptualized as an invisible, nonphysical structure in space that binds energetically encoded information into a cohesive arrangement.

A thought field is conjectured to contain energetic information about real, imagined, or remembered experience that has a direct effect on an individual's physical, emotional, and energetic state of being. The thought field can be accessed voluntarily or involuntarily. Callahan and Callahan (1996) described the thought field as similar to the electromagnetic pattern of information on videotapes, which can be instantly accessed or erased. Every thought field may have specific and overlapping patterns of electromagnetically stored information that impact the individual in definable ways. In performing EvTFT diagnosis and treatment it is essential that the patient be attuned to the problematic thought field. Additionally, in our opinion, *a thought field is an energetic bridge between thought, memory, and emotional experience that reaches beyond conscious awareness.*

The concept and use of the term *thought field* is a unique and essential aspect of the Callahan Techniques™. The generic descriptor *thought field therapy* was derived from the way this concept is used to facilitate the diagnosis and treatment of psychological problems. When we ask a patient to think about a problem, or if he or she is already experiencing emotional upset, we believe that the patient has specifically attuned to the thought field relevant to the problem. Although having a patient think about his or her problems during psychotherapy is far from novel, the specific use, necessity, definition, and role of a thought field in Callahan's techniques are clearly new to the discipline.

Perturbations: Active Information in the Thought Field

Bohm and Hiley incorporated their understanding of quantum theory into their description of *thought*. They wrote, "It seems clear . . . that at least in the context of the processes of thought, there is a kind of active information that is operating which is in key ways rather similar to that which operates in the action of the quantum potential. . . . [And for this purpose] it is convenient to introduce the notion that consciousness shows or manifests on two sides . . . the physical and the mental" (1993, p. 384). Bohm and Hiley also suggested that active information serves as a link or interface, although, the question arises of whether the two sides are truly separate or whether the bridge is essential and a part of the system. Having said that, there is a basic similarity between the quantum behavior of a system of electrons and the behavior of mind. Bohm and Hiley proposed that, in essence, the two are the same, and they describe a layered system that includes what we experience as mind, moving down to the level "of the 'dance' of the particles," with no unbridgeable gap or barrier between levels. "At each stage some kind of information is the bridge" (1993, p. 386).

Are we in essence at the bridge of the mind-body interface when doing EvTFT? As Bohm and Hiley wrote, "The content of our own consciousness is then some part of this overall process. It is thus implied that in some sense a rudimentary mind-like quality is present even at the level of particle physics, and that as we go to subtler levels, this mind-like quality becomes stronger and more developed" (1993, p. 386). This view also creates possibilities for overcoming the particular brain design deficits referred to by Koestler by suggesting that for human beings a wholeness is thus implied, in which mental and physical sides work closely, and intellect, emotion, and body are in sync. "Thus, there is no real division between mind and matter, psyche and soma" (Bohm & Hiley, 1993, p. 386).

In order to distill the model for practical usage, we may begin to think of active information as the conjectured perturbations, elaters, and other operational material in the thought field. Although the active information may be small relative to the thought field, it might be more useful to conceptualize the active information not as a bridge metaphor, but rather in a form that is somehow influencing a larger entity or an entire thought field. Such a metaphor may be likened to sour dough bread. A small amount of the dough is kept from each batch to add to and thus form the next batch of bread. The amount, although small, transforms the larger mass of ingredients. In some similar manner, it might be hypothesized that the active information influences and perhaps forms the entire thought field.

Callahan and Callahan portrayed a thought field as "an imaginary scaffold upon which one may project or imagine causal entities such as perturbations" (1996, p. 109).

Building on the writings of Bohm and Hiley (1993), Callahan conceived *perturbations* as minute "microstate" energy forms in a thought field that contain the active information to trigger all negative emotions related to the specific thought field (Callahan & Callahan, 1996). In Callahan's model, perturbations are the fundamental energy-generating structures that determine and influence brain chemistry, and the hormonal, neurological, cognitive, emotional, and behavioral responses usually associated with negative emotions. Accordingly, perturbations are the active ingredient to the sum of our negative emotional and physical responses. Simply put, if there are no perturbations in a thought field, there will be neither experience of negative or disturbing emotions nor undesirable changes in body chemistry and physiology.

Perturbations are the operational materials that reside in the thought field that create the uncomfortable and undesirable emotional and somatic states (see Figure 7.1). If there were no perturbations, there would be no problem. Perturbations may be likened to wrinkles in a sheet. The perturbations have no existence outside of the qualities of the fabric in conjunction with the environment, yet they surely have existence. Therapy may be likened to an iron that removes the wrinkles. In diagnosis and treatment in thought field therapy, perturbations may function as catalysts that cause a detectable disruption in the meridian system whenever the thought field is engaged. In this regard Gallo stated, "we might conclude that the thought (field) holds within it or has attached to it an electromagnetic, photoelectric, or other energetic marker that initiates or generates the imbalance" (2000, p. 10). See Chapter 15 for a detailed account of the hypothetical energetic underpinnings of thought field-meridian interactions.

The concept that emotional disturbance is mediated by subtle energetic forces (perturbations) in a person's thought field, which can be identified and treated via the acupuncture meridian system, is a novel and paradigm-challenging notion posited by Callahan. According to *Webster's* (1966), the noun *perturbation* is derived from the verb *perturb*, which

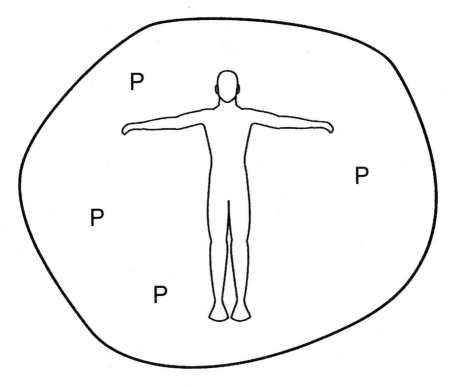

Figure 7.1 Thought field with perturbations (P)

relates to being the source or cause of alarm or agitation and, hence, the source of emotional disquietude.

The origin and purpose of perturbations, as the hypothetically fundamental causative agent for negative emotions, is open to speculation and verification. Perhaps perturbations can be compared to tiny energetic beacons that receive and transmit powerful energetic signals (information) when an individual experiences distress and trauma. The more severe (e.g., life threatening, painful, unbearable) the individual perceives or experiences the threat, the more alarming, frequent, and intense the signals become. We speculate that such signals trigger the experience of negative emotions to warn and alert the individual so he or she may take necessary action or precaution in the future. When proper protective action follows, or the traumatic event has ended, the perturbing signals quiet and eventually terminate, and the beacons return to an active state of readiness. Should a new threat occur, the energetic beacons would again emit their powerful signals of warning. But what if these tiny energetic beacons transmitted their warning signals to exclusively imagined or remembered danger in the absence of an immediate threat of danger? Would this constitute a malfunction of the signaling system? We think not. Since people can and do respond emotionally to memories, both intended and triggered, it appears more likely that this response style serves as an *energetic* reflection of how, and the degree to which, the individual has adjusted to the threatening experience.

Consistent with the above analogy, when an upsetting thought field is attuned, symptoms of alert or distress become evident by just thinking about the event. Although this response style might be considered a breakdown in the system because the upsetting response persists despite actual contextual information to the contrary (e.g., the traumatic event transpired many years earlier and the person is currently safe, yet he or she feels highly distressed or panic-stricken), it more likely indicates that individuals do respond emotionally to energetically encoded information. Accordingly, "it can be reasoned that thought, perception, sensation, and memory are energetically linked" (Diepold, 2002, p. 14). Therefore, when an individual has not yet resolved the impact of an upsetting experience *on an energetic level*, the perturbations will continue to function as an upsetting or disruptive influence whenever activated. Such emotional upset may also involve biochemical, neurological, muscular, and general physical sequelae because the body-mind-energy relationship is indivisible.

Anxiety, fear, panic, anger, rage, shame, and depression exemplify perturbation-driven emotions for which individuals seek psychotherapy. The impact of perturbations is disturbing, unwelcome, and seemingly uncontrollable.

SUBSUMPTION

Successful treatment, according to Callahan, would subsume the perturbations, thus neutralizing or eliminating their disruptive influence. Perhaps the image of ironing away the wrinkles (perturbations) in a tablecloth (thought field) is analogous to successful treatment whereby perturbations are subsumed according to some yet unknown law of nature. Stated another way, the process of subsumption disarms the perturbation's active information and neutralizes a previously experienced negative emotion.

Recall that negative emotions can be operationally defined as an uncomfortable affect that serves no current beneficial purpose for the individual. It is important to realize that even though there is complete relief from the negative emotion (via subsumption), the memory of the event remains intact and is frequently enhanced. It is as if negative emotions are debris on a window; as the debris is cleared away the patient obtains a clearer perspective, but without the agitation. Another outcome that frequently occurs with the elimination of upsetting emotions using EvTFT is a phenomenon that we call *cognitive clarity*. Either spontaneously or in response to inquiry, patients often report that they now think about the targeted thought field in a healthier way and in a manner that they were unable to achieve previously. In essence, there is a cognitive processing which is free of abreaction that occurs simultaneously during the treatment.

Holons

In the Callahan Techniques[TM], the term *holon* is used to indicate and describe the level or layers of complexity of the interrelated perturbations and the treatment required to resolve the negative emotion in the targeted thought field. The word *holon* is not identical to the term *treatment sequence*. *Treatment sequence* refers to the structure of the treatment, but *holon* carries with it all the theoretical possibilities of the architecture of the thought field. The term *holon* comes from the Greek words *holos*, meaning "whole," and *on*, meaning "part" or "particle." *Holons* are self-contained, autonomous units that follow a prescribed set of rules. The holon has a "self-assertiveness tendency" (wholeness), as well as an "integrative tendency" (part). This duality is similar to the particle/wave duality of light (Koestler, 1967). A *holarchy* is a hierarchy of holons.

Koestler wants us to understand that wholes and parts in the absolute sense do not exist anywhere in the domain of living organisms or of structural organizations. Any selection of one domain must have an artificial cutoff point. He suggests that all members of a hierarchy have two faces, like the Roman god Janus. One side faces the subordinate levels and is thus the master of those levels, and the other faces the apex and is servant to the higher level (Koestler, 1967).

The depth of meaning of *part* and *whole* is intriguing. Holons are two-directional: They can receive and send signals. A holon at one level of a system is not necessarily the same as a holon at a different level of the system. Holons are not rigid and can allow for modification and adaptability; they are open-ended and not absolute (Koestler, 1967). The idea that freedom increases as we move up the holon hierarchy will become important when we translate these energy concepts into more traditional psychotherapeutic constructs, such as transference and counter transference.[2] The pattern of interactions and relationships between the different components of a system are only limited by the vision of the person analyzing the system.

These concepts become important when one begins to consider sequence of points in treatment. Callahan asserts that diagnosis will reveal only one true treatment sequence, but if the treatment sequence is indeed a holon, there may not be a singular treatment sequence. More information on treatment sequence can be found in Chapter 15.

As shown in Figure 7.2, the holon can be perceived as a treatment subset of the thought field involving the identified perturbations evident in the acupuncture meridians, which were involved in all or part of the treatment as revealed by a particular therapist at a particular moment. Part A illustrates a holon with three treatment points. Parts B, C, and D illustrate additional or successive holons, with new and independent sets

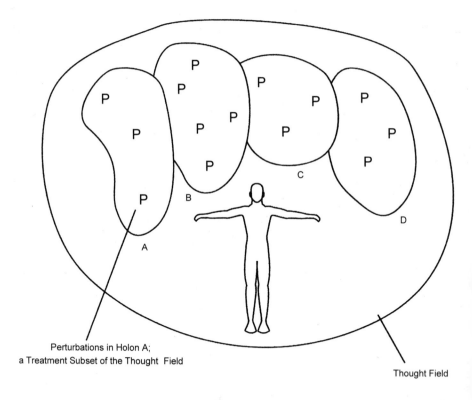

Perturbations in Holon A;
a Treatment Subset of the Thought Field

Thought Field

Perturbation/Meridian Treatment Sequence with Multiple Holons

A: e, a, c → ISq → TxSq
B: GV, if, a, c, CV → ISq → TxSq
C: ie, oe, e → ISq → TxSq
D: r, e, t → ISq →TxSq

Figure 7.2 The concept of holons as a treatment subset of the perturbations (P) in the thought field

of treatment points, that emerged after the preceding holon was completed. There is usually a reported decrease in the patient's subjective units of distress (SUD) level after completion of each holon. (When the patient's SUD level fails to drop, we recommend that the therapist evaluate for a psychological reversal (PR) or a belief related block (BRB) before proceeding; once corrected or cleared, the therapist should repeat the treatment of the same points of that holon—now the SUD level will decline.) The actual number of holons, or treatment points within a holon, are mostly descriptive at this time in the evolution of EvTFT and they simply represent the emerging pattern. As therapists, we continue diagnosing treatment points and holons until the patient's reported SUD level is zero. Perhaps the metaphor of having to clean an undetermined number of dishes will aid understanding. Therapists simply identify what needs to be washed; therapists assist the patient in washing away perturbations. Sometimes one plate is all there is and sometimes many plates, which all came from the same meal (the same thought field), are stacked up and in need of cleaning.

Many clinical cases involve a single holon, as revealed through the diagnostic process, to resolve the emotional upset related to the targeted thought field. It should be noted that treatment involving only one holon is very powerful and hypothetically reflects the manner in which the patient's energy system organized the information relevant to the thought field. On the other hand, more complex cases involve multiple holons containing either single or multiple treatment points and may reflect a more layered or convoluted synthesis of the issue. Perhaps such complexity stems from associations the patient has made to earlier or similar experiences that are further mediated by resulting beliefs of attribution. Additionally, there may be an immediacy factor that equates literally with the time needed by the individual to "let the dust settle" and permit the body's energy system to assimilate and accommodate the new event. In other words, the therapist may find that traumatic events that occurred recently (several days to several months ago) may entail more holons, which would reflect the current degree of flux in the bio-energy system involving both thought and emotion.

There are no clear-cut rules regarding the number of treatment points or the number of holons required to neutralize the upsetting emotions and sensations. What the therapist discovers most likely reflects the interaction of the patient's and the therapist's bio-energy patterns and the resulting linearly-determined sequence of treatment points when performing diagnosis. The therapist must learn to appreciate the unexpected and learn from what the patient reveals in the process of using EvTFT. Clinical experience has clearly shown that an issue may appear to be easy to treat with EvTFT but may in fact turn out to be surprisingly complex. Likewise, a severe traumatic experience from years past may resolve surprisingly fast.

To recap, the number of holons and the number of treatment points within each holon will vary, depending on the patient, the targeted thought field, and the influence and approach of the therapist. Sometimes the numbers of both holons and treatment points may become quite lengthy due to the inherent complexity of how the patient's bio-energy system dealt with the targeted problem. It should be noted that the use of the algorithm treatments (see Chapter 13) consists solely of a single holon approach with a limited number of predetermined treatment points, which contributes to limitations in treatment success with the algorithm method. Callahan reported that his algorithms are approximately "75 to 80 percent" successful (2001, p. 12). However, with diagnosis, the success rate approaches "98 percent, even with the most difficult cases" (p. 12), which allows for tailoring of the treatment points of the holon(s) the patient requires to neutralize or eliminate the upsetting emotions and sensations.

IMPLICATE AND EXPLICATE ORDER

In the process of performing a diagnosis, Callahan maintains that there is a single sequence of treatment points resulting from diagnosis. Consider Callahan's special emphasis on the exact order of the treatment points, which he describes as the bio-energetic code of nature or the combination required to open a lock, in light of what is known as *implicate* and *explicate* order.

Our knowledge of order comes from our common experience and intuition. The overt indicators come from the motion of objects, pressure, temperature, and color. The more subtle forms come from the order in language, the order of logic, the order in music, and the order of sensations and thought. "The notion of order as a whole is not only vast, but is also probably incapable of complete definition, if only because some kind of order is presupposed in everything we do, including... the very act of defining order" (Bohm & Hiley, 1993, p. 353). Physicists David Bohm and Basil J. Hiley suggested that such a notion of order should not be daunting and we should explore it to further our understanding of the "ordering phenomena."

To aid understanding about the complexity of decisions about order, we pass along the following parable. There were two Swiss watchmakers who made comparable watches, yet one prospered and one failed. The reason lay in the way the watches were made. The watches consisted of about one thousand parts each, but the two rivals used different methods to assemble the parts. The unsuccessful watchmaker assembled his watches as if each piece in the assemblage was distinct from every other piece. Thus, if the watch being assembled dropped or suffered some mishap, as was bound to occur in such a complicated assemblage, all was lost and the watchmaker would have to start from scratch. On the other hand, the successful watchmaker had learned to construct watches using units of assembly. One hundred units of 10 parts would be assembled. Next 10 units made up of the 100 units would be assembled, followed by one unit of 10 parts. If a watch dropped at any time, only a small portion of the watch would be lost, most of which could be easily recovered and reassembled from the units (Koestler, 1967).

One can extend this metaphor to the assemblage of the physical systems of human beings, such as the cardiac, respiratory, and neurological systems. But even more interesting, the metaphor might explain how order is operative for psychological systems when diagnosed using EvTFT methods.

It is suggested that the development of better measurement devices might further our experience and intuition. For example, the development of devices like the lens supported the Cartesian idea of order, which applied correspondence of separate points of an object to separate points of an image. The development of the hologram, however, has made available a new type of image that is unlike the Cartesian order in that the points of the image correspond to the whole image but the totality does not resemble the object until suitably illuminated. "The hologram seems, on cursory inspection, to have no significant order in it, and yet there must somehow be in it an order that determines the order of points that will appear in the image when it is illuminated" (Bohm & Hiley, 1993, p. 354). The idea is that the order is *implicit*, and the whole object is *enfolded* in each part of the hologram; the enfolded order is essentially similar, but does not correspond point-to-point to the object.

Bohm and Hiley do not see this enfoldment as a metaphor, and they relate it to many ordinary human experiences. For example, when one stands in a room, the whole order of the room is enfolded into each small region of space to the pupil of the eye. "This [enfolded] order is unfolded onto the retina and into the brain and nervous system, so as to give rise somehow to a conscious awareness of the whole room" (Bohm & Hiley, 1993, p. 354). They call the process of enfolding, *implicate order* and the process of unfolding *explicate order*.

Bohm and Hiley further suggested that within this concept of enfoldment and unfoldment, the Cartesian or explicate order, although extremely useful, is too limiting to be applied to laws of nature. As an illustration, a device is described that consists of two concentric glass cylinders filled with a viscous fluid, such as glycerine, into which is inserted a droplet of indelible ink. They go on to describe the appearance of the ink drop when the cylinder is rotated. At some point, the droplet is drawn out so finely as to be invisible, but when the rotation is reversed, the droplet reforms. Adding a droplet of ink of a second color and spinning the cylinder will further complicate the study. The readers are told to imagine that the ink particles will eventually intermingle, so that in a given region we could not say that the ink droplets were really separate. Then, when the cylinder is counter-rotated, we once again see separate colored drops. In this model, what appear to be separate ink drops is deceiving; actually these apparently separate droplets are internally related to one another (Bohm & Hiley, 1993, p. 359).

In describing the EvTFT protocol, we describe by necessity an implicate process in its explicate form. We might think of explicate order as a subset of the implicate order and useful in our daily life, just as Newtonian theory suffices in our daily lives. Unfortunately, it is difficult to go from the manifest level of ordinary experience based on the classical notions of form and order when attempting to explain theoretically the basis of energy psychotherapy. As explained in Chapter 2, a shift is required from Cartesian point by point correspondence to the conceptualization of an unbroken wholeness in an enfolded order that, once unfolded, is no longer representative of the entire experience. We can only step into the order at some arbitrary point and the perspective from that point may be different than were we to have chosen some other arbitrary point in which to begin. The explicate order can only be a limited expression of the implicate order (Bohm & Hiley, 1993). Therefore in describing EvTFT protocol, we must by necessity use an explicate form to describe sequence or steps in treatment. We acknowledge that there can be a different diagnostic sequence with a different observer or therapist, but we can only conjecture as to how a sequence might differ (see Chapter 15). Our steps are described in classical form and order because we have no other basis to unfold this process. We are certainly aware of the enfoldment when we do surrogate work (see Chapter 14) especially when the action is at a distance (see example 25 in Chapter 14). Once we experience such phenomena we look to explanations that allow for them.

Bohm and Hiley explained that it is easy to develop the mathematics for a second-level implicate order and, having done that, one could go on indefinitely to higher levels and "order of implicate orders" (Bohm & Hiley, 1993, p. 380). Thus, "it takes only a little reflection to see that a similar sort of description [one that includes a constant process of unfold-ment and re-enfoldment] will apply more directly and obviously to con-sciousness, with its constant flow of evanescent thought, feelings, desires, urges, and impulses" (p. 382).

ELATERS AND THE EMOTIONAL
SIGNALING MECHANISM

Diepold (2000, 2002) has speculated that perturbations constitute only one of a variety of information-bearing signals within the individual's subtle energy system, which are content and thought field specific. Cal-lahan conjectured that perturbations occupy the domain of the control-ling mechanisms of negative or disturbing emotions. However, the Callahan Techniques™ deal solely with the subsumption of these per-turbations. In our opinion, this perturbation-only model is incomplete in both clinical application and cognitive speculation.

Since we also experience positive and joyful emotions, Diepold hy-pothesized that there is a complement, which he called *elaters*, that trig-gers these feelings. According to *Webster's* (1966), the word *elate* means "to bring out, lift up; to raise the spirits of; make proud, happy, or joy-ful." Elaters would therefore occupy the domain of the controlling mecha-nisms related to positive or enjoyable emotions. Perturbations and elaters would account for two of the components of the *emotional signaling mecha-nism* (ESM) within individuals, which first and foremost influences the chemical, hormonal, neurological, cognitive, affective, and behavioral correlates of our life experiences.

It is plausible that perturbations and elaters both receive and emit energetic information to which we respond emotionally. Such special-ized information likely acts as a bio-energetic indicator of our life experi-ences for present and future reference; the indicator is reactivated when a thought field is engaged. For example, positive emotions (signaled by elaters) teach us that certain people and activities are safe, enjoyable, and rewarding or that we are proficient and comfortable. On the other hand, negative emotions (signaled by perturbations) teach us that certain people and activities are harmful, unpleasant, and to be avoided or that we are defective and shameful. The interplay of life events and the experience of our resulting emotions form the foundation of our core cognitive beliefs about ourselves and others. Formation of these beliefs most likely begins at birth, or in utero, and they are energetically en-coded within our neurological and subtle energy systems, which shape enduring patterns and perceptions of the world.

Successful EvTFT energetically resets the ESM whereby perturbations and elaters are returned to their quiescent state of readiness in that categorical thought field until they are needed again. Diepold further hypothesizes that this stable state of readiness is achieved via attainment of *frequency resonance coherence*, which is described in Chapter 15. We also believe that emotions, both negative and positive, exist for the purpose of teaching us about the world and are not intended for suffering or self-satisfaction. Accordingly, we consider EvTFT an ecologically safe psychotherapy.

HARMONIZERS
IN THE THOUGHT FIELD

Perturbations and elaters hypothetically comprise the subtle energetic controls for our respective experience of negative and positive emotions. However, Diepold (2002) further hypothesized that there is at least one other microstate element, the *harmonizer*, that controls or influences our neutral feelings related to calmness, tranquility, peacefulness, and unconditional love. The choice of the word *harmonizer* arose from Diepold's conversations with Gallo in 2001 in which they discussed their observations of patients and their own feelings when states of calm and harmony are experienced. The concept of harmonizers in the thought field implies the process or entity that facilitates harmony, which is reflected in our energetic, emotional, and physical states. When our thought fields are not encumbered by active perturbations and elaters, harmonizer signals in the thought field produce harmony and congruence in our feeling, action, thought, and health.

The influence of harmonizers can be both subtle and profound. Often the experienced state is so deep that words cannot do justice to the magnitude of the experience. Such events or opportunities literally take one's breath away, which leads to descriptors such as *breathless* and *awesome*. The state of "being in the zone," where performance just happens with little conscious intent, is perhaps another example of harmonizers. Recall, for example, the experience and feeling that accompanied the first time you saw your newborn son or daughter, a miracle without words, so precious it seemed time stood still. This is the "stuff" of harmonizers, the most natural core of harmonious existence. We are afforded only glimpses of these states, and only when perturbations and elaters are absent. Diepold suspects that individuals or groups (e.g., Tibetan Buddhist monks) have spent lifetimes learning ways to engage and sustain the experience of harmonizers.

Perturbations, elaters, and harmonizers together constitute a more complete emotional signaling mechanism (ESM) impacting the thought field (see Figure 7.3). Individually or in combination, perturbations, elaters, and harmonizers serve to create, balance, and shift the experience and intensity of emotional experience. However, the more sensitive and knowledgeable we become regarding the bio-energy aspects of our experiences, the more information-bearing signals we may find to further compliment the ESM.

Perhaps a gate theory is also applicable to the ESM. Diepold suspects that the signals emitted by perturbations and elaters serve to block or otherwise interfere with our reception of the signals from harmonizers. He believes that the deepest, healthiest, and truest form of emotional

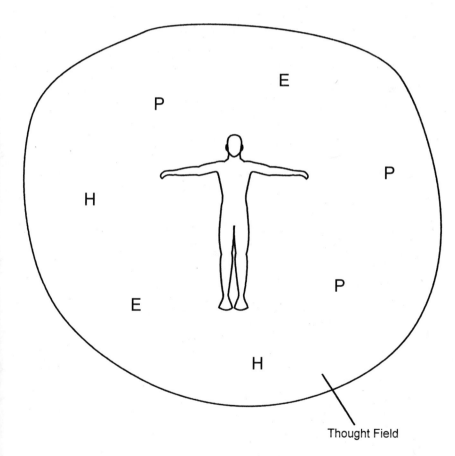

Figure 7.3 Perturbations (P), elaters (E), and harmonizers (H) in the thought field: The emotional signaling mechanism

and physical health results from the experience of harmonizers alone. Harmonizers may have their origin in the chi that flows in meridians and chakras. Harmonizers may also positively correlate with elevated alpha and theta brain waves as observed in meditation and trance states (Wise, 1995).

Chapter 8

THE STRUCTURAL
COMPONENTS OF EvTFT

Anyone who isn't confused really doesn't understand the situation.

—Edward R. Murrow

In this chapter we discuss the structural components of Evolving Thought Field Therapy (EvTFT) in historical and contemporary terminology and usage. Specifically, treatment points, the treatment sequence, therapy notation for treatment points, integration sequence, subjective units of distress (SUD), the ground to sky eye-roll, and therapy note documentation are described.

At its best, therapy is an evolving process with observations and conclusions derived from clinical experience, research, and patient feedback. To evaluate the effectiveness of this process it is important to have a uniform and reasonably straightforward structure so that treatment can be delivered in a consistent and orderly form, and results can be recorded in a standardized format. This uniform approach enables the practitioner to deliver treatment, to keep track of the patient's progress, and to assess treatment efficacy. It also renders the entire diagnostic and treatment modality teachable and amenable to research.

Structure in psychotherapy is traditionally quite variable. For example, gestalt therapy sessions, which are usually open and free flowing, would appear to some as offering little structure beyond the flow of the therapy issues. A behavioral desensitization session or a more structured eye movement desensitization and reprocessing (EMDR) session would probably be perceived as representing the opposite end of the structural spectrum. At this point in its evolution, we present EvTFT as a highly structured form of psychotherapy with procedural guidelines, methods, and sequences that are used to facilitate and evaluate the diagnostic and treatment process.

131

THE ACUPUNCTURE MERIDIAN
TREATMENT POINTS

Roger J. Callahan (Callahan & Callahan, 1996) referred to the sequential pattern of the fourteen specific acupuncture treatment points used in parts of a thought field therapy session as the *majors*. Specifically, the *majors* are the meridian treatment points that are determined via the diagnostic methods. They constitute a specified treatment sequence to be followed (e.g., inner eye, under arm, collar bone, under nose). Callahan called the points of this treatment sequence *majors* because they constitute what he conceived as the major or most fundamental part of the treatment; the term differentiates these points from treatment points used in other thought field therapy procedures (e.g., correction of psychological reversal). We might also speculate that the concept of majors stems from the use of the 12 major meridians in acupuncture when using the Callahan Techniques™.

However, some terms have historical value, but do not necessarily have consequence for additional or beneficial meaning over time. In this regard, the term *majors* as used by Callahan refers to certain acupuncture treatment points in much the same way that certain points of the musical scale are called *majors*. For ease of understanding, however, we have chosen to refer to the diagnosed meridians and their treatment points simply as *treatment points*, rather than *majors*. The pattern of one or more meridians and their corresponding treatment points, which have been diagnosed and treated while the patient is attuned to the thought field, is referred to as a *treatment sequence* (TxSq; see Chapters 7 & 15).

A TxSq can consist of a single point or multiple points. In the process of performing a diagnosis, there may be only a single treatment point indicated, or there may be multiple treatment points that comprise a sequence resulting from the order in which the treatment points were diagnosed. The number of meridians involved in a treatment sequence is not necessarily proportional to the complexity or the severity of the problem. Indeed, some very difficult issues may be resolved with surprisingly few treatment points in a single holon, while a seemingly straightforward problem may evidence many more treatment points and multiple holons than anticipated.

Treatment Point Notation

The notation for the treatment points has historically been connected to the location on or near the body part being treated. We continue this tradition because it is easier for the patient to remember physical treatment sites without having to learn acupuncture terminology. This may also simplify recall and enhance compliance for out of office self-treatment or homework. The following list specifies the 14 meridian and vessel points used in treatment, along with the neurolymphatic reflex (NLR) area.

inner eye (bladder-1)
outer eye (gall bladder-1)
under eye (stomach-1)
under nose (governing vessel-26)
under lip (conception vessel-24)
collarbone (kidney-27)
under arm (spleen/pancreas-21)
rib (liver-14)
little finger (heart-9)
middle finger (circulation/sex-9)
index finger (large intestine-1)
thumb (lung-11)
side of hand (small intestine-3)
back of hand (triple heater-3)
Neurolymphatic reflex area on upper left side of the chest

THE NINE GAMUT TREATMENTS

The *nine gamut* (9G) treatments are a sequential treatment exercise conceived by Callahan. He used the word *gamut*[1] because "a wide range of treatments are performed" while the triple heater-3 meridian point which he called the *gamut point*, was stimulated (Callahan with Trubo, 2001, p. 83). The 9G treatments are also perceived as the most unusual of Callahan's techniques in light of the different components. Callahan conjectured that "the theory behind the gamut treatments is that we are balancing various functions of the brain with each treatment in regard to the particular problem we are treating. . . . It is as if the brain must be tuned to the right frequency for each problem for the treatment to work" (1990, p. 15).

The 9G treatments are based in part on an applied kinesiology testing technique known as *eyes into distortion* (EID) developed by George J. Goodheart, Jr. Goodheart was apparently intrigued by his finding that "muscles test differently when a patient's eyes are oriented in different directions" (Walther, 1988, p. 43). While experimenting with this discovery Goodheart noticed that if the eyes are moved into distortion[2] then "subclinical problems" can be uncovered. The EID testing procedure is routinely used in certain techniques in applied kinesiology and, most notably, in the *beginning-and-ending* (B and E) technique. The B and E technique employs therapy localizing to determine the involved meridian for any particular disturbance and then treating that meridian by tapping vigorously at both the beginning and ending points (Walther, 1988). The eyes are then put into distortion to ascertain if the treatment holds, after which the initial treatment is repeated.

Callahan, a student of applied kinesiology, took note of Goodheart's observations and included the concept of EID into the formulation of the 9G treatments. For example, Callahan wrote, "The eye is an extension of the brain, and I believe that each eye movement may access a different area of the brain. Some research shows, for example, that when the eyes are open, the back of the brain receives relatively greater stimulation; when they are closed, the front of the brain is more stimulated. . . . In my own TFT research, I recognized that the position of the eyes could diagnostically reveal a hidden perturbation" (2001, p. 81). Like Goodheart's EID testing, each of the nine components of the 9G treatments can be therapy localized while the patient is attuned to the problem to ascertain if all nine steps are needed. However, since it is more efficient to simply have patients treat themselves in all nine conditions, most therapists do not routinely evaluate the need for each step of the 9G treatments.

The entire 9G treatment sequence consists of performing nine steps while simultaneously tapping on the gamut point, which is located on the back of the hand at the third point in the triple heater meridian, as the patient is attuned to the problem. The nine steps are: close eyes, open eyes, look down right, look down left, rotate eyes in a complete circle, rotate eyes in the opposite direction in a complete circle, hum a tune, count to five, and hum a tune again (e.g., Callahan, 1991). The 9G treatments are completed immediately following treatment of a diagnosed sequence or the use of a predetermined sequence called an *algorithm*.[3] Upon completion of the 9G treatments the treatment sequence is repeated, thus creating a 9G "sandwich." For example, after a patient has treated the diagnosed points of under eye, under arm, and inner eye, he or she would then perform the 9G treatments, and then repeat the treatment of under eye, under arm, and inner eye.

These nine steps are presumably stimulating, integrating, and balancing different areas of the brain to accommodate the "learning" (i.e., info-energy changes) from the initial treatment sequence. It appears that this exercise may integrate the meridian treatment into the neural pathways in some way and help the brain either to make new associations or to reinforce or enhance the treatment. According to the research of neurophysiologist and educator Carla Hannaford, the eyes need to move in order for learning to occur. "In any active learning situation, the external eye muscles are constantly moving the eyes up and down, side to side and all around.... As the eye muscles strengthen and move more in concert with each other, more connections to the brain are developed and available" (1995, p. 102). Hannaford's research is, in part, built upon Walther's (1981) writings on applied kinesiology, which describe several of the possibilities for these assumptions. For example, circling the eyes may take its form from the hypotheses offered by neurolinguistic programming wherein each position of the eye represents an organizing principle for accessing, processing, and utilizing sensory information. For the majority of right handed persons the following eye patterns are associated with specific sensory connections (when looking at the person): eyes up and to the right for visually constructed images; eyes directly right for auditorily constructed sounds; eyes down and to the right for kinesthetic, smell, and taste sensations; eyes up and to the left for eidetic visual images; eyes directly left for auditory memory; and eyes down and left for auditory self-talk (e.g., Walther, 1981; Bandler & Grinder, 1975).

In the 9G treatments the sequence of eye movements is followed by three activities designed to stimulate or activate specific brain hemisphere involvement. Callahan posited that having the patient hum a few notes of a tune, then count from one to five, and then hum again provides stimuli that "activate the right and left brain, respectively" (2001, p. 81). Through clinical observation Callahan noticed that some patients could not achieve the maximum benefit of the treatment by simply doing a single left-brain and right-brain activity. He conjectured that either the left or right hemisphere must be activated first, and he chose the hum-count-hum sequence to engage the right, then left, then right hemisphere again. Callahan could just as easily have chosen the count-hum-count sequence and achieved the same results of having activation of one hemisphere precede the other.

Goodheart observed that sometimes a malfunction in an organ could not be therapy localized except when combined with a one-sided brain activity. Humming a tune without thought to the words of the tune is conjectured to activate the creative side of the brain, whereas counting a series of numbers, doing mathematical computations, or describing an object is thought to activate the verbal part of the brain. Walther further wrote that "prolonged therapy localization of a point while activating one side of the brain may temporarily eliminate the positive therapy localization initially present with the activity" (1981, p. 108). Walther drew from this an indication of potential therapeutic activity in therapy localization, especially when combined with specific types of activity, such as humming or reciting multiplication tables, which independently activate the two sides of the brain.

Although we do not know exactly why or how the 9G treatments work, we have come to realize through clinical experience and observation that it is a beneficial part of the structure of EvTFT. Gallo wrote that the 9G treatment sequence was developed by Callahan as "a *fine tuning* device that likely activates various areas of the brain so as to enhance the therapeutic results obtained by the major treatments" (2000, p. 109). This is quite possibly the case, although research on the topic would prove extremely valuable.

The mechanisms of the brain continue to intrigue and elude us. We do know that certain parts of the brain seem to be compromised in trauma and a random or a seemingly random pattern of firing is obtained in functional magnetic resonance imaging (fMRI) as a subject undergoes therapy toward a resolution of post-traumatic stress disorder (Bender et al., 2000). It is unclear whether such patterns represent a jump-start process or an actual sequencing of events. It is also unclear whether the consequences are represented through hormonal changes or actual neurological structural changes.

THE COLLARBONE POINT
VERSUS THE GAMUT POINT

Since the inception of the Callahan Techniques™, the triple heater-3 (TH-3) treatment point has been used in conjunction with the eye movements and the hemisphere activation of the 9G treatments. Callahan wrote that "tapping the gamut point while moving the eyes in particular ways could contribute to a collapsing of a perturbation, immediately minimizing or eradicating a psychological problem" (2001, p. 81). However, aside from Callahan's stating that the use of the TH-3 treatment point "was found through numerous empirical tests" (Callahan & Callahan, 1996, p. 9), we have found no evidence to support the selection of this treatment point in publications about either applied kinesiology or traditional Chinese medicine regarding the purported brain balancing treatments.

There are, however, reasons for engaging the kidney meridian at the K-27 points to facilitate this treatment. The K-27 points are the standard points used in applied kinesiology to correct neurologic disorganization (Walther, 1988) and in other treatments having to do with the brain and performance. From an acupuncture perspective, Woollerton and McLean underscored the important role of the kidney meridian in influencing body function when they wrote, "yuan ch'i, which is stored in the kidneys, and kidney energy in general are regarded as catalysts or motivating forces for the rest of body" (1986, p. 49). Donna Eden wrote that K-27 points are "juncture points that affect all of our energy pathways. Working them sends a signal to your brain to adjust your energies so you can feel more alert and can perform more effectively" (1998, p. 64). Our own interest and experience with using the K-27 points is promising. In fact we use K-27 points exclusively for facilitating the EvTFT brain integration treatment. We also exclusively use the touch-and-breathe treatment method in our amended version of Callahan's 9G treatments, which we have renamed the *integration sequence.*

THE INTEGRATION SEQUENCE

The integration sequence (ISq) begins with the patient simultaneously touching his or her bilateral collarbone points (K-27) with two or three fingertips of each hand while taking one full respiration. Then, while maintaining contact at the K-27 treatment points, and breathing normally, the patient performs nine activities. The nine steps in the ISq are the same as those used by Callahan with the nine gamut treatments. However, we use the collarbone treatment points (K-27) while Callahan uses the gamut spot (TH-3). Further, we use TAB rather than tapping. The nine activities are as follows:

1. Close eyes.
2. Open eyes.
3. Look down right.
4. Look down left.
5. Rotate the eyes in one full circle.
6. Rotate the eyes in one full circle in the opposite direction.
7. Hum a tune for approximately three to five seconds.
8. Count from one to five.
9. Hum a tune again for approximately three to five seconds.

Please note that there is nothing hard-and-fast about the order of the first six activities; they can be performed in any order, although following a routine makes learning easier for the patient. The final three activities may also be successfully completed following a count-hum-count order if so desired. From a clinical standpoint, there are infrequent occasions when a patient is self-conscious about humming or refuses to hum altogether for personal reasons. (For example, a patient refuses to hum because he or she associates humming with an abusive situation the patient experienced in childhood.) In these instances we recommend, in lieu of humming, that the therapist invite the patient to "Think of hearing music without words" or "Think of listening to an orchestra," or "Imagine looking at a beautiful painting." Any of these options will serve to engage the right hemisphere of the brain.

SUBJECTIVE UNITS OF DISTRESS

Emotions, like physical pain, are subjectively experienced by individuals and therefore require a subjective frame of reference. *Subjective units of distress* (SUD) is a scaling method whereby the patient can rate his or her level of emotional distress using an 11-point scale from 0 to 10. Zero represents an absence of emotional distress or a neutral feeling, and 10 represents the highest level of emotional distress, when the patient is attuned to his or her problem (thought field). The SUD level is a convenient scaling method; it is a modification of the 0 to 100 point scale introduced by Joseph Wolpe in the 1960s.

The SUD level is a measure of what the patient is experiencing at the *present* moment; it does not attempt to measure how the patient felt at the time of the identified problem. The incident may have occurred months or years earlier, however when the patient thinks about it now there remains current resonant upset, which is why the person is seeking treatment.

This quantified measure of subjective distress is a useful tool to gauge the level of patient upset before, during, and after treatment. Most adults can readily provide a SUD level. The SUD levels can also describe the patient's emotional response style. For example, some patients may verbally report how upset they feel about the identified problem, and it may be mirrored in his or her voice intonation and body language, even though they report a low SUD level (e.g., 2). We have observed this situation, which appears indicative of repression, to occur more frequently with men. On the other hand, some patients frequently report SUD levels of "10 plus," or higher, to many targeted issues, which seems to reflect a more sensitive or hysterical response to his or her life problems. In any event, the reported SUD level is usually not challenged; it is accepted as a statement of the patient's present subjective feeling of distress.

There are, however, some instances when a patient will say that he or she simply cannot equate the upset with a number. This is an acceptable response. A verbalized SUD level serves only as a guide for both therapist and patient, and it is not essential for successful treatment results using EvTFT methods. One option is to determine the SUD level by using muscle-testing procedures. Muscle testing involves asking the patient to state what he or she thinks the SUD level might be, and then muscle testing the indicator muscle. When the muscle test is strong to a specific number, it is usually interpreted as the current SUD level. When the muscle test is weak to a specific number, it is usually interpreted as not being the current SUD level and the therapist must evaluate another number. Another method involves performing diagnosis and treatment based solely on the patient's muscle-test responses during the treatment protocol, which is described in Chapter 12. In these instances we are clearly using the body as an exquisite biofeedback instrument.

Children sometimes require a modified approach to acquire the equivalent of a SUD level. Many therapists simply draw a series of progressively sad to happy faces to represent the 0 to 10-point scale. The child is then asked to point to or draw a circle around the picture that matches how he or she is feeling when thinking about the targeted problem. Another approach is for the therapist to make a space between his or her two open hands and ask the child how much of a space should be between the hands to represent the amount of distress the child is experiencing.

Subjective Units of Elation: The SUE Level

Subjective units of enjoyment or *elation* (SUE) is similar in concept and operation to the SUD scale. The SUE scale is used when working with problems that are in part experienced as pleasurable by the patient but are ultimately recognized as problematic or compromising in some way. An example would be an addiction problem. The SUE level is also based on a 0 to 10-point scale where zero indicates no pleasure or enjoyment at all and ten indicates the highest degree of pleasure the patient can derive. This scale and its use are covered more completely in Chapter 11.

The Ground to Sky Eye-Roll

The eye-roll (ER) is traditionally used at the conclusion of an EvTFT treatment session, as it is in the Callahan Techniques™, when the SUD (or SUE) level is either a one or zero. Completion of an ER will usually drop the SUD level from a one to a zero because the ER appears to complete, anchor, and help solidify the treatment results. The ground to sky ER is similar to a test used by clinically trained professionals in hypnosis to assess an individual's degree of hynotizability (Spiegel & Spiegel, 1978); this test uses a pattern of eye movements that appear to facilitate relaxation by increasing alpha waves in the brain (Wise, 1995).

In EvTFT, the patient touches the bilateral collarbone points (K-27) with several fingertips of both hands and then takes one full respiration. While maintaining contact at the K-27 points and breathing normally, the patient does the following: Closes then opens his or her eyes, lowers the eyes to the ground while holding the head straight forward, and then slowly raises the eyes from the ground to the sky, taking approximately five to seven seconds. When the therapist thinks a patient did the upward ER too rapidly, the therapist can demonstrate the preferred length of time by having the patient follow the therapist's hand with his or her eyes as the therapist slowly moves it from ground to sky. It seems that both the integration sequence previously described and the ER engage and utilize eye and brain activity in concert with brain meridian energy.[4]

RECORD KEEPING IN EvTFT

As in all psychotherapy sessions, careful documentation regarding history, presentation of the problem, assessment methods, and treatment is an important part of an EvTFT session. In addition to our regular clinical case notes, we also record the actual diagnostic and treatment information of the EvTFT session. We encourage this careful note-taking for several reasons. First, it is much easier to read back the diagnosed treatment sequence from notes than it is to rely on memory alone, especially when the treatment sequences become lengthy. Second, many patients reveal patterns of involved meridians, or of needing (or not needing) treatment for neurologic disorganization or generalized psychological reversal; such information is more readily ascertained when written notes are reviewed. Third, should the patient or situation warrant the need for follow-up work at home, the exact treatment regimen is instantly available. Finally, in the interest of research, documentation of this type will prove invaluable in evaluating treatment outcome. Not only will good record keeping demonstrate precisely what transpired from session to session, but, more importantly, exactly what transpired during each session.

Table 8.1
Treatment Notations

ie	inner eye (bladder)	ISq	integration sequence
oe	outer eye (gall bladder)	ER	ground to sky eye-roll treatment
e	under eye (stomach)	SCB	simplified collarbone breathing
un or GV	under nose (governing vessel)	NOTx	neurologic organizer treatment
ul or CV	under lip (conception vessel)	OEC	over energy correction
c	collarbone (kidney)	BEC	brief energy correction
a	under arm (spleen/pancreas)	+/−	strong/weak
r	rib (liver)	−/+	weak/strong
lf	little finger (heart)	+/+	strong/strong
mf	middle finger (circulation/ sex)	−/−	weak/weak
if	index finger (large intestine)	GPR	generalized psychological reversal
t	thumb (lung)	ISPR	issue-specific psychological reversal
sh	side of hand (small intestine)	PSPR	process-specific psychological reversal
bh	back of hand (triple heater)	Future BRB	future belief related block
NLR	neurolymphatic reflex area	Safety BRB	safety belief related block
SUD	subjective units of distress	Deservedness BRB	Deservedness belief related block
SUD "9"	quotes indicate a Verbalized SUD level from the patient	PS/BRB	process-specific belief related block (indicate whether safety, future, or deservedness)
SUD 9	an underline indicates a muscle-tested SUD level	UB	unknown block
SUE	subjective units of enjoyment or elation	TAB	touch-and-breathe
TxSq	treatment sequence	HW	homework
→	go to the next step of the process	FPII	future performance imagery index

Table 8.2
Example of Record Keeping in a EvTFT Session

Although there is no typical EvTFT session, the following serves as an annotated description of what an entry in your notes might look like.

ENTRY	EXPLANATION
TF: Event at age 12	The thought field (TF) was specifically identified
SUD "8"	This is the SUD level at the beginning of treatment. The quotation marks around the number signify the patient's verbal report.
Polarity –/+: (BEC)	The patient's polarity was found to be reversed using the hand-over-head test. This was corrected using the brief energy correction. When the polarity is found to be properly polarized, the notation is "polarity OK."
No GPR	The patient was free of a generalized psychological reversal. If a GPR were evident the notation would be "GPR Dx and Tx @ NLR," indicating that a GPR was diagnosed and successfully treated at the neurolymphatic reflex area.
Permission OK	The patient gave permission to do the work, which was also reflected in an affirmative muscle response.
ISPR Dx and Tx @ NLR	The patient was diagnosed to have an issue-specific psychological reversal. It was successfully treated at the neurolymphatic reflex area after it failed to correct at the primary treatment point at the side of the hand (SI-3).
TDdx: arm/deltoid	Thought directed diagnosis was the diagnostic method used, and the indicator muscle was the deltoid using the extended arm.
ie, c, mf, c → ISq → TxSq	The notation on the left side of the first arrow represents the order of the corresponding meridian treatment points that were diagnosed in this holon. In this case they were inner eye (bladder), collarbone (kidney), middle finger (circulation/sex), and collarbone (kidney) again. After treating these points, the patient completed the integration sequence (ISq) and then repeated the diagnosed treatment sequence (TxSq) again (ie, c, mf, c).
SUD "5"	After completion of this holon, the patient reported a SUD level of five.

Table 8.2
Continued

Although there is no typical EvTFT session, the following serves as an annotated description of what an entry in your notes might look like.

ENTRY	EXPLANATION
PSPR Dx and Tx @ sh	The patient was diagnosed to evidence a process-specific psychological reversal, which was successfully treated at the primary treatment point at the side of the hand (SI-3).
TxSq → ISq → TxSq	After correction of a PSPR, it is automatic that the patient must repeat treatment of the entire holon that preceded diagnosis of this reversal.
SUD "3"	The patient now reported a SUD level of three.
	(At this point the patient was again weak to the thought field, so diagnoses of the meridians in the next holon was required.)
un, lf, e → ISq → TxSq	The notation on the left side of the first arrow represents the order of the corresponding meridian treatment points that were diagnosed in this second holon. In this case they were under the nose (governing vessel), little finger (heart), and under the eye (stomach). After treating these points, the patient completed the integration sequence (ISq) and then repeated the diagnosed treatment sequence (TxSq) again (un, lf, e).
SUD "0" / 0	The patient now reported a SUD level of zero, which was confirmed via muscle testing.
ER	The patient completed the ground to sky eye-roll treatment.
No HW	Homework was not indicated. When a situation requires homework, the specific times and duration would be recorded here (e.g., twice a day for three days).

The Process of Record Keeping

Whenever we do an EvTFT intervention, every step is identified and recorded. Therefore, using the system of treatment notations, shown in Table 8.1 can simplify the process. As will be clarified in Chapter 10, we begin recording by specifying the targeted thought field. As the diagnoses and treatments proceed, we record the SUD level before treatment and all the changes in SUD that occur on the way to obtaining a SUD level of zero. Often the SUD records reflect both the verbal report and a muscle-tested report as needed. We specify the measure of body polarity at the beginning of diagnosis, and we record which intervention(s) was used and proved successful when polarity problems were found. We note the presence of a generalized psychological reversal (PR) or an issue-specific PR, and we record the correction procedures used and the degree of effectiveness of the correction procedure(s). We note the confirmation of permission to do the treatment on the designated thought field. When diagnoses of specific treatment points begin, every treatment point is recorded in the order in which it was diagnosed. Use of the integration sequence and the results of testing for and treating a process-specific PR are also recorded. Similarly, the results of testing for and treating belief related blocks (BRB) and recurrent PRs are recorded along with the correction points used with the associated affirmations. Should time expire in the therapy session before a SUD level of zero is achieved, the ending point is recorded and it becomes the starting point when treatment is resumed. Basically, as shown in Table 8.2, every step along the way is documented for ease of review.

Table 8.2 is by no means a complete representation of what may be involved and recorded in an EvTFT session. For instance, the example did not include BRBs, recurrent PRs, or situations where a neurologic organizing treatment was required. In addition to the above the therapist may also note statements made by the patient during treatment, which may reflect a newly emerging thought field to be treated. Depending on the case, changes in body posture, the number of respirations taken at some treatment points and reported body sensations may also be of interest to record. At the end of each session we usually ask if the patient notices any changes in his or her thinking regarding the targeted issue just treated. Often the patient will describe a shift in cognition, indicating a *cognitive clarity* about the problem that was not evident before treatment.

Chapter 9

EvTFT DIAGNOSTIC METHODS

A man of courage flees forward in the midst of
new things.

—Jacques Maritain

This chapter defines and describes the term and concept of *diagnosis* as it is practiced in thought field therapy. We also present a historical overview and a description of the evolution of the three distinct diagnostic methods utilized in Evolving Thought Field Therapy (EvTFT): *contact directed diagnosis-patient* (CDdx-p), *contact directed diagnosis-therapist* (CDdx-t), and *thought directed diagnosis* (TDdx). Each diagnostic method is energetically connected to the next and progressively provides for flexibility, efficiency, and match of therapist and patient characteristics. Although all three diagnostic methods will be described in this chapter, the actual protocol steps, which are basic to all three methods, are presented in Chapter 10.

DIAGNOSIS IN THOUGHT FIELD
THERAPY VERSUS TRADITIONAL
PSYCHOTHERAPEUTIC DIAGNOSIS

The conception and role of diagnosis in thought field therapy is markedly different from its traditional use in psychotherapy, where diagnosis involves the identification and classification of symptoms. The traditional way of thinking about diagnosis in psychotherapy involves assessing the patient using the fourth edition of the American Psychiatric Association's *Diagnostic and Statistical Manual of Mental Disorders* (2000), more commonly referred to as *DSM-IV*. This conventional type of diag-

145

nosis is descriptive and serves to classify the psychological, behavioral, cognitive, and affective symptoms that accompany a problem. Although the symptom patterns allow for a nosological classification of symptom complexes (e.g., post-traumatic stress disorder, major depressive disorder, specific phobia, etc.) that is useful for insurance and educational purposes, and can serve as a beginning guide to case conceptualization, the symptom patterns are frequently too global and do not lead directly to the small steps of a precise treatment methodology. Diagnosis in EvTFT is more similar to the dynamic assessment process used in family systems work, where treatment and assessment coevolve.

The traditional method of diagnosis is static and may be conceptualized as a noun, whereas in EvTFT diagnosis is conceptualized as a transitive, active verb. Diagnosis in thought field therapy is described as causal rather than descriptive.[1] By this we mean that within the thought field therapy framework, diagnosis is a method that provides specific meridian-based "energetic information" for direct and immediate treatment of the identified problem. That is, once a meridian or treatment block is identified via diagnosis as involved in a patient's problem, that meridian is immediately treated by touch-and-breathe (TAB).

HISTORY OF
MERIDIAN-BASED DIAGNOSIS

In the Callahan Techniques[TM], Roger Callahan presented a method of using therapy localization procedures, as gleaned from applied kinesiology, to treat psychological problems. Although John Diamond preceded Callahan in the treatment of psychological problems by engaging the meridian system (Diamond, 1979), Callahan endeavored to muscle-test the meridian alarm points as a way to determine perturbations in the thought field. Once a meridian is identified as being "causally" related to the experience of emotional upset within the targeted thought field, suggesting the presence of perturbations, that meridian is treated at a specified meridian point. After treatment (Callahan uses tapping and we use TAB), the patient is muscle-tested again while attuned to the problematic thought field to determine if additional meridians need to be diagnosed. This process of diagnose-treat-check continues until the patient muscle-tests strong to the thought field. Sometimes a single meridian treatment is all that is required, although multiple treatment sites are more common.[2]

As the Diamond and Callahan procedures developed and changed over the years, students of these pioneers added variations. For example,

James V. Durlacher, an early student of Callahan's work, presented his Acu-POWER diagnostic and treatment procedures in *Freedom From Fear Forever* (2000). Fred Gallo, a student of both Callahan and Diamond, formulated Energy Diagnostic and Treatment Methods (EdxTM) in the late 1990s.

The authors, who jointly teach workshops as The BDB Group, are continuing the tradition of method development stemming from the work of Callahan and Diamond and have modified and expanded the procedures in a number of ways. For example, the EvTFT treatment protocols use the patient-friendly TAB method, and we emphasize the incorporation of meridian-based psychotherapy into traditional psychotherapy, instead of promoting it as a stand-alone therapy. We have also clarified and extended the basic protocol and have added helpful details where the original protocols were vague or unclear. In addition, the diagnostic and treatment methods have been expanded to include diagnosis and treatment of positive emotions that drive self-sabotaging behavior, and issues of future experience and performance, which are addressed in separate protocols. Lastly, we instituted language changes to help clarify various concepts and procedures in a more orderly and consistent fashion.

THE SIGNIFICANCE OF ORDER
IN DIAGNOSIS

Callahan has made bold claims pertaining to his method of diagnosing perturbations that are subject to controversy and debate. For example, he has written that "our diagnosis reveals the specific perturbations in the thought field in the precise order in which they occur and in correct order for proper treatment" (1998, p. 19). Callahan compares his diagnosis to the work of a safecracker, who must determine the precise order of the required combination of numbers to unlock the safe. Callahan maintains that the treatment sequence revealed through diagnosis is equivalent to a natural code that supplies the only correct treatment to completely alleviate the negative emotion. However, given the reported effectiveness of Gary Craig's Emotional Freedom Techniques[TM] (Craig & Fowlie, 1997), which is a repetitive, algorithmic, non-diagnostic meridian treatment approach, as well as the findings by The BDB Group that different diagnosed treatment patterns are equally effective in eliminating emotional upset, it is more likely that different diagnostic procedures reveals *a* code or pattern for treatment and not *the* code. In Chapter 15 we address this issue of treatment sequence in detail and offer a hypothetical framework from which to view treatment effectiveness regardless of the method used.

DEFINING A THOUGHT FIELD
FOR CLINICAL USE

In thought field therapy the patient is directed to "tune into" or "attune" the thought field of the problem being diagnosed and treated. In most cases, asking the patient to think about or remember the situation that is causing them distress serves to attune the thought field. We speculate that every thought field contains energetically encoded information relevant to an individual's specific experience; this encoded information includes the patient's associated feelings, both positive and negative, as well as other related details (e.g., visual memories, auditory recall, bodily sensations).

The concept of "tuning in" to a thought field is similar to the definition of the term as used in electronics: "adjusting a receiver to receive signals at a particular frequency." The verb can also mean "make or become aware or responsive" (*Webster's*, 1996). Thus, attuning a thought field is analogous to tuning in a radio station. When we tune in, the receiver locks on to a specific frequency, which carries specific information denoting the radio program's style of music, disc jockeys, and advertisers. When we change a radio station we change the tuner to lock on to another frequency and thus change the information we receive because different frequencies carry different information. Similarly, attuning a thought field targets the patient's specific memories, experiences, and feelings that are relevant to the problem being addressed and that have been energetically encoded. The encoding mechanism is a challenging concept to define, but for our purposes we conceptualize it as bound energy and refer to it as operating at the interface of mind and body.

Diepold hypothesizes that successful EvTFT culminates in "field-shifting" of embedded bound energy within the thought field in a way that had not previously occurred. Accordingly, the patient not only retains the memory of the event after treatment, but he or she does so without emotional distress and is usually able to think about the event quite differently. We call the experience of the patient now being able to think differently about the previously disturbing event *cognitive clarity*. Cognitive clarity is frequently observed and spontaneously reported by patients after successful neutralization of the interfering emotions (positive or negative). It can also be elicited by the therapist asking directly, "What comes to mind now when you think about (the targeted thought field)?" and perhaps, "Were you able to think that way before?" Accordingly, thought field influences from EvTFT extend beyond the notion of restoration or rebalancing of meridian activity.

When we ask our patients to "tune in" to a problem we go beyond just "thinking" about the problem because a patient's attention to the issue is often more than purely cognitive. Knowing this, we may ask the patient to attune to whatever makes the memory or experience of the problem most pronounced at this moment. For example, if a patient is working to resolve the psychological effects of a car crash, he or she could simultaneously tune into any one, a combination of, or all of the following aspects, depending upon how the patient has catalogued the event: the felt sense (Gendlin, 1996) of the negative emotions experienced when remembering the event, the sound of screeching tires and the crash, the visual memory of an oncoming vehicle or an injured passenger, the smell of rubber tires or gasoline, or the strong emotions of fear and terror that accompanied the accident. Sometimes the therapist may only need to treat the accident as a single thought field, while at other times, all of the aspects may need to be diagnosed and treated as individual thought fields depending upon how the patient has filed away the experience. The patient will guide the therapist.

It is imperative that the patient attune and remain with the same thought field during the treatment process to allow consistent assessment of the energetic information embedded in the thought field, which resonates with the meridians. When we intentionally change a thought field (i.e., think or recall something different), the specific memories, experiences, and feelings also change to match the new thought field.

SPECIFYING THE THOUGHT FIELD
FOR CLINICAL USE

The therapist may need to assist the patient in selecting and identifying the most appropriate thought field. While some targeted thought fields may be straightforward (e.g., a specific trauma or simple phobia), others can be more complex and require assistance to isolate (e.g., complex post-traumatic stress disorder, physical pain, and depression). An accurate determination of the thought field serves to address the identified problem in the most direct way. In most instances the actual event is the primary thought field. The rationale is that there would be no upset if that event had never occurred. Some beginning EvTFT therapists may initially want to lock in on the feeling state reported by the patient (e.g., anger, fear, embarrassment) because working with feelings has been a major focus of traditional psychotherapy. When the patient is able to focus on the primary event, rather than one isolated feeling, all of the disturbing emotions stemming from that event are more likely to be neutralized. For example, a patient who is angry because the boss yelled at him or her in front of co-workers may also have experienced feelings of embarrassment, shame, guilt, frustration, and perhaps some unnamable emotion that could go untreated if only the feeling of anger were targeted. As stated earlier, sometimes there is no language for the felt experience; this rationale applies to the felt sense in which the patient can experience many different and distinct sensations while recalling an event. However, these unpleasant experiences can still be neutralized because the triggering components are isolable in the thought field.

It is also important that a thought field not be too global. For example, if a patient presents with a fear of flying, rather than the therapist saying, "Tune into your fear of flying," it would be more productive initially to isolate the specific aspects gleaned from the history-taking. Was there a prior trauma involving flying? Or perhaps there is a particular concern about a condition like turbulence, fear of crashing, fear of dying, claustrophobia, or anticipatory anxiety at the moment of take-off, which may have culminated in the patient's fear of flying. The presenting issue may not be the most productive starting point, especially if there is a history of similar experiences. The background information the patient provides and the therapist's clinical assessments remain important components in utilizing EvTFT.

A potential problem to recognize and address when utilizing EvTFT is a patient switching thought fields during the diagnosis or treatment process. This can occur when the patient becomes aware of other related aspects (e.g., memories, sensations, comments) of the original thought field. The intruding thought field might be repressed material that has been released as a result of the work to that point or it may be the next layer of the therapeutic onion. Clues that this is occurring are spontaneous comments by the patient or a reported increase in SUD level instead of a decrease. For instance, a patient who has suffered through a day of severe trauma may first recall one part of the day and later another part, which serves to shift the thought field. When this happens, and the patient does not spontaneously report it, the SUD level will spike upwards and serve as a signal to the therapist to inquire about the possibility of a shift in the patient's thought field. When the patient acknowledges that he or she was thinking about different parts of the trauma, the therapist should accept the new information as a communication from the patient that those aspects may also be in need of treatment. Having assured the patient that he or she will work on these other aspects later on in that or another session, the therapist redirects the patient to again attune the original thought field. At this point the SUD level will continue to decline as the treatment process continues, and it will reflect the shift in this thought field as the negative emotions abate. Therapists need to pay careful attention when there are switches in the thought field because sometimes it may be necessary to work on what the patient has switched to before continuing with the original thought field. Although this appears to be an infrequent occurrence, it can easily be determined by muscle testing the patient and saying, "I need to work on issue B before I can continue with issue A" or "I can finish the work on issue A now."

A minor but important point regarding targeted thought fields pertains to any beneficial purpose the patient may have attached to the associated feelings. Even though the therapist may clearly recognize the need to treat a particular thought field and the corresponding emotions, the patient may not be ready. One way to assess this possibility is to ask the patient, "When you think about (the specific issue), do the feelings you experience serve any beneficial purpose?" Most often the patient will momentarily reflect and state that there is no beneficial purpose, which further clears the path for treatment. However, sometimes surprisingly, a patient will state that he or she wants to keep his or her feeling (e.g., anger) for the time being because the patient uses it as a motivator in some way. Our recommendation is to respect the patient's decision at that time and perhaps comment that, "When you are ready to resolve that issue and the feelings please let me know. Until then, what else would you like to work on?"

OBTAINING PERMISSION TO BEGIN TREATMENT

The EvTFT model postulates that the mind-body-energy system has an "inner wisdom" or innate capacity to move toward healing that is engaged during the diagnostic and treatment process. We prefer to conceptualize this process as akin to what traditional psychotherapeutic formulations refer to as communication of information from an *unconscious aspect* of the patient. However, in psychodynamic models this unconscious aspect is frequently labeled *resistance*; it is considered a system compromise and resultant efforts to treat the patient are deemed nonproductive. In EvTFT, we operate from the stance that, in addition to the nonproductive or resistant possibility, there is also a cooperative possibility. We interpret this as the system guiding and directing treatment with a knowledge of not only how and what to heal, but also when to heal. It is not possible to distinguish between the negative and positive efforts of the system, so we must be sure that cooperation is never mistaken as corruption. We ask permission early in the treatment process so that we are assured any error is in favor of the possibility that cooperation—and not disruption—is involved.

This method of communication is easily established through use of a yes/no set of muscle responses. Specifically, the therapist asks the patient to "think *yes*," then muscle-test the indicator muscle. Then the therapist asks the patient to "think *no*," and muscle-tests again. The two responses should be different; if they are not, the therapist should check for polarity problems and correct as needed. Each respective muscle response can be interpreted as a *yes* or *no* response. This method allows for assessment of verbal and nonverbal congruence. Most often the verbal and nonverbal muscle response are congruent.

There are times when a patient is not yet ready to address a specific problem for a variety of reasons, both conscious and unconscious. For example, there may be another problem that needs to be treated before the proposed issue can be successfully addressed. It is therefore prudent to honor this wisdom and obtain permission to work on the identified problem by muscle-testing the patient to verify verbal and nonverbal permission. As the protocols in the following chapters illustrate, we ask whether it is "okay to work on this problem now." We have found that a muscle response that denies permission is rare; however, when the response is *no*, it is imperative to respect that "inner wisdom" and explore what it means and what else may need to be treated first.

We have found in our clinical work that there is often a good (legitimate) reason for denied permission. Accordingly, we recommend a few specific follow-up questions. First, we might ask the patient "Is there something else that has come into your mind right now?" If there is, then it needs to be discussed in view of the problem or issue to be addressed. The therapist might also ask the patient what they think the objections might be to working on the problem now or if there is something else to be worked on first. If unsure, the therapist might muscle-test the patient regarding "Is there a problem that we need to work on first?" If the response is yes, then exploration is needed. The therapist might even consider muscle testing to learn if the patient knows consciously what the issue is, and if the patient does not, whether it is necessary for him or her to know consciously to complete the treatment. It may be prudent to keep open the possibility of working on the original problem in the future by muscle-testing the patient to the statement "It will be okay to work on this problem in the future."

This process of obtaining and verifying permission may also help the patient become more clear about the nature of his or her problem and the degree to which it interferes in other areas of living. Getting permission to proceed in treatment with a patient diagnosed with a dissociative disorder requires some modifications in the protocol; these are discussed in Chapter 12.

THE THREE DIAGNOSTIC METHODS IN EVTFT

We classify our diagnostic methods based upon how the therapist elects to therapy localize to determine the treatment sequence. EvTFT involves two methods that we call *contact directed diagnosis*, and a third method that we call *thought directed diagnosis*. The three methods are interrelated and interchangeable. The therapist is free to use one method exclusively or to mix methods, depending on the clinical situation and the comfort level and experience of the therapist with meridian-based diagnosis. The methods are intended for use in the clinical setting where the patient and therapist share a one-on-one interaction. Although applicable, it is beyond the scope of this chapter to address how these methods could be used for diagnosis and treatment when a patient is not physically present, or only available via the telephone. However, these procedures would be applicable for diagnosis using a third party as a surrogate for another person. The consideration and use of surrogates will be discussed in detail in Chapter 12.

Contact Directed Diagnosis-Patient

The first method, *contact directed diagnosis-patient* (CDdx-p), is based on the work of Callahan (1998). As will be explained in the protocol steps of Chapter 10, the indicator muscle typically tests weak at the beginning of diagnosis when the patient is attuned to the problem. With CDdx-p, the patient is directed to touch a meridian alarm point while attuned to the thought field, as the therapist tests the response of an indicator muscle. As can be seen in Figure 9.1, the patient is touching the stomach alarm point. In this manner the therapist endeavors to diagnose (i.e., discover) an *active* meridian alarm point by therapy localizing and muscle testing the patient. (By *active* we mean that there is resonance of a per-

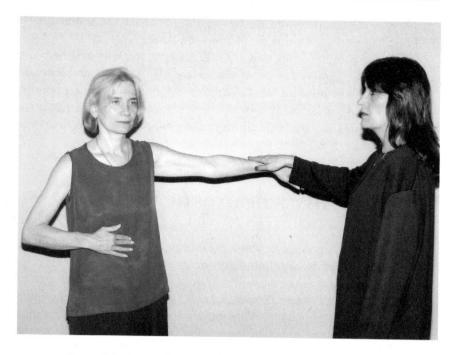

Figure 9.1 Testing the stomach meridian alarm point (CDdx-p)

turbation or elater evident in the tested acupuncture meridian that contributes to the experience of distress when the patient is attuned to the
thought field.) In the thought field therapy model, an alarm point is
considered active when the patient is attuned to the problem and the
indicator muscle tests strong when the patient is touching that alarm
point. When a strong response is obtained, the patient then self-treats
the corresponding meridian treatment point using touch-and-breathe
(TAB). Figure 9.2 shows a patient doing TAB on the bladder meridian
treatment point (BL-1). When a weak response is obtained, the therapist
then redirects the patient to touch another meridian alarm point and
muscle-tests again. This process of testing alarm points continues until
an active alarm point is identified and the meridian treated.

After treatment of the identified meridian at the designated acupoint,
the indicator muscle is retested while the patient is attuned to the target
thought field. If the muscle tests weak it is hypothesized that another
perturbation or elater is active at this time in maintaining the experienced distress. The therapist then directs the patient in therapy localizing (i.e., touching another alarm point and muscle testing) to determine
the next meridian in need of treatment.

The process of diagnose-TAB-retest is repeated as many times as necessary until the indicator muscle tests strong to the thought field. It is almost as if the body says "stop" so we can proceed to the next part of treatment as directed in the protocol.

Contact Directed Diagnosis-Therapist

The steps in using *contact directed diagnosis-therapist* (CDdx-t) follow the same principles used with the CDdx-p method (i.e., physically touching an alarm point to assist with therapy localization). However, contact directed diagnosis-therapist is a bio-energetic extension of CDdx-p because this method obtains the bio-energy information about the patient *through the therapist*. With CDdx-t, the *therapist touches* the acupuncture alarm points on his or her *own* body while simultaneously muscle testing the patient. Figure 9.3 shows the therapist checking the spleen meridian alarm point. The resulting sequentially diagnosed acupuncture meridians involved in treatment will be identical in both the CDdx-p and the CDdx-t methods. Because a free arm or hand is required for the thera-

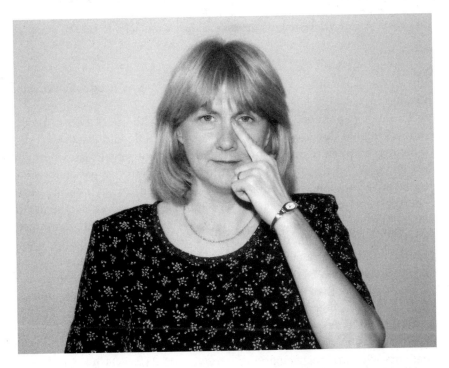

Figure 9.2 TAB treatment of the bladder meridian treatment point (BL-1)

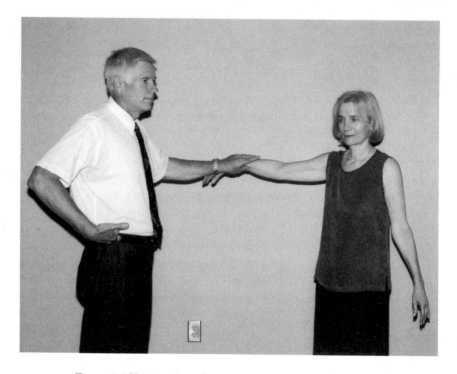

Figure 9.3 Testing the spleen meridian alarm point (CDdx-t)

pist to touch his or her own body, CDdx-t cannot be used when muscle testing fingers.

Through experience and experimentation with the CDdx-p procedures, Diepold developed the CDdx-t method. Diepold discovered that touching his own alarm points yielded the same results as when the patient touched his or her own alarm points when the patient was attuned to a problem. This observation supported the hypothesis of an energetic connection between patient and therapist, which can be useful in facilitating psychotherapy. CDdx-t is actually a first-degree surrogate model. The CDdx-t method is helpful when working with patients who are uncomfortable touching their own body, or who have difficulty locating the alarm points. From a practical standpoint, CDdx-t progresses more efficiently than CDdx-p because the therapist can quickly progress from one alarm point to the next with little delay.

With the CDdx-t method the therapist can also perform the hand over head polarity test on him or herself for the patient if needed (e.g., with patients who are incapacitated or very young). However we do not routinely advocate doing the polarity checking this way with most patients.

We believe it is important for patients to participate in their therapy, regardless of what we might be able to do as therapists.

As will be explained in the protocol steps of Chapter 10, the indicator muscle typically tests weak at the beginning of diagnosis when the patient is attuned to the problem. With CDdx-t, the patient is directed to tune into the thought field as the therapist touches his or her own alarm point and simultaneously tests the response of the patient's indicator muscle. In this manner the therapist endeavors to diagnose an active meridian alarm point by therapy localizing and muscle testing the patient. In this EvTFT diagnostic method, an alarm point is considered active when the indicator muscle tests strong when the patient is attuned to the problem and the therapist is therapy localizing his or her own alarm points. When a strong response is obtained, the patient then self-treats the corresponding meridian treatment point using TAB. When a weak response is obtained, the therapist then touches another of his or her own meridian alarm points and muscle tests again. This process of testing alarm points continues until an active alarm point is identified and the meridian treated.

After treatment of the identified meridian at the designated acupoint, the indicator muscle is then retested while the patient is attuned to the targeted thought field to ascertain whether another perturbation or elater is active in maintaining the experienced distress. If the indicator muscle tests weak, the therapist continues therapy localizing (i.e., touching another alarm point and muscle testing) to determine the next meridian in need of treatment. The process of diagnose-TAB-retest is repeated as many times as necessary until the indicator muscle tests strong to the thought field.

Thought Directed Diagnosis

Thought directed diagnosis (TDdx) in EvTFT involves the same principles and procedures used in CDdx-p and CDdx-t. However, TDdx acquires sequential bio-energy information about which meridians require treatment without the need for either patient or therapist to physically touch the meridian alarm points. Instead of physical contact at the meridian alarm points during muscle testing, the therapist focuses his or her attention and thinks, using either visual imagery or words, about the specific alarm point to be tested while muscle testing the patient. In other words, *diagnosis is directed or guided by the therapist's use of imagery and thought*. As with CDdx-p and CDdx-t, the patient is required to attune to his or her problem or issue throughout the procedure.

TDdx is a bio-energetic extension of CDdx-t. TDdx also makes a quantum leap in harnessing the subtle energies of visual imagery, thought, and intuition as the therapist resonates with the patient's energy fields. The therapist's initial use of visual imagery, thought, intuition, or some combination thereof will most likely vary depending on the sensitivities and prior training of the therapist in developing his or her skills in these realms. The treatment points that are acquired by using TDdx will match treatment points obtained using CDdx-p and CDdx-t with the same therapist and patient.

TDdx began as an innovative procedure developed independently by The BDB Group. Diepold observed from experience and experimentation with CDdx-t that merely thinking and imagining (visualizing) the touching of his own alarm points while muscle-testing the patient worked just as well as actually touching them. Britt and Bender observed that if the therapist simply thought of the name of the meridian (e.g., bladder) while the patient was attuned to the thought field, that this worked equally well. In addition, all three observed that sometimes thoughts and images of alarm points would "pop into mind," or the phenomenon of simply "knowing" would occur while performing the diagnostic procedures, thus serving to assist and direct the process by intuition. Diepold often experiences a rapid visual and kinesthetic scanning of his alarm points during diagnosis, as if the alarm points had tiny "lights," along with a sensation of being drawn to that point. The lights appear to sequentially "flicker" as he ponders the next alarm point to check, and they will often stop on a more brightly "lit" area with a stronger feeling and clarity of image. The "lit" alarm point then becomes the next one tested, which is often, although not always, found to be the next meridian in need of treatment.

Both Britt and Bender report that they use less visualization than Diepold when doing TDdx. They often report that all they need to do is think something such as "Is it the stomach meridian?" and then they muscle-test the patient without directly visualizing the alarm point. This approach also works, suggesting that there is more than one way to acquire the bio-energy information needed to complete a meridian diagnosis. However, Britt and Bender already know the location of the alarm point of each meridian in question, which may be simultaneously engaged when they muscle-test the patient.

Whatever the manner in which thought, imagery, intention, and intuition successfully enable the therapist to identify the meridians to be treated, the TDdx method is clinically effective. Perhaps a line from the *Physicians' Desk Reference* pertaining to the often prescribed and clinically effective antidepressant medication, Serzone® (nefazodone), is applicable here: "The mechanism of action of nefazodone, as with other antidepressants, is unknown" (2001, p. 1018). Accordingly, it appears it is more important to recognize that a particular intervention or procedure is clinically effective than it is to know precisely how it works.

TDdx relies heavily on recognizing and utilizing the energetic connection between the therapist and patient. We hypothesize that this bio-energetic connection forms the basis of all successful rapport in psychotherapy. In addition, in concert with the intention of the therapist, the bio-energetic connection utilized with TDdx becomes a powerful diagnostic and psychotherapeutic tool engaging and affecting the acupuncture meridians.

The advantages of using TDdx incorporate and go beyond those described for using CDdx-t. The time required to complete the diagnostic procedures using TDdx is clearly reduced to the minimum and provides for quick access to evaluate meridians, psychological reversals and blocks, and other therapy issues.

As will be explained in the protocol steps of Chapter 10, the indicator muscle typically tests weak at the beginning of diagnosis when the patient is attuned to the problem. With TDdx, the patient is directed to tune into the thought field as the therapist visually imagines touching his or her *own* alarm point or thinks about a specific meridian, and simultaneously tests the response of the patient's indicator muscle. Any indicator muscle can be used with the TDdx method. In this manner, the therapist endeavors to diagnose an active meridian alarm point by therapy localizing and muscle testing the patient. In this EvTFT diagnostic method, an alarm point is considered active when the indicator muscle tests strong when the patient is attuned to the problem and the therapist is therapy localizing by using TDdx. When a strong response is obtained, the patient then self-treats the corresponding meridian treatment point using TAB. When a weak response is obtained, the therapist then visually imagines touching another of his or her own meridian alarm points or thinks about another meridian, and muscle-tests again. This process of testing alarm points continues until an active alarm point is identified and the meridian treated.

After treatment of the identified meridian at the designated acupoint, the indicator muscle is retested while the patient is attuned to the target thought field. If the muscle tests weak it is hypothesized that another perturbation or elater is active at this time in maintaining the experienced distress. The therapist then continues therapy localizing (i.e., visually imagining touching another alarm point or thinking about another meridian, and muscle testing) to determine the next meridian in need of treatment. The process of diagnose-TAB-retest is repeated as many times as necessary until the indicator muscle tests strong to the thought field.

CLOSING NOTE

Since the late 1990s, all three authors, as independently licensed and practicing therapists, have used TDdx almost exclusively in treating patients when employing thought field therapy. The reasons for this become more evident after practice and experience. However, we recommend that therapists start at the beginning with CDdx-p, as we did, to understand the mind-body-energy connection and the relationship to the acupuncture meridians, and to truly appreciate the power of the therapist-patient relationship in psychotherapy. After the therapist has gained experience using all three diagnostic methods, the therapist can use the method that suits him or her best, or mix and match the methods as the patient-therapist circumstances warrant.

Chapter 10

THE BASIC DIAGNOSTIC
AND TREATMENT PROTOCOLS

Yikes, do I have to learn all this?
—Anonymous

During our workshop trainings we have found it necessary to give a substantial level of detail in order to provide the beginning EvTFT therapist with a solid map of options to facilitate a successful diagnostic process. For most, the diagnostic models are different from any previously learned procedure in psychotherapy. While the protocol may seem complex at first, it can be mastered with continued use and familiarity with procedures. Even the modest level of competence that all beginners show will mature into an elegant and powerful approach that can be used to resolve many psychological problems in a brief period of time.

The *basic protocol* is a user-friendly and detailed procedural outline that simplifies the steps of EvTFT diagnosis and treatment; it applies to each of the three diagnostic methods described in Chapter 9. The protocol begins with identifying a thought field and preparing the patient for meridian-based diagnosis and treatment. It ends with an application for enhancement of treatment effectiveness beyond the office setting (when applicable). A diagrammed flowchart of the basic protocol appears in Appendix 3.

THE BASIC PROTOCOL

Let's take a brief walk through the protocol before addressing the individual steps. Steps 1 through 9 describe acquiring patient permission and preparing the patient for meridian diagnosis and treatment of the disturbing thought field. These initial steps incorporate many of the procedures detailed in the previous chapters regarding muscle testing, polarity, and assessment of psychological reversals or other blocks to successful diagnosis and treatment. The remainder of the steps (10 to 23) can be summed up as: diagnose-TAB-retest. Many of the steps in the basic protocol can be viewed as decision points to guide the therapist toward successful diagnosis and treatment. Steps 12 and 13 are repeated three times in the protocol to reflect the differences in the three diagnostic methods. All other steps remain the same.

1. Obtain verbal permission to touch and to muscle-test the patient

Be sure to inquire about the possibility of any physical problems that would preclude your using any particular indicator muscle to test.

2. Select and qualify the indicator muscle (IM)

Choose which muscle or muscle group you will be testing. Now proceed to calibrate the response of that muscle by asking the patient to clear his or her mind and to "hold" or "hold strong" while you muscle-test. If you are using an outstretched arm, you may exert about 7 to 10 pounds of pressure (less when testing the fingers). Remember to clear your mind as you muscle test.

3. Notice and get a feel for the patient's muscle response style

Do this by testing various true and false statements (about, for example, names, math facts, day of week) or asking about positive versus negative thoughts and feelings. The response pattern you are looking for is a strong muscle response to correct, accurate, and pleasant thoughts or feelings, and a weak muscle response to incorrect, false, and unpleasant thoughts or feelings. If the response pattern of the patient is other than this, a polarity issue may be evident. See step 4.

4. Do a hand over head polarity check on the patient

Muscle-test the patient while he or she holds a hand one to two inches over the center of his or her head. The correct polarity is shown when the patient's muscle response is *strong* when the hand is held *palm down*, and *weak* when *palm up*. Correction is needed if the patient shows an opposite response or a nonpolarized strong/strong (locked) response. Correct by having the patient do one of the energy correction procedures described in Chapter 4. Usually the brief energy correction will suffice. If the patient shows a weak/weak response, have him or her drink two to eight ounces of water. If a correction was needed, verify the correction by retesting and write down the results, noting which correction was used. It may be necessary to recheck polarity during the course of treatment with some patients if they show a pattern of nonpolarized responses.

5. Obtain permission, via muscle testing, to work on the problem

Muscle-test the patient to the statements "It is okay to work on this problem now" (response should be strong) and "It is not okay to work on this problem now" (response should be weak). If you get the opposite result, then you and your patient need to explore how to continue with the session. Often there is something else that needs to be addressed first.

6. Check for generalized psychological reversal (generalized PR)

Muscle-test the patient to the statements "I want to be happy" and "I want to be unhappy." Usually the patient will test strong to the first statement and weak to the second. If this occurs, go to step 7. If the patient reveals a reversed muscle response (being weak to "I want to be happy" and strong to "I want to be unhappy"), have him or her correct this generalized PR by rubbing the neurolymphatic reflex (NLR) area ("sore spot") in a clockwise direction while stating three times, "I deeply (and profoundly) accept myself with all my problems and limitations." (An alternate correction statement for the GPR could be, "I deeply (and profoundly) accept myself with all the problems and limitations that contribute to my being unhappy.") Verify the correction by retesting and write down the results. Occasionally, rubbing the NLR spot does not work. In this case you may have the patient TAB on the side of the hand (SI-3) while repeating the above affirmation. Verify the correction.

7. Have the patient tune into the thought field

The patient can achieve this by thinking about, remembering, or experiencing the specific issue in some way. Get a subjective unit of distress (SUD) level rating from 0 to 10. Write down the SUD level; this is the subjective starting point. It may be helpful to explain the SUD level range each time by asking, "On a scale from 0 to 10, with 0 being no disturbance or neutral and 10 being the most disturbed you can feel, how upset do you feel right now as you think about the problem?"

8. Muscle-test the patient while he or she is thinking about the problem

For example, you might say, "Tune into the problem and hold" [or "resist" or "hold strong"]. The muscle response should be *weak* when attuned to the problem. If weak, go to step 10. If strong, go to step 9.

9. Muscle-test for a belief related block (BRB)

If the muscle response is strong, when the patient is attuned to the problem, muscle test for the influence of a BRB (see step 17). (The hallmark of a block is that it thwarts treatment progress, and the block can manifest anywhere in the process.) Correct the identified BRB, and verify the correction by muscle testing again to the thought field. Correction is evident when the muscle response is weak to the upsetting thought field. Go to step 10.

10. Check for an issue-specific psychological reversal (issue-specific PR)

Muscle-test the patient to "I want to be over this problem (its cause and all that it means and does to me)" and then to "I want to keep this problem (its cause and all that it means and does to me)." When the patient tests strong to "I want to be over this problem . . . " and weak to, "I want to keep this problem . . . ", proceed to step 11.

When the patient's muscle-test responses are reversed (i.e., weak to "I want to be over this problem . . . " and strong to "I want to keep this problem . . . "), this is indicative of an ISPR, which must be corrected. Have the patient TAB on the small intestine treatment site (SI-3 on the side of the hand) and then repeat three times, "I deeply (and profoundly) accept myself even though I have this problem (its cause and all that it means and does to me)." Verify the correction by repeating the assessment questions and muscle testing. Write down the results. If there is no change and the patient is still reversed, repeat the procedure using the NLR area. Once again, always verify the results. In the vast majority of cases the issue-specific PR will clear using these two correction points. If not, you will want to therapy localize the point(s) needed for correction (as described in Chapter 12).

11. Diagnose alarm points

At this point, you are ready to begin diagnosing the alarm point(s), which will indicate the meridians involved in the emotional disturbance. As you begin to decide which meridian alarm point(s) to diagnose, think about the identified problem and consider the following questions. This information can help guide your alarm point selections.

a. **Where does my intuition lead me?** It is important to give yourself permission to open your awareness to the subtle energies at work during the diagnosis and treatment process. Like many therapists, you are already *unconsciously* using your intuition during the course of a traditional psychotherapy session. However, in EvTFT, we encourage you to *consciously* and willfully open yourself to the possibility of receiving and being aware of subtle energetic communication, which can guide the course of diagnosis. Learn to trust yourself, your instincts, and your gut feelings because they may turn out to be surprisingly on target.

b. **What meridians are thought to be correlated with these emotions?** Consider using the meridian-emotion chart found in Table 3.2. Remember, these correlations are speculative and serve only as a reference to occasionally guide the selection of a meridian. If you use this method at the beginning, then the following questions also need to be considered.

c. **What negative emotions has the patient revealed when thinking or speaking about his or her problem?** As you proceed with the information gathering and observation portions of the treatment session, it is helpful to note what feelings the patient experiences in relation to this problem (e.g., anger, guilt, anxiety).

d. **What inferences can you make by watching and listening about the negative emotions the client is experiencing when attuned to the problem?** Sometimes patients are unaware of, or cannot articulate, which emotions they are feeling at the present time. Some patients are even "numb" or void of the feelings, which can be true of patients with dissociative disorders. Therefore, it is prudent to carefully observe the behavior of the patient as he or she communicates about the problem. For example, in the case of a traumatized patient, notice the times when the patient seems to be unable to articulate: Is this an example of frozen terror? Does anger, rage, or anxiety seem to lie just beneath the surface of a very controlled exterior? Although this is informed guesswork on the part of the therapist, and can be extremely useful, it should not become an exercise in projection on the part of the therapist.

e. **What thought field therapy algorithm might apply to this problem?** Familiarity with the algorithms (Chapter 13) provides the therapist an option to "think algorithmically" about which meridians he or she may want to test. For instance, if the presenting problem is a phobia, it might be helpful to know that using a stomach, spleen, and collarbone combination successfully treats many simple phobias and anxiety issues.

f. **What minimal cues have you observed in the session?** Often patients will nonverbally and unconsciously communicate through minimal cues which meridian to treat next. For example, the patient may unwittingly touch a specific treatment or alarm point in between the prescribed procedures while attuned to the thought field. Although a patient's gestures do not always lead to the next meridian, it happens often enough to warrant your observations. Also recognize your own minimal cues. We have observed ourselves and other EvTFT therapists also unconsciously touching an alarm or treatment point during treatment sessions.

g.   **Does the patient have a previous treatment pattern that is applicable?** When working with a patient across a number of problems, you may notice that some treatment sequences tend to follow specific patterns. For example, you might notice that a patient's treatment sequence often begins with the bladder meridian or the governing vessel, immediately followed by the stomach meridian, when working on incidents that occurred in his or her youth. It would follow that you might consider starting with those meridians when treating similar issues.

Steps 12 and 13 are repeated three times to reflect the differences in the three diagnostic methods. All other steps remain the same. Go to the appropriate heading for the method you are using.

12. Contact directed diagnosis-patient

Say to the patient, "Tune into your problem" or "Think about the problem." As the therapist, clear your mind of expectations. Now have the patient touch the alarm point (therapy localize) you have selected while you muscle-test.

a.   If the indicator muscle (IM) is weak, then this alarm point is inactive at this time. Now have the patient touch another alarm point. Keep checking alarm points until you get a strong IM response while the patient is attuned to the problem. Now go to 12b.

b.   If the IM is strong, have the patient TAB on the corresponding meridian treatment site. Record the treatment site. You have now diagnosed the first treatment point in the holon. There may or may not be other meridians involved. Go to step 13.

13. Say again, "Tune into your problem" or "Think about the problem."

Do this while you muscle-test the patient.

a.   If the IM is weak, then there are more meridians involved with perturbations in the thought field that contribute to or sustain the problem. Now have the patient touch another alarm point as he or she thinks about the problem, and muscle-test. When the IM tests strong on the specified alarm point, have the patient TAB on the corresponding treatment site. When completed, say, "Tune into your problem," and muscle-test. When the muscle response is strong, go to 13b. If the muscle response is weak again, keep repeating this step to diagnose and treat all of the involved meridians until the muscle response is strong when the patient thinks about the problem. Now go to 13b. Remember to write down every treatment site as it is diagnosed.

b. If the IM is strong, while the patient is attuned to the thought field, you have completed the sequence of treatment points for this holon. Now, have the patient do the integration sequence (ISq) using the collarbone treatment points. When the ISq is completed, have the patient once again TAB on the entire sequence of treatment point(s) you just diagnosed. (Your notes at this time should look something like this: ie, e, c, a → Isq → ie, e, c, a. In lieu of rewriting all the treatment points again after the ISq, you may simply note TxSq [treatment sequence] in its place. In this case your notes would look like this: ie, e, c, a → Isq → TxSq. Go to step 14.

12. Contact directed diagnosis-therapist

Say to the patient, "Tune into your problem" or "Think about the problem." As he or she does, clear your mind of expectations and touch an alarm point on YOUR body while you muscle-test the patient.

a. If the indicator muscle (IM) is weak, then this alarm point is inactive at this time. Touch another alarm point on your body as you muscle-test the patient, who is attuned to the problem. Keep checking alarm points until you get a strong IM response while the patient is attuned to the problem. Now go to 12b.

b. If the IM is strong, have the patient TAB on the corresponding meridian treatment site. Record the treatment site. You have now diagnosed the first treatment point in the holon. There may or may not be other meridians involved. Go to step 13.

13. Say again, "Tune into your problem" or "Think about the problem"

Do this while you muscle-test the patient.

a. If the IM is weak, then there are more meridians involved with perturbations in the thought field that contribute to or sustain the problem. Now touch another alarm point on your body as the patient thinks about the problem, and muscle-test. When the IM tests strong on the specified alarm point, have the patient TAB on the corresponding treatment site. When completed, say again, "Tune into your problem," and muscle-test. When the muscle response is strong, go to 13b. If the muscle response is weak, keep repeating this step to diagnose and treat all of the involved meridians until the muscle response is strong when the patient thinks about the problem. Now go to 13b. Remember to write down every treatment site as it is diagnosed.

b. If the IM is strong, you have completed the sequence of treatment points for this holon. Now, have the patient do the integration sequence (ISq) using the collarbone treatment points. When the ISq is completed, have the patient once again TAB on the entire sequence of treatment point(s) you just diagnosed. (Your notes at this time should look something like this: ie, e, c, a → Isq → TxSq.) Go to step 14.

12. Thought directed diagnosis

Say to the patient, "Tune into your problem" or "Think about the problem." As they do, clear your mind of expectations and imagine (visualize, think, feel) touching an alarm point on YOUR body while you muscle-test the patient. Alternatively, clear your mind of expectations and think, "Is it the _____ meridian?" as you muscle-test the patient.

a. If the indicator muscle (IM) is weak, then this alarm point is inactive at this time. Once again, visualize or think of another meridian alarm point as you muscle-test the patient, who is attuned the problem. Keep checking alarm points until you get a strong IM response. Now go to 12b.

b. If the IM is strong, have the patient TAB on the corresponding meridian treatment site. Record the treatment site. You have now diagnosed the first treatment point in the holon. There may or may not be other meridians involved. Go to step 13.

13. Say again, "Tune into your problem" or "Think about the problem."

Do this while you muscle-test the patient.

a. If the IM is weak, then there are more meridians involved with perturbations in the thought field that contribute to or sustain the problem. As the patient is tuned into the problem, visualize or think of another alarm point and muscle-test the patient. When the IM tests strong on the specified alarm point, have the patient TAB on the corresponding treatment site. When completed, say again, "Tune into your problem," and muscle-test. When the muscle response is strong, go to 13b. If the muscle response is weak, keep repeating this step to diagnose and treat all of the involved meridians until the muscle response is strong when the patient thinks about the problem. Now go to step 13b. Remember to write down every treatment site as it is diagnosed.

b. If the IM is strong, you have completed the sequence of treatment points for this holon. Now, have the patient do the integration sequence (ISq) using the collarbone treatment points. When the ISq is completed, have the patient once again TAB on the entire sequence of treatment point(s) you just diagnosed. (Your notes at this time should look something like this: ie, e, c, a → Isq → TxSq.) Go to step 14.

14. Re-evaluate the SUD level

Ask the patient to re-rate his or her level of upset *now* on a scale from 0 to 10, and write it down.

- If the SUD level is 0 or 1, go to step 15.
- If the SUD level has dropped 2 or more points but is not yet down to 0 or 1, go to step 16.
- If SUD level fails to drop, or if there is a pattern of the SUD level dropping one point at a time, go to step 17.

15. Ground to sky eye-roll treatment

If the SUD level is 0 or 1, have patient complete the treatment with the ground to sky eye-roll treatment sequence. After completion of the ground to sky eye-roll, have the patient re-rate his or her SUD level. *When the SUD level is 0, you have completed the basic protocol.* (However, you may want to check for a recurrent PR [see step 21], or make use of the future performance imagery index [FPII] when appropriate. [See step 22.]) If the SUD level is not yet 0 after doing the ground to sky eye-roll, check for a BRB (see step 17), or a process-specific PR (step 16), if applicable, and correct accordingly. If no BRB is evident, have the patient attune the targeted thought field, and muscle-test. There may still be one or more meridians involved that require treatment. If the muscle response is weak, you will need to diagnose another treatment point(s) following the procedures outlined in step 12. However, in some instances (e.g., experience of pain) there may be a delay of several minutes or hours before complete relief is reported. (See modified protocol for pain management in Chapter 12.)

16. Muscle-test for process-specific PR

If the SUD level has dropped two or more points, but is not yet down to 0 or 1, muscle-test the patient for process-specific PR. Muscle-test the patient after he or she says, "I want to be completely over this problem (its cause and all that it means and does to me)," and then muscle-test to "I want to keep some of this problem (its cause and all that it means and does to me)." If the patient tests strong to the first statement and weak to the second, go to step 12 (no process-specific PR) and resume diagnosing. When the muscle response is reversed (i.e., strong to "keep some . . . "), a process-specific PR is evident and requires correction. Correct by having the patient TAB on the side of the hand (SI-3) while saying three times, "I deeply (and profoundly) accept myself even though I still have some of this problem (its cause and all that it means and does to me)." Verify the correction by repeating the test procedures described above. Write down the results. If there is no change, repeat the correction statement while rubbing the NLR area. In the vast majority of cases, using these two treatment sites will correct the process-specific PR.

After the correction of a PR, you must always repeat the diagnosed meridian point treatment sequence that came immediately before the process-specific PR using TxSq → Isq → TxSq. Then re-rate the SUD level. If the SUD level is now 0 or 1, complete treatment with the ground to sky eye-roll treatment. If the SUD level is 2 or more, repeat steps 12 through 14.

17. Further possibilities for evaluation

When the SUD level fails to drop (see a, b, c, d, and f below), or when there is a pattern of 1 point drops (see e below), you have several possibilities to evaluate.

a. Check for a future BRB. Muscle-test the patient after he or she has said, "I *will* be over this problem (its cause and all that it means and does to me)," and then muscle-test to "I *will never* be over this problem (its cause and all that it means and does to me)." If the muscle response is strong to the first and weak to the second statement, then there is no evidence of a future BRB interfering at this time. When the muscle responses are reversed or nonpolarized, have the patient TAB under the nose (GV-26) and say three times, "I deeply (and profoundly) accept myself, even if I will never get over this problem (its cause and all that it means and does to me)." Verify the correction. If the patient is still reversed, have the patient repeat the correction this time using the small intestine treatment point (SI-3) at the side of the hand, or therapy localize by diagnosing other specific treatment point(s) and treat as above. After correction, repeat treatment of the diagnosed treatment sequence in the holon that came immediately before this BRB. Then have the patient provide a SUD level. If the SUD level is 0 or 1, go to step 15; if it is 2 or greater, repeat steps 12 through 14.

b. Check for a safety BRB. Muscle-test the patient after he or she has said, "It is *safe* for me (for others) to be over this problem (its cause and all that it means and does to me)," and then muscle-test to "It is *unsafe* for me (for others) to be over this problem (its cause and all that it means and does to me)." If the muscle response is strong to the first statement and weak to the second, then there is no safety BRB interfering at this time. When the muscle responses are reversed or nonpolarized, have the patient TAB under the nose (GV-26) and say three times, "I deeply (and profoundly) accept myself, even if it is unsafe for me (for others) to get over this problem (its cause and all that it means and does to me)." Verify the correction. If the patient is still reversed, have the patient repeat the correction this time using the small intestine treatment point (SI-3) at the side of the hand, or therapy localize by diagnosing other specific treatment point(s) and treat as above. After correction, repeat treatment of the diagnosed treatment sequence in the holon that came immediately before this BRB. Then have the patient provide a SUD level. If the SUD level is 0 or 1, go to step 15; if it is 2 or greater, repeat steps 12 through 14.

c. Check for a deservedness BRB. Muscle-test the patient after he or she has said, "I *deserve* to be over this problem (its cause and all that it means and does to me)," and then muscle-test to, "I *deserve* to keep this problem (its cause and all that it means and does to me)." If the muscle response is strong to the first statement and weak to the second, then there is no deservedness BRB interfering at this time. When the muscle responses are reversed or nonpolarized, have the patient TAB under the lip (CV-27) and say three times, "I deeply (and profoundly) accept myself, even if I deserve to keep this problem (its cause and all that it means and does to me)." Verify the correction. If the patient is still reversed, have the patient repeat the correction this time using the small intestine treatment point (SI-3) at the side of the hand, or therapy localize by diagnosing other specific treatment point(s), and treat as above. After correction, repeat treatment of the diagnosed treatment sequence in the holon that came immediately before this BRB. Then have the patient provide a SUD level. If the SUD level is 0 or 1, go to step 15; if it is 2 or greater, repeat steps 12 through 14.

d. Check for an unknown BRB. When checks for the future, safety, and deservedness BRB are negative, ask the patient if he or she is aware of any blocking thoughts that may be obstructing the resolution of the problem. If the answer is *no*, say to the patient, "tune into whatever it is that is blocking you from completing this treatment, which you may or may not be aware of with words (consciously)," and then muscle-test the patient. An unknown block is indicated when the muscle response is weak. When an unknown block is present, test the patient for an issue-specific PR for the unknown block. To do this ask the patient to say, "I want to be over this (unknown) block (its cause and all it means and does to me)." Then muscle-test him or her. Then ask the patient to say, "I want to keep this (unknown) block (its cause and all that it means and does to me)." If the muscle response is weak to the first statement and strong to the second, or strong to both, correction is needed.

Correction procedures are the same as for any issue-specific PR. To correct an issue-specific PR for an unknown block, have the patient TAB on the small intestine treatment spot on the (karate chop) side of the hand (SI-3) while saying aloud three times, "I deeply accept myself even though I have this (unknown) block (its cause and all that it means and does to me)." As usual, verify the correction. You should now get a strong muscle response to the statement about wanting to be over this unknown block, and a weak muscle response to wanting to keep the unknown block. Most issue-specific PRs regarding an unknown block will be corrected in the above manner. If this correction fails, the second option is to have the patient gently but with deep pressure rub the neurolymphatic reflex (NLR) area on the upper left side the chest in a clockwise direction, while repeating three times, "I deeply accept myself even though I have this (unknown) block (its cause and all that it means and does to me)." Again, verify the correction as described above. There are instances when neither of these corrections is effective. In those cases, the specific treatment point(s) will need to be diagnosed. The protocol for diagnosing treatment points for issue-specific PR and unknown blocks is found in Chapter 12.

When the patient's muscle response is weak to thinking about the unknown block, begin to diagnose the required treatment points to resolve that unknown block by using the same EvTFT diagnostic procedures in steps 12 through 14. You do not need a SUD level for this. After the treatment point(s) are identified and the patient now shows a strong muscle response to thinking about the unknown block, have the patient do the integration sequence, and repeat the treatment sequence you just diagnosed. Now check for a possible process-specific PR to the unknown block, and correct if needed using the previously described procedures. If the patient still muscle-tests *weak* to the unknown block, then you need to diagnose more treatment points in the next holon. When the patient muscle-tests *strong* to thinking about the unknown block, consider this block successfully corrected and repeat the treatment sequence, integration sequence, and the treatment sequence (TxSq → Isq → TxSq) of the preceding holon. Have the patient re-rate the SUD level, and resume at step 14.

e.   Check for neurologic disorganization and the need for a simplified collarbone breathing (SCB) treatment or a neurologic organizer treatment (NOTx). This assessment option ought to be considered with some patients who initially show a greater degree of neurologic disorganization. When treatment is indicated, have the patient complete the SCB treatment or the NOTx procedure as previously described in Chapter 4. After the patient has completed the corrective breathing exercise, have him or her tune into the problem and re-rate the SUD level; often it will have decreased. If SUD or SUE level is 0 or 1, go to step 15; if it is 2 or greater, repeat steps 12 through 14.

f.   Check for process-specific PR forms of the BRBs (as described above). This form of block can only be considered if a previous BRB of this type has been treated earlier in the process. For example, if a safety BRB was diagnosed and treated the therapist might suspect that a safety process-specific PR is now evident. Although less frequent, this form of a BRB does need to be checked, especially when the SUD level stalls when getting close to 2 or below. An example of a process-specific BRB test statement for safety would be, "It is safe for me (for others) to be completely over this problem (its cause and all it means and does to me). Aside from the language adjustment to reflect the form of the BRB, treatment procedure and treatment points are the same as for the process-specific PR.

18. Repeat treatment sequences from the preceding holon after correcting any treatment block

Then, continue with steps 12 through 14. Do so, if necessary, until the SUD level drops to 0 or 1.

19. Ground to sky eye-roll treatment sequence

When the SUD level has dropped to 0 or 1, have the patient do the ground to sky eye-roll treatment sequence. Often it is helpful to get both a verbal and a nonverbal (muscle-checked) SUD level for verification and confirmation. Many patients find this muscle-check verification affirming. However, some patients are not sure that their emotional distress has gone all the way down to 0, despite what the muscle check suggests. When the muscle checks a SUD level of 0, but patient's self report is greater than 0, check for a likely belief related block. This may also be suggestive of the apex problem, which is discussed in the section following the protocol (p. 179 of this book).

20. Prescribe "home treatment" as needed

Although in many cases a single EvTFT treatment in your office is sufficient for successful treatment of a problem, there are occasions when the treatment protocol needs to be repeated outside the office by the patient. The need for home treatment will be based on clinical judgment and the problem being treated. When benefit from home treatment is a consideration, use muscle testing as a guide to gain insight into the need and the frequency of additional treatment. See the section on home treatment (p. 175 of this book) for a more complete discussion of how to determine home treatment.

21. Check for a recurrent PR

Muscle-test the patient after he or she says, "I want to be over this problem (its cause and all that it means to me) once and for all," and then muscle-test to "I want this problem (its cause and all that it means to me) to keep coming back." When the patient tests strong to the first statement and weak to the second, then no recurrent PR is indicated.

When a reversed muscle response is found, have the patient rub the NLR area while saying three times: "I deeply (and profoundly) accept myself, even though this problem has come back." Verify the correction. If the correction did not take, therapy localize by diagnosing the specific treatment point(s). After correction is verified, repeat treatment of the prior holon.

22. Use the future performance imagery index (FPII)

Use the FPII when appropriate to assess how clearly the patient can imagine (e.g., see, hear, feel) himself or herself successfully and comfortably behaving or performing in a future situation, which was the focus of the treatment. See Chapter 12 for details.

23. Always follow-up your work at the next session

Inquire about the problem that was treated and check how the patient has been managing the issue. You can get a SUD level rating as a confirmation of completion or to determine if more work needs to be done. If symptoms reappear, evaluate for recurrent PR and treat if needed, or explore other related thought fields that may have become evident.

ADDITIONAL CONSIDERATIONS

Although in many cases a single EvTFT treatment in your office is sufficient for successful treatment of a problem, there are occasions when the treatment protocol needs to be repeated outside the office by the patient. The need for home treatment will be based on clinical judgment and the nature of the problem being treated. Most often cases involving addictive urges, obsessive-compulsive disorders, neurologic disorganization, energy or allergen-like toxins, pain management, and some of the anxiety disorders (e.g., panic disorder) benefit from home and in vivo treatment. Performance issues (e.g., athletic competition, performing arts, test taking) also lend themselves to additional treatments as needed.

Home Treatment

The therapist may use muscle testing as a guide to the need and frequency of home treatment. When the SUD or SUE level is 0, use the following steps:

1. Muscle-test the patient after he or she says, "This treatment is complete," and then muscle-test to "I need to repeat this treatment." If the patient tests strong to the first statement and weak to the second, then no additional treatment appears to be needed. If the patient tests weak to the first and strong to the second, then home treatment is indicated. Go to step 2.

2. You now need to ascertain how many times the patient may need to repeat the treatment for it to be complete. This can be accomplished by asking a series of questions designed to narrow a homework assignment. First establish a *yes/no set* if you have not already done so (see Chapter 4). Then, for example, muscle-test the patient after the patient says, "I need to repeat this treatment only one more time." If the muscle response is *no*, then muscle-check to "I need to repeat this treatment more than once," and the muscle response ought to be *yes*.

   Now you need to find out how many times and for how long the treatment should be repeated. At this time you muscle-check the statement "I need to repeat this treatment two to five times a day" and so on until you arrive at a definitive number. Then you might ask and muscle-check "I need to repeat this treatment everyday for one week (two weeks, etc.)" until a definitive time frame is acquired. You and your patient now know how many times per day and for how many days the treatment should be repeated to complete the work.

3. Give the patient a "home treatment" assignment sheet (see Appendices 4 & 5) to take home. This sheet will have the *entire* treatment protocol you have diagnosed and written down, including the reversals and polarity corrections, if applicable. The patient simply has to follow the steps.

4. Some patients may assume that it will take as long to do the home treatment as it did to diagnose and treat the problem in the office, and thus may be reluctant to do the follow-up. To encourage compliance, assure the patient that the assignment will only take a few minutes since no time is required for diagnosis.

Muscle-Testing the SUD Level

As described in Chapter 8, the subjective units of distress (SUD) scale is a method whereby the patient can verbally rate his or her level of emotional distress. There is, however, another method of obtaining a SUD level via a nonverbal response derived by muscle-testing the patient. Most times a muscle-tested SUD level is not necessary, and in the majority of cases the verbal and muscle-tested SUD levels match in value. Although the reasons for different verbal and muscle-tested SUD levels are unclear when they occur, we conjecture that the verbal and non-verbal expressions are two avenues of communication the patient uses to convey information about his or her emotional experience. Patients who are unable to report a verbal SUD level or report a very low or very high SUD level relative to his or her described degree of distress, or who evidence discord between the verbal and muscle-tested SUD levels, are providing clinical information about how they cope. Often such patients are more dissociated from their emotional or physical self as evidenced in cases involving repression and hysteria.

There are times when a non-verbal check of the SUD level is helpful to clarify direction in treatment or to affirm attainment of zero SUD levels. In addition there are times when a patient is unable to verbally express a SUD level, which therefore can be assessed by the non-verbal muscle-testing method when the clinician judges this information to be helpful. (While the SUD level is a helpful guide with EvTFT, it is not necessary to have a SUD level to successfully treat a problem. The skillful EvTFT clinician uses information gleaned from the patient's muscle-tested responses [e.g., when diagnosing an unknown block] as described in Chapter 12.) To assess a non-verbal SUD level, or to verify whether verbal or non-verbal SUD levels match, muscle-test the patient after he or she says, "My SUD level (or distress level, or upset level) is a seven (whatever number the patient states)." If the muscle response is strong, then the verbal SUD level is considered accurate because both avenues of communication are in accord. If the muscle response is weak, then there is discord in communication about felt emotional distress. This difference in verbal and muscle-tested SUD levels is neither good nor bad; it just is. Both concordant and discordant verbal and non-verbal SUD levels are important for the purposes of EvTFT diagnosis and treatment. Some might be drawn into thinking that the muscle-tested SUD level is "more true" than the verbal SUD level. However, we caution that to truly understand the intricacies of the mind-body-energy interface, clinicians ought to be free of this potential bias and pay attention to how the discord resolves as the EvTFT session progresses.

Verifying the patient's verbal report of a zero SUD level at the conclusion of a session by muscle-testing lends face validity and a sense of confirmation to the patient's experience of emotional and physical relief from the disturbing emotions. It has been our clinical experience that most patients are accurate in their reporting of SUD levels. Accordingly, we emphasize that discrepancies deserve attention to assure success of the EvTFT intervention.

The SUD level (verbal and nonverbal) is a baseline for the patient and therapist when beginning treatment of a thought field. Sometimes patients are unsure what their level of disturbance is after treatment has begun. For example, a patient might say, "Well, it feels somewhere around a six or seven; I'm not exactly sure." In most cases this uncertainty is not a concern requiring a muscle-tested SUD level because the verbal SUD level is greater than two indicating more diagnostic work needs to be done. However, if the therapist suspects a discrepancy based upon patient report and observation, then a muscle-test for a SUD level can provide useful information. For example, if the SUD level is reported to be unchanged or to decrease by only 1 point but the affect and degree of visible upset is considerably decreased, the therapist might muscle-test a SUD level. Often such discrepancies are indicative of a BRB, often a process-specific BRB.

Determining a SUD level through muscle-testing is generally a simple process of elimination. One way is to select a starting point and muscle-test the patient to the statements, "My level of distress is five," or "My upset level is more than five," or "My level of distress is less than five." (The language can be adjusted to the patient. One can also say, "My SUD level is . . . .") If, for example, it is less than 5, proceed to muscle-test to individual numbers until you get a strong response for a particular number. This number now becomes the non-verbal measure of communication. If a patient is unsure of one of two numbers, as in the case of the patient saying, "It's either a one or a two," muscle test him or her for both numbers. When a patient cannot distinguish between a SUD level of 1 or 2 it is recommended that a muscle-tested SUD level be obtained. How the EvTFT therapist proceeds will differ with a SUD level report of 2 (i.e., check for a process-specific PR and diagnose treatment points in the next holon) compared to a 1 (i.e., complete the ground to sky eye-roll).

Aside from confirming a SUD level of 0, or clarifying uncertainty between a report of 1 or 2, we typically do not recommend constant muscle testing to confirm every verbal report. Some exceptions might be when a therapist suspects that the patient is either trying to please him or her or is trying to hurry the process along. For research purposes, it is important to verify the patient's verbal report of the SUD level when beginning and ending the treatment.

For a variety of reasons, some patients may find it difficult to quantify their distress level with a number. In these cases it is helpful to be able to physically quantify their level of upset. Some reasons for an inability to quantify a SUD level include the following: (1) The patient may not generally think in terms of a 0 to 10 scale regarding the experience of emotions, and it may be difficult for him or her to adapt to this way of thinking; (2) The patient may be initially too distressed to come up with a number and will sometimes state "twenty" when asked for a 0 to 10 rating; (3) Even though the problem is reportedly disturbing to the patient while he or she is experiencing it, the patient may not be able to connect with those feelings of disturbance while in the therapist's office, and this cannot accurately rate his or her distress level; (4) The patient may be too young or not competent enough to grasp the concept of the scale.[1]

The Apex Problem

There is an interesting phenomenon that sometimes occurs after a successful thought field therapy session. It involves how the patient viewed the cause of the emotional change. Patients may attribute the resolution of their problems to causes other than the EvTFT treatment, or they deny, forget, or minimize the fact that they had a problem to start with. Another telltale sign is when a patient states, after achieving complete relief of his or her emotional upset, "So, how long will this last?" Callahan (1995) named this the *apex problem* and described it as follows:

> APEX PROBLEM. The robust tendency, it could be called a compulsion, for treated clients or observers of therapy, to give "explanations" of the treatments which are totally inappropriate and irrelevant. . . .

Mental work at the apex of the mind is required to grasp and understand these new treatments. Most of us attempt to avoid such work and erroneously attempt to fit it into something we believe we understand. (pp. 71–72)

One clinical example of this was a patient who was successfully treated with EvTFT for a lifelong fear of heights. In the follow-up session, the patient claimed that during the interim week he had seen a television program in which the protagonist had acrophobia. The patient told the therapist, "I saw what was happening to him and it didn't make sense; so I decided that I wouldn't be afraid any more." Other explanations can be that the patient suddenly "outgrew the problem," made a conscious decision to give it up, was convinced by a third party's intervention, the medication finally started to work, hypnosis or distraction was used "with all that counting and humming stuff," or that the problem really was never that bad or was nonexistent. Callahan's hypothesis that the "dramatic change" (1995, p. 71) effected by this therapy cannot be readily integrated into existing frames of reference is certainly worth examining.

Chapter 11

DIAGNOSIS AND TREATMENT OF ELATERS

The diseases which destroy a man are no less
natural than the instincts which preserve him.
—George Santayana

This chapter will introduce an experimental method for diagnosis and treatment of positive emotions, sensations, and thoughts that drive unwanted and self-sabotaging behaviors. As briefly described in Chapter 7, it is hypothesized that the experience of positive feelings are triggered by tiny information-bearing signals emitted from *elaters* in our thought field. These signals are received and amplified in our meridian system, then resonate in our body and pave the way for our emotional and physical experience of these positive emotions. There is usually no reason to extinguish or subsume elater signals because we, and society in general, have a high tolerance and desire for happy and joyous emotions. Smiles, good cheer, and gracious behavior are usually well received.

Most people want to feel good. Good feelings help sustain us and even teach us about life and ourselves. We have been encouraged to be with people and do things that foster these good feelings. In this regard, positive emotions are usually welcomed with open arms and hearts. These desired good feelings increase the probability that we will continue or repeat the behavior that feels so good. But what do we do when the desired good feelings lead to bad outcomes?

We have observed in our clinical practices that there are times when unwanted or self-defeating behavior can be initiated and maintained by positive emotions, sensations, and thoughts. When something feels good or tastes good, there is a greater likelihood that the behavior that promotes these feelings and tastes will continue. Accordingly, positive emotions may also serve to maintain self-defeating behaviors that accompany conditions like overeating, addictions, and compulsions.

Traditional psychotherapy has concentrated on negative thoughts and emotions when treating unwanted or self-defeating behaviors. As we have described, the treatment or elimination of perturbations are targeted and defined as the singular cause of disturbance in the thought field by the Callahan Techniques™ and other energy psychology methods. The absence of treatment for positive emotions may account for why many forms of psychotherapy struggle the hardest with addictive or repetitive disorders and personality disorders. We suggest that the impact of positive thoughts and emotions as potential sources of disruptive and self-sabotaging behaviors require careful scrutiny. It has been our opinion, and our clinical experience, that the positive aspect is also a viable component for treatment of psychopathology with certain conditions (e.g., addictions, obsessions, compulsions, personality traits).

Why are behavior patterns involving eating disorders, substance dependencies and addictions, obsessive-compulsive patterns, and personality disorders so challenging to change? The most likely explanation is that these behavior patterns are related in some way to making the individual feel better. We hypothesize that these types of patterns are not *dis-orders* but rather *in-orders*. The person adopts and maintains his or her self-defeating pattern *in order* to improve his or her experienced emotional state or physical condition. Accordingly, it would be prudent to also address the positive, elater-influenced dimensions in a person's thought field when providing psychotherapy.

As clinicians we all have had numerous patients say that the reason they continue to drink alcohol or smoke cigarettes, despite protests from loved ones and physicians, is because "I like it. It tastes good. I want to. I like how it makes me feel." We also hear thoughts that deny the validity of information, so the patient may say, "I've got to die of something," or "My doctor smokes (or is overweight) so it can't really be true." Or patients may acknowledge that they know the behavior is not healthy or good for them and they would like to stop but are unable. After the fact, many of these patients lament and question their behavior. However, when they are actively engaged in a triggered thought field, they feel powerless to control their emotional response and behavior. The pattern is similar to a patient who presents upsetting symptoms of post-traumatic distress when attuned to a trauma. However, with elaters, it is the reverse side of the emotional coin that tickles the affect and drives the self-defeating behavior. Elater involvement also appears to contribute to suicidal ideation, especially when the depressed patient reports a belief that there will be peace and calm connected to dying. Even undesirable characterological traits can be evaluated for elater involvement and treated to foster desirable changes.

We propose that the energetic formulations that describe the underlying inability to control addictive, compulsive, or obsessional behavior are similar to those underlying phobias or post-traumatic stress disorder, with one important difference. If we conceptualize the "negative" associations to an event as *perturbations* in the thought field, we need to have a means to distinguish them from the "positive" associations to an event in the thought field. Therefore, in addition to perturbations, we introduce into the treatment protocols the concept of *elaters* as another potential disruption in the thought field.

Elater involvement ought to be considered in any self-defeating or sociopathic situation in which the person is engaged *in-order* to escape or relieve himself or herself of distress and to momentarily "enjoy" an undesirable or later unwanted activity. Elater involvement is obvious in addictions, obsessions, and compulsions, but elaters may also play a role in the traditional concepts of *secondary gains*. The desired emotional outcome (e.g., enjoyment, attention) may also come from the response of others to the patient's behavior. For example, psychopathology that involves exhibitionism relies on a response from others in order to experience the desired "positive" emotion whereas voyeurism does not. Perhaps impulsive violent crime (e.g., rape, torture) is also elater driven since sadistic satisfaction is derived in part from the victim's response. In the paradoxical realities of emotion and behavior, corrupted core beliefs may twist reason in strange ways that are unfamiliar to healthier individuals. In such pathological conditions, for example, inflicting pain (to self or others) may equal relief, revenge, or some other "positive" feeling for coping, which is distortedly justified as warranted and good.

As clinicians, not only do we need to treat the negative thoughts and emotions that drive problem behavior, we need to identify and treat the positive emotions that drive, and maintain problem thoughts and behavior. However, this is not to say that the treatment of elaters is a self-standing panacea, because clearly it is not. We recommend that identification and treatment of positive emotions (elaters) become an integral part of any method of psychotherapy, which also includes identification and treatment of perturbations, cognitive core beliefs, and other emotional and behavioral change methods.

THE ELATER APPROACH

Similar to perturbations, elaters can be diagnosed and treated using the meridian system. This experimental protocol for the treatment of elaters (Diepold, 2000, 2002) involves the following changes from the standard protocol presented in Chapter 10.

In place of a SUD level, have patients rate their subjective units of enjoyment or elation (SUE) level. The SUE level uses the same 0 to 10 point scale, where 0 is the absence of enjoyment (or neutral) and 10 the highest degree of enjoyment, derived benefit, or secondary gain. Have patients attune his or her problematic thought field, and to their positive benefit (elater). For example, you might ask the patient to "Tune into your feeling of enjoyment[1] when you (smoke a cigarette, take a drink, eat chocolate, pull your hair, etc.), even though you know it is not good for you (and/or your body)."[2] When you muscle-test to this thought field, the patient's indicator muscle should go weak. The inner wisdom of the body-mind-spirit, or unconscious, "knows" the cost of this problem. If the indicator muscle is strong, then there is an issue-specific psychological reversal (PR) that needs to be corrected before continuing. Self-sabotage and persistence of a negative behavior pattern, despite knowing better, is an indicator of PR.

To test for an issue-specific PR pertaining to an elater, muscle-test to the statements "I want to be over my enjoyment of X because I know it is not good for me (and/or my body)," and "I want to keep my enjoyment of X even though I know it is not good for me (and/or my body)." (Or you might have the patient say, "I want to be over my enjoyment of X because I know the cost to me and others" and "I want to keep my enjoyment of X despite the cost to me and others.") A strong indicator muscle response to the latter statement indicates an issue-specific PR, which needs to be corrected. Have the patient correct this by using touch-and-breathe (TAB) on the side of the hand (SI-3) while saying three times, "I deeply accept myself even though I enjoy (or derive benefit from) X, which I know is not good for me (and/or my body)." Or you might have the patient say "I deeply accept myself even though I enjoy (or derive benefit from) X, which I know comes at a considerable cost to me and others.") Muscle-test again to verify the correction. If an issue-specific PR is still evident, you may try rubbing the neurolymphatic reflex area (NLR) ("sore spot" on the left side of the chest between second and third ribs) or use a diagnostic method to identify the required correction point(s).

The procedure and language adjustment for diagnosing and treating other elater related blocks to treatment (e.g., process or belief-related PRs) would follow the same format as above. All procedures are completed as the patient is attuned to his or her problem of enjoying X, while simultaneously aware that X is not good for them or comes at considerable cost to the patient or others.

There are currently no known algorithms for the treatment of elaters. Although a comprehensive algorithm or the emotional freedom techniques (Craig & Fowlie, 1997) could be used in the treatment of elaters, our clinical preference is to individually diagnose and treat the indicated meridians. In keeping with the diagnostic model, when an alarm point tests strong, treat the corresponding treatment point for that meridian. Continue diagnostic procedures until the indicator muscle responds strong to the thought field. Follow with the integration sequence treatments, and then repeat the diagnosed treatment sequence again. Now re-rate the SUE level. If the SUE level is 0 or 1, complete the ground to sky eye-roll treatment. If the SUE level is 2 or above, follow the same diagnostic procedures described in the diagnosis and treatment of perturbations in Chapter 10 to finish treating the energetic underpinnings of the remaining positive benefit (elater) until the SUE level is 0 or 1. Then finish with the eye-roll treatment.

The above elater approach to diagnosing and treating meridians that respond strong to an alarm point test is consistent with how we diagnosis and treat perturbations with negative affect. Some colleagues have questioned why the indicator muscle would test weak when the patient is attuned to a pleasant or enjoyable thought field. That possibility stems from observations that the indicator muscle will usually test strong when people think of something pleasant. However, emotions are experienced within a context (thought, memory, experience); it is the positive emotion in relation to the context (the unwanted behavior) that we are attempting to change in using this elater approach.

Chapter 12

SUPPLEMENTARY AND
MODIFIED PROTOCOLS

Necessity inspires creativity to adjust to the individual needs of our patients.

—The BDB Group

This chapter describes nine supplementary and modified protocols that build on the basic diagnostic and treatment protocol described in Chapter 10. These protocols should be used in conjunction with the basic protocol by clinicians whose patients present with the issues addressed by these methods. It is preferable that the clinician be proficient with the basic protocol since the following protocols work in concert with the basic protocol and extend the application of Evolving Thought Field Therapy (EvTFT) to more specific clinical populations and conditions.

The supplementary and modified protocols pertain to the following:

1. Diagnosis and treatment of known (e.g., psychological reversals) and unknown blocks (e.g., beliefs or events).
2. The future performance imagery index (FPII).
3. Peak performance issues.
4. Pain and pain management.
5. Diagnosis and treatment of patients with dissociative identity disorder (DID) and other dissociative disorders.
6. The use of a cluster technique to treat multiple thought fields.
7. Recognition and treatment of energy disrupters.
8. Ways to muscle-test and diagnose oneself.
9. Use of surrogates for diagnosis and treatment.

DIAGNOSIS AND TREATMENT OF PSYCHOLOGICAL REVERSALS, KNOWN AND UNKNOWN BLOCKS, AND BELIEF RELATED BLOCKS

In Chapter 6 we described the basic assessment and the algorithmic correction point with concomitant affirmation for various categories of treatment blocks (e.g., psychological reversal and belief related blocks). Often a second correction point was listed for instances when the first treatment site proved ineffective. Although usually successful, there are times when neither of the suggested treatment sites are effective and it becomes necessary to diagnose the needed treatment sites to correct the treatment blocks. As necessary, this diagnosis is done as part of the EvTFT process and blends smoothly with the other procedures.[1]

Protocol for Diagnosing Treatment Points for Psychological Reversals or Known Blocks

The need to diagnose treatment points to correct a psychological reversal or a consciously known block arises after both the standard and the alternative treatment points (if provided) fail to correct the problem. In these instances the patient continues to show a reversed polarized muscle response to the test statements, or a nonpolarized muscle response (e.g., strong/strong); that is, he or she tests *weak* to a positive statement (e.g., "It is safe to be over this problem (its cause . . .)," and *strong* to its negative counterpart (e.g., "It is not safe to be over this problem (its cause . . .)", or strong to both statements.

There are two ways of conducting the diagnosis, which are based on the muscle response of the patient: (1) When there is reversed polarity, the patient is asked to tune into the positive statement as the thought field; and (2) when there is a strong/strong nonpolarized muscle response, the patient is asked to tune into the negative statement as the thought field. (The occurrence of a nonpolarized weak/weak muscle response in this phase of the EvTFT protocol is rare. When it does occur, it is almost exclusively found when working with patients who have a diagnosis involving dissociation [e.g., DID].) The reasons for these differences will be explained below. These diagnoses are essentially simplified versions of the basic protocol, with many of the steps eliminated, such as a taking a SUD level. For the sake of clarity, we shall use a safety belief related block for the example protocols.

Tuning in to the Positive Statement

After having assessed that the patient demonstrates appropriate polarized muscle responses regarding true and false items, using the positive statement as the thought field is the method of choice when the patient muscle-tests weak to the positive statement on a check for a psychological reversal. When using this method of diagnosing the necessary treatment site(s) to correct the block, we treat the meridians whose alarm point(s) muscle-test *strong* as the patient is attuned to the positive statement. This is the same format used in the basic diagnosis protocol.

The following steps are offered to assist the clinician when the patient's muscle response is weak to the positive statement when checking for a psychological reversal:

1. Have the patient tune into the statement, "It is safe for me to be over this problem (or block). . . ." With a clear mind, muscle-test an alarm point using one of the three diagnostic methods.

    a. If the indicator muscle (IM) is *weak* when you muscle-test, then this meridian is inactive at this time and does not require treatment. Keep checking alarm points until you get a *strong* IM response while the patient is attuned to the positive statement. Then go to step 1b.

    b. If the IM is *strong* when you muscle-test, have the patient touch-and-breathe (TAB) on the corresponding meridian treatment site. Write down the treatment site. You have now diagnosed the first treatment point. There may or may not be other meridians involved. Go to step 2.

2. Have the patient again tune into the positive statement while you muscle-test him or her.

    a. If the IM is *weak*, then there is at least one more treatment point to be diagnosed in this holon. Continue diagnosing using alarm points; when the IM responds *strong* on an alarm point, have the patient TAB on the corresponding treatment site. Again have the patient tune into the positive statement while you muscle-test him or her. Repeat this step of diagnosing and treating meridians until the muscle responds *strong* when the patient is attuned to the positive statement.

    b. If the IM is *strong*, you have completed the treatment sequence for this holon. Now have the patient do the integration sequence (ISq) and then repeat the treatment sequence (TxSq).

3. Since there is no subjective units of distress (SUD) level to guide you, you must always check next for the possibility of a process-specific psychological reversal (process-specific PR). If one is found, correct it in the usual way at the side of the hand (SI-3) and then repeat TxSq → ISq → TxSq. (Remember, the affirmation statement with a process-specific PR involves using the word *completely*, as in, "It is safe for me to be *completely* over this problem . . . ").

4. Recheck the IM by muscle-testing the patient as he or she is attuned to the thought field (i.e., thinking or saying the positive statement of the psychological reversal check or the block). As long as the IM responds weak, continue diagnosing the needed treatment points by repeating steps 1, 2, and 3 until the reversal is corrected and the IM response is strong to the positive statement or block. To verify, the muscle response should be strong to the positive statement and weak to the negative statement.

5. When the psychological reversal or block is corrected and verified, resume the diagnosis of the presenting problem. Remember to repeat treatment of the holon that came immediately before the psychological reversal or known block, and then re-check the SUD or SUE (subjective units of enjoyment) level. When the SUD or SUE level is 0 or 1, complete the treatment with the ground to sky eye-roll treatment. If the SUD or SUE level is 2 or higher, return to the basic protocol and resume diagnosis and treatment of additional holons or blocks for the presenting problem based upon the muscle response (i.e., if the muscle response is weak to the thought field then diagnose the next holon; if the muscle response is strong to the thought field then evaluate for another belief related or unknown block).

Tuning in to the Negative Statement

Using the negative statement as the thought field is the method of choice when the patient muscle-tests strong to *both* the positive and negative statements when checking for a psychological reversal. Again, this is of concern because the patient demonstrates appropriate polarized muscle responses regarding true and false items not related to the test for psychological reversal. When using this focus of diagnosing the necessary treatment site(s) to correct the polarity block, we treat the meridians whose alarm point(s) muscle-test *weak* as the patient is attuned to the negative statement. This is an inverse format compared to the basic diagnostic protocol. In other words, instead of looking to find which meridian makes the indicator muscle strong, we look to identify the meridian that makes the IM appropriately weak.

The following steps are offered to assist the clinician when the patient's muscle response is strong to both the positive and negative statements when checking for a psychological reversal:

1. Have the patient tune into the negative psychological reversal statement ("It is not safe for me to be over this problem [or block] . . ."). Then, with a clear mind, muscle-test an alarm point using one of the three diagnostic methods.

   a. If the IM is *strong* when you muscle-test, then this meridian is inactive at this time and does *not* require treatment. Keep checking alarm points until you get a *weak* IM response while the patient is attuned to the negative statement. Then go to step1b.

   b. If the IM is *weak* when you muscle-test, have the patient TAB on the corresponding meridian treatment site. Write down the treatment site. You have now diagnosed the first treatment point. There may or may not be other meridians involved. Go to step 2.

2. Again have the patient tune into the negative statement while you muscle-test him or her.

   a. If the IM is *strong*, then there is at least one more treatment point(s) to be diagnosed in this holon. Continue diagnosing alarm points; when the IM responds *weak* on an alarm point, have the patient TAB on the corresponding treatment site. Again have the patient tune into the negative statement while you muscle-test him or her. Keep repeating this step of diagnosing and treating meridians until the muscle responds *weak* when the patient is attuned to the negative statement.

   b. If the IM is *weak*, you have completed the treatment sequence thus far. Now, have the patient do the ISq treatment and then repeat the TxSq.

3. Since there is no SUD or SUE level to guide you, you must always check next for the possibility of a process-specific PR. If one is found, correct it in the usual way at the side of the hand (SI-3) and then repeat TxSq → ISq → TxSq. (Remember, the affirmation statement with a process-specific PR involves using the word *completely*, as in, "It is safe for me to be *completely* over this problem . . .").

4. Recheck the IM by muscle-testing the patient as he or she is attuned to the thought field (i.e., thinking or saying the negative statement of the psychological reversal check or the block). As long as the IM responds strong continue diagnosing the treatment points by repeating steps 1, 2, and 3 until the reversal is corrected and the IM response is weak to the negative statement or block. To verify, the

muscle response should be strong to the positive statement and weak to the negative statement.

5. When the psychological reversal or block is corrected and verified, resume the diagnosis of the presenting problem. Remember to repeat treatment of the holon that came immediately before the psychological reversal or known block, and then re-check the SUD or SUE level. When the SUD or SUE level is 0 or 1, complete the treatment with the ground to sky eye-roll. If the SUD or SUE level is 2 or higher, return to the basic protocol and resume diagnosis and treatment of additional holons or blocks for the presenting problem based upon the muscle response (i.e., if the muscle response is *weak* to the thought field then diagnose the next holon; if the muscle response is *strong* to the thought field then evaluate for another belief related or unknown block).

The Diagnosis of Unknown Blocks

The concept of diagnosing and treating what we term an *unknown block* is unique to EvTFT. We found that using this approach eliminates the guesswork in which the patient and therapist frequently engage. We also hypothesize that this diagnostic approach invites the psyche of the patient to attune whatever is necessary to help resolve the targeted issue. A typical scenario goes something like the following: The diagnosis and treatment of a thought field is progressing well when, after treating at least one holon, the SUD or SUE level is reported to be 2 or greater. The requisite tests for a process-specific PR are negative but when the patient is muscle-tested as he or she attunes the thought field the muscle response is strong. Typically, when a patient attunes the thought field with a SUD or SUE level greater than 0, the IM will respond weak because he or she is still upset and more treatment is needed. If the IM is strong in the face of the reported distress, then a belief related block, which is generating a reversed polarized muscle response (strong instead of weak), is suspected.

In keeping with the basic EvTFT protocol, we then recommend that the patient be evaluated for the possibility of any of the three primary belief related blocks (i.e., future, deservedness, safety). If none of the three belief related blocks are present, then a check for evidence of neurologic disorganization could be done because of the polarity switch and treated with neurologic organizer treatment (NOTx) or simplified collarbone breathing (SCB) if indicated. Asking the patient what he or she thinks is blocking treatment, as well as checking lists of criteria-related beliefs that could interfere, could also be done. However, we find that the easiest and most effective way to continue is to simply invite the patient to "Tune into whatever it is that is blocking you now from completing this work, even though you may not know consciously what it may be." Then, while the patient is attuned to "whatever it is," muscle-test him or her. The IM should now test weak to this thought field. This thought field is the unknown block.

What is an unknown block? It could be a suppressed belief, or a repressed experience or trauma perhaps occurring at a preverbal developmental level. Maybe an unknown block results from interaction with Sheldrake's hypothetical morphogenic fields, the collective unconscious as proposed by Jung, or perhaps from a past life if the patient's culture or beliefs support reincarnation. The reality is that we may not ever know, and it really does not seem to matter. What matters is that when the unknown block is diagnosed and treated like any other thought field, the patient is able to again resume treatment of his or her initial issue and attain the desired emotional relief.

The following guidelines will assist the therapist in recognizing when an unknown block may be present, and will provide the steps involved in resolving its interference and in completing the work with the targeted thought field.

1. As described in the scenario above, an unknown block interferes with the ability to continue diagnosis and treatment. This form of block is adjudged only after proper body polarity has been established, all recommended checks for psychological reversal have been completed and found to be absent, and the SUD or SUE level is reported to be 1 or higher, but the IM responds strong when the patient attunes the thought field being treated. An unknown block could become evident at the beginning or during treatment with the basic EvTFT protocol.

2. When an unknown block is suspected, invite the patient to tune into this unknown block, even if they do not consciously know what it is, and muscle-test. The language we frequently use to invite the patient's involvement is, "Tune into whatever it is that is blocking you now from completing this work, even though you may not know consciously what it may be." When you muscle-test the patient as he or she attunes to "whatever it is," the IM will go weak as it would to any disturbing thought field.

3. Check for the possibility of an issue-specific psychological reversal (PR) using the statements, "I want to be over whatever it is that is blocking me from resolving this problem" and "I want to keep whatever it is that is blocking me from resolving this problem." At this point you can tell the patient that this is called an *unknown block*.

    a. When the muscle test is strong to the first statement and weak to the second, there is no indication of an issue-specific PR; therefore, proceed to diagnose alarm points and treat the indicated meridians per the basic protocol using the unknown block as the thought field.

    b. When the muscle response is weak to the first statement and strong to the second, an issue-specific PR is evident and requires correction. Use the recommended correction method of TAB at the side of the hand (SI-3) while the patient says three times, "I deeply accept myself even though I have this unknown block, its cause, and all that it means and does to me." As usual, verify the correction. The alternate treatment site is the NLR area on the upper left chest.

4. Proceed to diagnose alarm points and treat the indicated meridians per the basic protocol using the unknown block as the thought field. Follow the standard format of TxSq → ISq → TxSq. Since there is no SUD or SUE level to guide you, you must always check for the possibility of a process-specific PR to this unknown block. If a process-specific PR is evident, correct it according to the basic protocol. When a process-specific PR is not evident, muscle-test the patient again to the thought field (i.e., the unknown block). If the IM tests weak, diagnose the next holon for this unknown block. If the IM tests strong, the unknown block is cleared. (In a small percentage of cases the therapist may need to check for the possibility of future, deservedness, and safety belief related blocks regarding an unknown block. Use your clinical judgment and intuition.)

5. When the unknown block has been cleared, return to the original target thought field and re-rate the SUD or SUE level. We also recommend having the patient re-treat the entire holon that preceded the presentation of the unknown block as you would after correction of any other block or psychological reversal. If the SUD or SUE level is still 2 or higher, the patient should now muscle-test weak to the original thought field. Now complete the diagnosis and treatment. If the muscle response is again strong to the target thought field and the SUD or SUE level is 2 or higher, re-evaluate for another unknown block.

The Diagnosis of Nonpolarized Muscle Responses

A nonpolarized response is one in which there is no differentiation in muscle response to positive and negative statements. In these instances of treatment block, the patient will test either strong/strong or weak/

weak to the psychological reversal test statements after demonstrating appropriate and differentiated muscle responses to other true and false items. These nonpolarized responses are atypical, especially the weak/weak muscle response, which is almost always corrected by having the patient drink a little water. However, such responses occur frequently enough to merit attention and correction.

The therapist can consider the nonpolarized response as a block to further diagnosis and treatment, and therefore correct for it using the standard correction for that particular type of block. For example, if a patient demonstrates a strong/strong muscle response to the statements, "It is safe for me to be over this problem (its cause ...") and "It is unsafe for me to be over this problem (its cause ...)," then this may be considered a block which can be treated by having the patient TAB under the nose and say three time, "I deeply accept myself even if it is unsafe for me to be over this problem (its cause ...)" as per the basic protocol. In these instances the therapist should always perform the corrections on himself or herself because the interaction of the therapist's body polarity might be affecting the muscle-testing results. When the usual treatment procedures for blocks fail to correct the nonpolarized response to the thought field, the therapist can proceed to evaluate for an unknown block that is affecting treatment continuation.

THE FUTURE PERFORMANCE IMAGERY INDEX (FPII)

Often the work we do with our patients pertains to situations and events that will likely occur for them in the future: for example, riding in an elevator, driving in certain situations, seeing a family member or co-worker, flying in an airplane, and so on. While many times the basic EvTFT treatments in the office, and use of follow-up homework treatments as needed, are sufficient to maintain successful and comfortable performance outside the office setting, we have found it advantageous to "stack the deck" in the patient's favor by evaluating how he or she will respond to the event or situation in the future. This is a way of creating a future template for any future-occurring situation or activity that you have just successfully treated in the context of present or past, as indicated by attainment of a SUD or SUE level of 0. The index builds from concepts related to the use of positive imagery; if you can imagine yourself in the future being comfortable and acting successfully, then the intention and the corresponding feelings that resonate with that perception will increase the probability of a successful experience. The

Future Performance Imagery Index (FPII) originated as part of our peak performance protocol. However, we learned it had value in the basic protocol when working with many anxiety and panic provoking situations, interpersonal issues, and impediments to daily interactions.

The FPII is a 1 to 7 point scale used to assess how clearly the patient can visualize and imagine (i.e., see, hear, feel) himself or herself successfully and comfortably being in or performing in a future situation. The FPII is used with the treatment of perturbations and elaters whenever the patient will address (e.g., face, perform, confront) the focus or topic of treatment in the future. An FPII score of 1 represents a low ability to currently visualize or imagine successful and comfortable performance. An FPII score of 7 represents the highest and sharpest ability to currently visualize or imagine successful and comfortable performance. The FPII score will serve as a guide to both patient and therapist in knowing when the maximum results have been achieved. When the patient reports an FPII score that is lower than 7, treatment is warranted to enhance his or her future performance.

Using the FPII

The FPII is used when the patient has completed the treatment for the presenting problem and reports a SUD or SUE level of 0. We believe it is helpful for the patient to create a positive mental and physical experience in which the patient imagines himself or herself in the future addressing the situation or event while being free of emotional distress. For example, if, after an EvTFT treatment intervention, a patient has resolved her anger at her husband, she can then imagine herself in the future interacting with him and being as comfortable (i.e., anger-free) as she is during the therapy session, thus creating a pattern for future communication and comfortable affect. Other examples would be patients who completed an EvTFT intervention to resolve emotional upset from a driving trauma, a performance problem, or a phobia. In these instances we would invite the patient to imagine himself or herself in the future (e.g., driving through that same intersection, performing in an upcoming event, or being in the presence of the prior phobic stimulus). Then we ask the patient to rate his or her subjective ability to clearly imagine or visualize achieving their goal with comfort.

The following steps are provided as a guide to using the FPII:

1. After completing diagnosis and treatment on the targeted thought field(s) as confirmed by a reported and verified SUD or SUE level of 0, invite the patient to imagine himself or herself *in the future*

addressing (e.g., facing, performing, confronting) the resolved problem situation.

2. Ask the patient to rate how clearly he or she is able to imagine himself or herself in this future situation using a scale from 1 to 7. For example, say to the patient, "How clearly can you now imagine yourself in the future engaging in this situation and feeling as comfortable as you do at present? Please rate your experience using a one to seven point scale where one equals no or low ability to currently imagine successful and comfortable performance, and seven represents the highest and sharpest ability to currently imagine successful and comfortable performance." Or you might say, "How clearly can you see and imagine yourself in the future doing [the target issue], and feeling as comfortable and confident as you do now? Use a scale from one to seven where one is 'not very clear' and seven would be 'as clear as it gets' when you can imagine yourself doing [the target issue]."

3. When the FPII score is reported to be 7 there is usually no need for additional treatment. If, however, you sense what Diepold terms a "soft seven," as suggested by a delay in response, uncertainty in voice or face, or an unconvincing affect, then treatment is worth pursuing.

4. When the FPII score is reported to be less than 7, additional treatment is recommended as follows. Invite the patient to again imagine achieving the desired outcome and instruct him or her to "TAB under the arm (SP-21) while taking three respirations, or more if you like, until the image is maximized." Then have him or her "TAB on the inner eye (BL-1) while taking three respirations, or more if you like, until the image is maximized." Note whether the left or right arm or eye was used. Now have the patient do the ISq and repeat the TxSq, this time using the opposite arm and eye.[2] Complete the treatment with an eye-roll. Recheck the FFPII score. When the FPII score is 7 (a "solid 7"), treatment is complete.

5. When the FPII score remains below 7 after treatment, inquire about any additional issues (thought fields) that might be keeping the patient from imagining their goal more clearly. Perhaps a new memory or concern has come to the fore that needs to be diagnosed and treated. At this point it is usually easier to ask the patient to "tune into whatever it is that is keeping you from imagining your desired outcome more clearly," and muscle-test. The muscle response will usually be weak. When weak, diagnose and treat as an unknown block to remove any remaining obstacles to imagining the future

more clearly. If the muscle response is strong, evaluate for possible blocks—at this point, there could be a future or another belief related block; be sure to check and treat for these when present—and treat accordingly.

PEAK PERFORMANCE ISSUES

We define *peak performance* as the ability of a person to perform at his or her optimum potential in a given activity in which he or she already has some degree of ability. This is a performance enhancement methodology; a beginning performer with no prior experience would not be appropriate for this protocol. (This protocol uses visual and felt experiences and related circumstances relevant to the actual performance of the activity.) For example, if a person has just decided to take up golf and requests help to maximize his or her performance, it would be premature to use this protocol. The protocol would be appropriate after he or she has taken golf lessons, learned the game, played for a period of time, reached a plateau in performance level, and desires to improve. Peak performance issues can apply to many situations in which the patient is proficient but has reached difficulty in advancing. These situations may include job function, artistic or creative endeavors, sport or fine art performance, or goal-oriented achievements of any kind.

Blocks to peak performance can be obvious or mysterious to patients. Frustration is often the driving force that leads them to the therapist's office. By the time they seek help it is probable that they have tried many other avenues offered by coaches, teachers, friends, books and articles, co-workers or teammates, and even various superstitious rituals, all to no avail. Often the patient is looking for a quick fix, a band-aid of sorts, to put him or her back on track as quickly as possible. High anxiety is a close cousin to frustration, and often spills over into feelings of self-anger, embarrassment, shame, and sometimes depression. Most who seek assistance for performance enhancement are highly competitive and intense individuals who are driven to excel; they expect to excel and need to excel. Obstacles are to be conquered and beaten before they themselves are conquered and beaten. Helping the patient see the bigger picture of performance enhancement, as well as the various forms and sources of potential obstacles, is essential in the early phases of establishing rapport, information gathering, and treatment formulation.

Sometimes the origin of the difficulties that impede higher performance can be traced to current circumstances or, more often, to events in the past. Previous difficulties or traumatic experiences often dictate the presenting behavior patterns and create the template for the patient's performance difficulties. For example, a rivalry issue with a co-worker might be traced to a similar unresolved sibling relationship, or a high school wrestler's inability to perform in a match (like he does in practice) may relate to unresolved childhood experiences when performing in front of others. Mindful of this, it is important to carefully assess the broader scope of possible impediments to better performance during the assessment phase of the protocol. Inquiries should be made regarding

1. when the difficulties began,
2. the circumstances around the initial incident,
3. how the patient (and others) responded,
4. the duration of the current situation,
5. what has been tried to remedy the situation,
6. when specifically does the problem occur and under what circumstances,
7. what does the patient think is involved or needed,
8. what does the patient think and feel before, during, and after the situation,
9. when have similar things happened in the past, and
10. do the circumstances involve another person and does this replicate another relationship from the past.

We recommend a thorough history with specific emphasis on the presented performance issue. It has also been our experience that many who seek treatment for performance enhancement find comfort and trust in a therapist who has participated in his or her activity or has experience treating others in similar situations. At the very least, having interest and knowledge about the patient's concern, sport, or activity facilitates a bridge for asking the needed questions and tailoring the needed interventions.

As is true in other clinical issues, the use of EvTFT methods with peak performance issues is not designed or intended to be a stand-alone treatment. Assessment of realistic goals, positive self-talk, and use of imagery are frequently included in treating issues of peak performance. Use of traditional clinical interviewing techniques will serve to identify pertinent thought fields and guide the use of EvTFT interventions. As a basic guideline, treatment of all earlier upsetting or traumatic experiences ought to be treated with EvTFT prior to addressing the current difficulties. Often the healing effect of neutralizing the associated negative affect of the earlier issues and traumas, especially the initial event(s), brings considerable relief and improvement with the current concern. Then, focus may be directed at assessing and treating the specific remaining performance issues.

The EvTFT Peak Performance Protocol

The peak performance protocol that follows is designed as a guide to assist the clinician in targeting and treating relevant thought fields that impact performance. It also includes provisions for incorporating positive self-talk and imagery to enhance accomplishment of the desired goals. The basic EvTFT protocol is used as the primary intervention to treat the cluster of related events and experiences connected to the performance goal(s). Notice, however, that select meridians or procedures are used differently in some steps of this protocol (compared to the basic protocol) to fortify attainment of the desired performance outside the office setting.

1. Evaluate the goals and obstacles as reported by the person. What fears, worries, or traumatic events are involved? In addition, are there past or current interpersonal problems with a boss, coach, teacher, teammate, opponent, coworker, or parent? Are there current or past problems with expectations or self-talk?

2. Using your choice of the three EvTFT diagnostic methods, diagnose the appropriate treatment sequence for each specified thought field (e.g., fear, worry, traumatic incident, previous issue affecting the problem as obtained in step 1). There are often several problems affecting difficulties with peak performance, and every thought field needs to be diagnosed and treated separately. (A case example would be a concert pianist who had trouble playing a particular piece. The patient revealed that she had played this piece badly in public a few years earlier and became anxious whenever she played it thereafter. Using an EvTFT diagnostic method, the therapist had her attune the memory of when she performed poorly in public, and then the therapist proceeded with the standard EvTFT protocol to treat that interfering memory.) This step may be lengthy, depending on the amount of history and the number of associated issues the patient presents.

3. After having diagnosed and treated the problems and situations affecting the patient's peak performance, have the patient focus on the specified goal(s) for peak performance and operationally define the goal(s) for clarity and ease of recognition. For example, if you are working with a baseball player struggling with hitting, the pa-

tient's goal of "I want to hit better" would be more accurately and objectively stated as "I want to make solid contact and drive the ball." List all goals for future reference and operationally define them as needed.

4. Muscle-test each peak performance goal for an issue-specific psychological reversal (ISPR). In this example, muscle tests would be performed to the statements, "I want to make solid contact and drive the ball," and then to, "I do not want to make solid contact and drive the ball." When the muscle response is weak to the first statement and strong to the second, correct for an issue-specific PR. The goal and purpose is to free the patient from any self-sabotaging or self-limiting beliefs that could block attainment of the performance goal.

5. Test for a possible future belief related block (BRB) by muscle-testing the statements, "I will be able to make solid contact and drive the ball" and "I will never be able to make solid contact and drive the ball." When the muscle response is weak to the first statement and strong to the second, correct for a future BRB by having the patient TAB under the nose and say three times, "I deeply accept myself even if I will never make solid contact and drive the ball." The alternate correction site is the side of the hand (SI-3).

6. After having completed the previous 5 steps, have the patient imagine himself or herself achieving the peak performance goal in the future. Ask how clearly he or she is able to imagine himself or herself accomplishing this goal using the future performance imagery index.
   a. If the FPII score is a 7, proceed to step 8.
   b. If the FPII score is less than a 7, proceed to step 7.

7. Invite the patient to again imagine achieving the peak performance goal and to "TAB under the arm (SP-21) while taking three respirations, or more if you like, until the image is maximized." Then have him or her "TAB on the inner eye (BL-1) while taking three respirations, or more if you like, until the image is maximized." Note whether the left or right arm or eye was used. Now have the patient do the ISq and repeat the TxSq, this time using the opposite arm and eye. Complete the treatment with an eye-roll. Recheck the FPII score. When the FPII score is 7, treatment is complete.
   a. If the FPII score is now 7, go to step 8.
   b. When the FPII score remains below 7 after treatment, inquire about any additional issues (thought fields) that might be keeping the patient from imagining more clearly. Perhaps a new memory or concern has come to the fore that needs to be diagnosed and treated. At this point, however, it can be easier to ask

the patient to "tune into whatever it is that is keeping you from imagining your desired outcome more clearly" and muscle test. The muscle response will usually be weak. When weak, diagnose and treat as an unknown block to remove any remaining obstacles to imaging more clearly in the future. If the muscle response is strong, evaluate for possible blocks and treat accordingly. (At this point, there could be a future BRB or another BRB. Be sure to check and treat for these when present.)

8. Finally, invite the patient to create a positive statement regarding his or her future performance (e.g., "I am capable and confident of making solid contact and driving the ball.") Then have the patient repeat the statement three times while doing TAB under the nose (GV-26). Additionally, you could ask patients where they notice the positive statement in their body, and have them focus both on the statement and on the body sensation while using TAB.

ISSUES OF PAIN AND PAIN MANAGEMENT

Working with patients who present with acute and chronic pain issues requires, in our opinion, a broader perspective on the nature of human experience and the interface of the mind-body-energy relationship. For effective treatment, the mind and body should not be considered separately, but must be addressed and treated as a whole. We know of no circumstances where a physical malady or injury is free of psychological response, or conversely, of psychological difficulties that are free of physiological response. The common denominator between the two is the mind-body interface, which we speculate contains the info-energy that effects thought, feeling, sensation, and physiological functioning. When used strategically, EvTFT can make vibrational info-energy changes that reasonate with both the mental and physical domains resulting in relief and management of the reported discomfort or pain.

Is the "Pain" the Most Appropriate Target?

When patients present with issues of physical discomfort or pain it is easy to be drawn into wanting to help relieve their reported suffering without having the necessary information to assess the best way to proceed. Pain issues can arise and result from multiple sources. Some sources are known and have a medical history and documentation of suspected physiological causes. However, some sources of pain and discomfort are unknown, or speculative at best, even after medical testing, and may run the gamut from soft tissue injuries, to reflex sympathetic dystrophy, to an absence of physical explanations. Regardless of the presenting pain issue, we highly recommend that the therapist evaluate whether the "pain" is the most appropriate or beneficial target. Often it is not.

Pain is a signal; it is a powerful signal that provides important information that can guide the path of treatment in the physical and psychological arenas. The pain of discomfort and suffering informs that "something is not right" and attention is directed to the location to promote assistance. Unfortunately pain may also function as a distraction that can interrupt and mislead the best intentions of the patient, physician, and therapist. Careful analysis of the patient's story regarding the history and development of his or her pain is mandatory before launching a treatment approach.

It is vital to check that the patient has sought appropriate medical intervention. Psychologists, social workers, and other psychotherapists need to be mindful that they are not licensed to practice medicine when working with this patient population. As non-physicians, our help is sometimes sought specifically because we do not prescribe medication with potentially unwanted and undesirable side effects and because we offer modalities of care that complement the existing physical protocol. For example, relaxation training, biofeedback techniques, and hypnosis have been effective complementary approaches in the management of pain over the past thirty years. Also, we in the mental health field are frequently "the court of last resort" for many patients (and physicians) because the standard medical treatments and interventions provided limited success. From these patient histories we can learn what was beneficial and what was not (so as not to repeat the same ineffective approach), and we can ascertain what is now needed to help mobilize the patient's resources to promote health, healing, and improved comfort.

What Conditions or Circumstances Preceded, Caused, or Sustain the "Pain"?

What is the patient's story? In detail, what happened from the beginning to the present? At the beginning of treatment, and after the customary social, medical, and psychological histories are acquired, it is essential to have the patient describe as specifically as possible what he or she believes was the cause of the current pain problem. Sometimes there is an obvious traumatic incident (e.g., a fall, car crash, work injury); other times the source or cause is not so apparent (e.g., stressors, intense unresolved feelings, attention and secondary-gain issues), and can even be convoluted (i.e., a physical event with concomitant psychological overlay). In event-connected situations, information is needed regarding what happened at the moment of the incident. Specifically, how did the patient experience it? What was he or she thinking and feeling immediately before, during, and after the incident? Was medical care sought and what was the outcome of the medical interventions? In all situations it is useful to know what the patient believes is the cause of their current pain and what the resulting impact on his or her life has been to date. What are his or her concerns and fears regarding the future? Can or will the patient recover, and to what degree? Does the patient experience flashbacks or dreams and nightmares about the event? The astute clinician will identify as much of the patient's physical and psychological reality as possible to discern the most beneficial targets for treatment.

Identifying and defining the thought field is critical to assisting patients with pain when using EvTFT. More often than not, treatment of the initial traumatizing event (physical and/or psychological) will be among the first targets of intervention. It is important that the event take priority over emotions or sensations. The rationale is that if that event or interaction had not transpired, then the patient would not be experiencing the reported emotions and sensations. To put it another way, if there were no injury, there would be no pain. Treating the unresolved emotions connected to the initial trauma will often bring a reduction in physical discomfort as the emotional components are relieved. In this regard, asking the patient to rate his or her level of discomfort (e.g., 0 to 10) at the beginning and end of the session can provide a barometer to assess baseline changes in the physical domain, even though you may not have worked directly on the "pain."

When Treating The "Pain"

After the trauma related emotional components have been addressed and treated as thoroughly as possible, focusing on the pain experience may be the next thought field to address. The physical injuries, and the extent of them, need to be considered in regard to what has been medically documented or is "known" about the patient's medical condition. We often must straddle the fence between providing hope and helping the patient accept the realities of certain injuries or conditions. Our treatments may at times appear "magical," but they are not.

In discussing the "pain" issues, it may be learned that the patient has acquired some limiting and negative beliefs about his or her medical condition. These beliefs can be acquired honestly via numerous sources:

comments made by treating physicians, family members, or friends; written information in magazines or on the internet; personalized attributions that he or she is being punished; "it's in the family"; "it's God's will"; or secondary gain issues involving fear of economic demise and specialized attention. In our opinion, when these limiting beliefs are identified they ought to be treated whenever possible to remove disrupting influences to attaining comfort and restoration of function. Frequently we need to assist the patient in beginning to think "outside the box" to instill hope and a realistic expectation for physical healing.

When the "pain" becomes the targeted thought field, we suggest two modifications in treating the diagnosed meridians: (1) bilateral TAB and (2) "breathing through" the area of discomfort.

When the pain becomes the targeted thought field for diagnosis and treatment first we recommend bilateral TAB on all acupoints requiring treatment. In other words, all treatment points ought to be treated on both sides of the body (e.g., under both eyes, both arms, on both hands and fingers). This can be done simultaneously or sequentially, depending on the patient and the treatment site (e.g., some individuals will need to TAB under the arm on one side, then under the other arm). The exceptions are the treatment of the governing and central vessels because these treatment points are on the midline of the body.

The rationale for bilateral TAB stems from an attempt to utilize as much of the patient's bio-energy system as feasible. This approach also incorporates Voll's observations that electrical activity in a meridian on one side of the body seems to correspond to electrical activity on one side of the organ related to that meridian. It therefore seems prudent to treat all experience of physical discomfort bilaterally in order to affect the entire organ system. The physical body is also likely to be more inertial in response to treatment compared to thought and emotional factors that have no physical mass. Accordingly, bilateral treatment may serve to reduce the delay in maximum relief possible with EvTFT, which is sometimes observed with physical pain. The slower response in treating some physical pain is thought to be related to inertia because it will take more time and energy to affect change when more solid mass is involved. Our physical body is composed of slower moving energy compared to cognitive and feeling states, whose energy moves more quickly.

Second, have the patient "breathe through" the area of discomfort whenever he or she takes each full respiration while treating each diagnosed treatment site. William Tiller, the physicist, researcher, and author, reported to Diepold that "breath is a carrier of intention" and that he uses directed breathing to manage his personal pain. It has been our experience that the patient's intentional focus and mindfulness regarding his or her pain issue is enhanced when combining treatment of the meridian point with intentionally directed breathing. Again, we are looking to stack the deck in the patient's favor to facilitate comfort and healing.

We underscore that we are not *directly* treating the physical problem. However, we do acknowledge and believe that treatments using EvTFT *indirectly* impact the physical domain so as to influence comfort and healing. We hypothesize that the diagnosed treatment sequence shifts the energy field (i.e., field-shifting) when the patient is attuned to the thought field. In so doing, and with every treatment thereafter at home, we surmise that the treatment re-shifts the energy field to a pattern that promotes comfort, health, and healing. Often the patient is required to complete follow-up treatment outside the office on a scheduled or as needed basis to facilitate comfort and healing. It is never stated or implied that the EvTFT treatments replace or supersede the patient's medical treatment protocols.

DIAGNOSIS AND TREATMENT OF PATIENTS WITH DISSOCIATIVE DISORDERS AND DISSOCIATIVE IDENTITY DISORDER

This section delineates the modifications to our basic diagnostic and treatment protocol when treating patients with dissociative disorders in general, and dissociative identity disorder (DID) in particular. EvTFT is an ideal treatment complement for patients with DID or dissociative disorder not otherwise specified (DDNOS) because of the contributory traumatic histories that predispose these psychological disorders. Dissociative amnesia, dissociative fugue, and depersonalization disorder round out the complete current spectrum of dissociative disorders in the American Psychiatric Association's *Diagnostic and Statistics Manual of Mental Disorders, Fourth Edition (DSM-IV)*, with which EvTFT can also be used beneficially. It is, however, beyond the scope of this section to review this challenging area of dissociation and its treatment. The interested reader is referred to the many books and journals devoted to this topic (e.g., Chu, 1998; Chu & Bowman, 2000; Kluft and Fine, 1993; Putnam, 1989; Ross, 1989; Spira, 1996).

Our combined clinical experience, and that of our colleagues who have trained in our methods, has allowed us to come to a number of conclusions regarding the treatment of this population with EvTFT. Let us begin with what we believe EvTFT can do in the treatment of dissociative disorders:

- *Rapid resolution of isolated and repeated traumatic events.* Traumatic experience is considered universal as a contributory component leading to the dissociative coping phenomenon. The ability of EvTFT to resolve and neutralize the negative emotions that linger from remembered events, dreams, or flashbacks serves to provide rapid relief and quickly stabilize this sensitive population.
- *Resolution of negative emotions toward past abusers and should-be protectors.* Because of the abuse histories typically found with dissociative disorders, these individuals often harbor intense and unresolved upset with the perceived abuser(s), as well as with individuals believed to have been in a position to prevent or stop the abuse. Resolving the negative interference from the past with EvTFT can prove comforting and serve to focus attention on current issues more effectively.
- *Resolution of negative emotions in the present toward abusers, spouse, children, and peers, which stem from projected or generalized concerns (e.g., transference and trigger issues) from the past.* EvTFT assists in resolving and neutralizing the evoked negative emotions toward individuals who are currently involved in the patient's life.
- *Resolution of negative emotions toward self.* A substantial number of patients with DID will, at some level of his or her perception, blame themselves for the events and incidents that transpired. Divided perceptions and experience of self often referred to as *alters*—or *resources*, as Diepold (1998) chose to reframe it—can be comfortably treated with EvTFT, which results in a more realistic perspective free of emotional upset (i.e., anger, shame) and self-blame.
- *Allowing patient privacy about his or her trauma or issue.* It is unnecessary with EvTFT for a patient to disclose the details of a flashback, traumatic memory, or the effects of the trauma. This is the simple eloquence of using a thought field. As long as the patient is attuned to the thought field the therapist can proceed with diagnosis and treatment. In this way the therapy process is respectful (e.g., patients are not required to reveal aspects of a trauma that is initially too shaming or upsetting to speak about) and frees patients from possible re-traumatization and abreaction, which can result from retelling his or her story.
- *All dissociated perspectives of the self (i.e., resources, alters, ego-states) can simultaneously attune the thought field for diagnosis and treatment.* With EvTFT the totality of the patient's experience of a traumatic memory can be addressed simultaneously. This advantage respects the whole

of the patient and provides a gestalt-like perspective when resolving the traumatic incidents.

EvTFT, like other forms of psychotherapy, has realistic limitations including:

- *EvTFT does not erase negative memories.* This, in our opinion, is positive because memory is retained without the negative emotion. Often patients unrealistically desire or request not to have to remember aspects of their past because it is painful. We have had patients say, "Can't you just hypnotize me so I can't remember anymore?" Memories are not reported to be distorted or erased with EvTFT; nothing is lost in the reality of the patient's history except the negative feelings that were previously associated to the memory. As described earlier in this book, there is often a cognitive shift toward clarity (cognitive clarity) after treatment is completed and the patient achieves a more objective understanding of the whole of the thought field because he or she is no longer encumbered by the negative feelings. However, very often after the treatment, patients do share and process the event, having been relieved of the uncomfortable feelings (e.g., sense of shame or guilt) that accompanied the thought field.

- *EvTFT cannot quickly resolve a lifetime of trauma.* While EvTFT can move the therapy process along more quickly, psychotherapy remains a long and hard process despite the rapid treatment effects.

- *EvTFT methods are not designed to directly fuse or integrate resources.* For years, many of us have used hypnotic and imagery techniques for the purpose of fusing resources or ego states to foster a state of integration as needed. Clinical experience using EvTFT with DID has demonstrated that fusion and integration occur spontaneously as a result of complete trauma resolution for the various resources. It appears that resources naturally fold back within the individual (in the same fashion as they unfolded when overwhelmed in trauma) when the purpose of the resource (e.g., to conceal or manage traumatic material) is no longer evident.

- *EvTFT is not a mechanistic approach.* To the contrary, EvTFT places a premium on the rapport between therapist and patient. The essentials of sound clinical skills and judgment, respect, and an understanding of the history that has brought the patient to this point in his or her life and the pain he or she suffers are part and parcel of the EvTFT method. Observation of subtle cues of behavior and affect assist in the diagnostic process and serve to confirm treatment effects.

We wish to emphasize that there is no single agreed upon method of psychotherapy with DID and dissociative disorders, and accordingly we suggest that EvTFT be utilized as part of a carefully conceived treatment plan. Psychotherapists will find that EvTFT is complementary to most traditional psychodynamic and cognitive-behavioral therapies, as well as hypnosis and eye movement desensitization and reprocessing (EMDR). However, appropriate caution should still be used if an EvTFT-trained therapist has never worked with DID before. Professionalism and ethical responsibility require that these cases be referred to a colleague with training and experience in treating patients with dissociative disorders, or that the therapist acquire the needed training and supervision to handle the case. In other words, we must caution any therapist who has never worked with this patient population to refer him or her to an expert in the area or get supervision and training.

Basic Considerations

Therapists who work with this population are sensitive to the fact that timing is perhaps even more critical than therapeutic technique. With all patients it is necessary to proceed only when the patient is ready, willing, and has a full understanding of the process. However, patients in this group may be so fragile and fragmented that they require additional time, support, and supplementary therapeutic skills on the therapist's part to stabilize and prepare the patient and build trust and safety. Therapy should proceed slowly because therapy often takes years; the more diminished the ego-strength the slower the therapy moves. The therapist should strive to develop a trusting relationship with the patient and to establish a safe environment in which he or she can prosper. The following considerations are offered as guidelines when working with this population:

- *Work with what the patient gives you.* Take a careful history including a detailed account of the patient's recall of his or her life experiences. Avoid any leaps of interpretation about cults and additional abusers. Also, assumptions about the types of trauma reported or experienced ought to be limited to what the patient reports. When using EvTFT, it is acceptable that the exact nature of the trauma or its details is not fully known to the patient or therapist. For example, an early medical trauma could be mistaken for a sexual trauma, in which case erroneous conclusions could be drawn.

- *Know your patient and his or her goal before beginning use of EvTFT.* This may involve development of a treatment plan with clear, attainable, and realistic goals. Use of assessment instruments will aid in understanding how and when the patient experiences dissociation. Trust and safety in the therapeutic relationship are essential with this population, as is respectfulness. This population appears to be more sensitive than any other group regarding attention to subtle physical, social, and environmental cues.

- *Be aware of concomitant personality disorders and patterns.* Evaluate for personality disorders, which are often a part of this clinical picture. Set boundaries and use written contracts as needed. Use appropriate caution and treatment strategies when there is a borderline personality diagnosis.

- *Work within your conceptual framework of dissociation.* EvTFT focuses on resolving negative emotions stemming from patient issues regardless of how they are conceived conceptually by the therapist. There is no need to conform to a particular framework to use EvTFT beneficially with your patients. Our recommendation is to also work within the context of the patient's unique presentation of his or her dissociative disorder.

- *Mapping techniques.* Mapping of the patient's inner system, which is done by the patient, can be helpful in understanding the patient's uniqueness involving the use and experience of dissociation. Patient mapping can also indicate areas of change (fusion/integration) resulting from resolution of traumatic experiences as therapy progresses. There are many styles of mapping, so let the patient lead you in his or her own way.

Using EvTFT in the Treatment of the Dissociative Disorders

There are many advantages to using EvTFT, which can rapidly remedy the sequelae of isolated and repeated traumatic events. EvTFT is effective in treating the symptoms that often accompany dissociative disorders, including panic, intrusive thoughts, anxiety, flashbacks, and nightmares. A major strength in using EvTFT with a DID patient is that the therapist can simultaneously work with all resources[3] involved in the targeted thought field (i.e., the traumatic event). Patients experience this advantage to be respectful of the whole individual regarding the event, as well as a time efficient therapeutic approach. This modification will be explained in more detail later in this section.

The diagnostic methods are, in our opinion, the preferred EvTFT approach in the treatment of DID. Given the unique history and complexities of patients with dissociative disorders in general and DID in particular, the diagnostic approach can quickly and precisely address the problem and stabilize the patient. Algorithms may be helpful in some situations; for example, teaching patients to use the trauma algorithms can help lessen emotional distress while providing self-care between psychotherapy sessions. Algorithm use may also prove effective during telephone contacts when direct muscle-tested diagnosis is not possible. However, we advocate use of the diagnostic methods during the psychotherapy session as the most efficient and direct manner of intervention.

Using EvTFT with DID patients may clearly demonstrate the uniqueness and complexity of this clinical population. While there are no set patterns or standards for the number of treatment points used in a holon, our clinical experience suggests that some patients with DID produce remarkably long, or unpredictably short, treatment sequences. This may result from the number of resources particpating in the diagnosis and treatment of the designated thought field. With a lengthy number of treatment points, 20 to 30 or more, it would suggest that resources take turns attuning the same thought field from their perspective reflecting the convolutions of dissociated experience that lay deep within the psyche of the patient. Diepold had a patient who produced frequent long holons, as high as 107 points in the TxSq, which gradually reduced in number as the traumatic memories were emotionally neutralized. Perhaps a longer TxSq is also related to very early childhood trauma where the perception of the experience(s) predated structured verbal or cognitive ability.

Another phenomenon occasionally observed with this patient population relates to the added time required (by some) between treatment of a meridian point and diagnosis of the next meridian. It seems some patients need more time for the energy fluctuation to settle (perhaps between and among resources or meridians) before another meridian can be accurately diagnosed. This becomes evident when all 14 alarm points test weak, but then an alarm point tests strong the second time around. Accordingly, the clinician may need to test alarm points a second time if none tests strong the first time after a treatment. Some patients may also take several respirations, taking even several minutes, while doing TAB on a treatment point. Postural changes have also been observed to occur with prolonged TAB, perhaps reflecting body memories.

Modifications to the EvTFT Basic Protocol When Working with Dissociative Identity Disorder

Necessity inspires creativity to adjust to the individual needs of our patients. Clinical experience is a wonderful teacher. In fact, our patients diagnosed with DID—previously know as multiple personality disorder—have taught us a great deal about using EvTFT over the past seven years. It is with gratitude and thanks to these men and women that we can offer the following modifications to the basic EvTFT protocol:

- Be more mindful about obtaining permission to touch when muscle-testing. Sometimes new resources, who are perhaps leery of another person's touch, are present (e.g., co-conscious). Although the presence of different resources is usually communicated before hand, it is always respectful and safe to seek permission. If overt switching of resources/alters occurs during treatment, you may want to ask permission again of the resource who has now come forward. Use your clinical judgment.

- As is standard protocol in all EvTFT treatment, when muscle-testing for a false name, allow the patient to provide it (e.g., "tell me a name that is not your own"). Strong muscle responses to "false" names are ways the patient is communicating. A strong muscle response to "a name that is not your own" can indicate an inner resource before it becomes "known" to the patient or therapist. For example, Diepold asked a patient to say her name, "Annie," and the patient muscle-tested strong to this name. When he asked her to say, "My name is Diane," which was not her name, she also tested strong. Later it was learned that one of her resources was named Diane. At other times patient's will offer names on their own and to which they muscle-test strong. When information like this is obtained it is clinically prudent to make a note of the name in the margin of your notes. Then ask the patient for another name, and muscle-test. There is never a reason to alarm a patient regarding his or her response to a name. In addition, just because someone tests strong to a name that is not their own, it does not necessarily mean that they have a DID. We have found that some people muscle-test strong to a name that is not their own because it was an old childhood nickname, a middle name, or a name they always wanted to have.

- After the thought field is identified ask the patient "Who is involved?" in the trauma or problem. This is a direct reference to the inner resources that were affected and need to be involved in the diagnosis and treatment at this time. The therapist's language ought to match the patient's descriptions of his or her inner resources. Accept whatever the patient offers in response; sometimes the patient can only provide partial or incomplete replies because of limited awareness. Then say, "As you think about that memory/flashback/event, permit all of you (all of your resources) who were involved and affected to participate." In this way all of the effected resources can simultaneously be involved in treatment without the need to treat resources one at a time.

- Be certain to ask, "Are there any objectors to doing this work?" An *objector* is a resource, known or unknown, that for some reason is resistant, fearful, or anxious about doing the work at this time. Verbal information about the possibility of objectors is acknowledged. However, the therapist can muscle-test this inquiry in the early stages of therapy when there are objectors, or when you or the patient are uncertain about the presence of an objector. When an objector is acknowledged, you will need to negotiate the opportunity to proceed. For example, you can invite the objector(s) to watch and not participate if they so desire. You can than obtain permission from the objector to allow the "others" to participate without interference from the objector. Invite the objector(s) to join in if they so choose as the treatment progresses. Most often the objector will agree to allow the treatment to go forward, to which a "thank you" is in order. Frequently objectors eventually join in. When an objector denies permission, then exploration and intervention with this objector must be done before proceeding. Often these objectors are not directly part of the thought field but are threatened in some way by that issue being treated. Permission to proceed must be unanimous.

- When diagnosing and correcting psychological reversals or belief related blocks, adjust the language to reflect the dissociative features. For example:

For generalized PR: "I deeply accept all of me, with all my problems and limitations."

For issue-specific PR: "I deeply accept all of me, even though I have this problem, its cause, and all it means and does to me."

For process-specific PR: "I deeply accept all of me, even though I still have some of this problem, its cause, and all it means and does to me."

Caution: Do NOT use these language changes with dissociative patients who are not DID because you could confuse or frighten them.

When diagnosing psychological reversal and belief related blocks, correct all strong/strong, weak/weak, or "mushy" muscle-test responses. These responses are what Diepold calls "dissension in the ranks," meaning that at least one resource is for and one is against the specific test statement.

All TAB treatment is bilateral. Clinical experience and feedback from patients have shown us that the treatment effect is more robust with DID patients when meridians on both sides of the body are treated. Perhaps this observation results from info-energy being processed differently when there are multiple perspectives (or amnesia) about life events. It may also stem from selective or alternative brain-hemisphere involvement when this population attunes thought fields.

The TAB treatment can be either simultaneous or sequential. For example, after a meridian is diagnosed, the patient needs to TAB on the meridian treatment points on both the left and right sides of the body. Treating the inner eye, eye, outer eye, collarbone, under arm, and liver points can be accomplished by doing TAB on both treatment points simultaneously. When treating the other bilateral meridian treatment points (i.e., little finger, middle finger, index finger, thumb, side of hand and hand) the patient needs to TAB first on one treatment point and then the other. Bilateral treatment also includes correction of belief related blocks and psychological reversal. For example, when correcting a process specific reversal ("I want to be *completely* over this problem . . ."), the patient first does TAB on the side of one hand (SI-3) and says the affirmations three times, then does TAB on the other hand and repeats the affirmations.

Minimize Risks When Using EvTFT

Sound clinical judgment is always paramount. In the early phases of treatment, when some patients are too fragile, fragmented, or untrusting to engage in trauma work, use your other therapy skills to stabilize him or her and build trust and safety. You might also begin by teaching your patient the neurologic organizing treatment (NOTx) and the simplified collarbone breathing (SCB) treatment as a grounding technique, which can be settling and soothing. Proceed with treatment of flashbacks and disturbing memories when the patient is ready.

Neutralization of traumatic memories is a core aspect in the treatment of patients with DID. Much has been written about the phenomenon of abreaction in the treatment of patients with PTSD and DID, as well as the origin, appropriateness, purpose, and historical and theoretical roots of abreaction (e.g., van der Hart & Brown, 1992). Most contemporary and nonpsychoanalytic therapists endeavor to avoid patient experience of abreaction because it can be emotionally draining, debilitating, and lacking in previously believed value in raw emotional discharge. Abreactions can also be disruptive to the therapy session and to the unsuspecting therapist. Abreaction had been defined by the American Psychiatric Association as "emotional release or discharge after recalling a painful experience that has been repressed because it was consciously intolerable" (1980, p. 1). Van der Hart and Brown italicized *that has been repressed* in the above definition to emphasize a key difference between abreaction and experiencing emotion when thinking about a past trauma. In general, experience of a distressing emotional response when attuning a thought field does not qualify as an abreaction.

Some patients are more prone than others to present an abreactive pattern. When using EvTFT, we have observed that this treatment approach is basically free of abreaction. In other words, EvTFT does not initiate an abreactive response in the patient. The authors have encountered only one incidence of abreaction when working with DID patients, and that occurred because an attempt was made to focus on an unwanted body sensation (fragment) without first having a context for the sensation. Accordingly, we caution that there is a risk of abreaction when attempting to treat body sensations without a context. Otherwise, treatment with EvTFT has been free of abreaction. Indeed, patients have been non-abreactive during EvTFT treatment, even when relating painful aspects of their history. This most likely occurs because the thought field can be quickly attuned so diagnosis and treatment can be quickly initiated. Abreaction-free does not mean that a patient is void of emotion; the patient may show mild upset even though he or she is not caught up in the memory or is not emoting as if the event were recurring. If a dissociative patient suddenly becomes abreactive to a flashback memory during a traditional psychotherapy session, EvTFT can quickly neutralize the negative emotions.

Perhaps EvTFT allows emotion in a way that the patient experiences as more controlled—emotion without fear so to speak. This managed emotional response, which can be interpreted as a reflection of increased ego strength, may result from all the resources having been invited to participate, thus increasing the probability of greater coping ability. From this gestalt perspective, the whole is calmer than the individual parts.

USING A CLUSTER TECHNIQUE
TO TREAT MULTIPLE
THOUGHT FIELDS

Up to this point, we have described treatment with EvTFT as targeting one specific thought field at a time. At the November 2002 Energy Psychology conference in Toronto, Canada, Gallo demonstrated a *container technique* by which several issues could be treated by putting them together in a metaphorical container and treating them with a preset treatment sequence (algorithm). Building on Gallo's demonstration, the following EvTFT *cluster technique* allows for multiple related thought fields to be bundled or clustered together and then diagnosed and treated as a single thought field. Use of the cluster technique is applicable when treating perturbations or elaters.

We have found that the option to use the cluster technique seems to emerge from the content of the patient's descriptions of his or her targeted problem. In particular the patient appears to attribute multiple but related aspects to a specific problem or concern. For an example regarding perturbations, a case study is described in Chapter 14 where a patient reported five specific comments frequently spoken by his mother that were a source of upset and performance failure throughout most of the patient's life. In lieu of treating each statement individually, all five statements were clustered and successfully treated collectively. With treatment of elaters, clusters are also formed involving the positive feelings and benefits of the identified behavior. For example, a patient may list three, four, or five reasons why they continue to engage in eating, drinking, or using a substance (e.g., "It tastes good, it makes me feel good, it's there, it helps me relax, . . ."). In a situation regarding procrastination, the patient may report several alternate behaviors he or she preferably enjoys doing to divert him or her from completing the needed behavior, which may be clustered and treated collectively.

Procedural Guidelines for the Cluster Technique

The following procedural guidelines will assist the clinician in using the *cluster technique*:

1. Identify several related thought fields to the presenting issue. This can be as few as two, or as many as five. Clinical judgment and muscle testing may assist in determining the number and the appropriateness of content.

2. Obtain a SUD or SUE rating for each thought field in the cluster.

3. Invite the patient to bundle and label the related thought fields or to imagine placing them in a container of his or her choosing and labeling it.

4. After the related thought fields have been clustered, EvTFT diagnosis is then performed using the basic protocol but without a SUD or SUE rating. In this regard, diagnosis and treatment progress as if treating an unknown block. The patient is asked to attune to the cluster or container without the need to attend to any of the bundled thought fields specifically. You do not need a SUD or SUE rating to successfully diagnose and treat a problem with EvTFT. The muscle-testing responses of the patient to the procedures in the basic protocol will provide all the information you will need to resolve the targeted issue. When diagnosing and treating psychological reversals or belief related blocks, remember that language modifications are required to reflect the multiple thought fields being addressed. For example, in testing for an issue-specific psychological reversal the test statement would be, "I want to be over *these problems, their causes,* and all that *they* mean and do to me." Continue EvTFT diagnosis and treatment until the patient's body is completely clear and muscle-tests strong the thought field cluster.

5. After completion of diagnosis and treatment, invite the patient to unbundle or remove the separate thought fields from the container and re-rate the SUD or SUE levels for each. In the majority of cases, the SUD or SUE level for each thought field will now be 0.

6. When one or more of the separate thought fields retain a SUD or SUE level above 0, diagnose each thought field separately to remove the residual unwanted component.

RECOGNITION AND TREATMENT OF ENERGY DISRUPTERS

In the course of utilizing the EvTFT diagnostic protocol, there are times when the clinician is unable to "unlock" nonpolarized muscle responses by use of the recommended polarity restoration treatments or the advanced diagnostic approaches discussed earlier in this chapter. There may also be occasions when patients, who have been treated successfully with EvTFT for a specific problem, return to the following week's session reporting a return of the same symptoms. Additionally, muscle testing indicates that symptom return is not due to a recurrent psychological reversal or lack of follow-up home treatment. Although these incidents are relatively infrequent in EvTFT, they happen often enough to merit attention and special consideration.

Applied kinesiologists call this locked, strong, nonpolarized muscle response *general hypertonicity* (Frost, 2002, p. 93). In speculating about the causes of general hypertonicity, applied kinesiologist Robert Frost wrote, "no mention is given in the early literature . . . One reason for this is that twenty years ago, there were few such cases. The phenomenon has emerged only recently as a widespread problem. The pollution of food, water and air plus the stress of modern lifestyles are suspected to be the major causes of this increase" (p. 94). Our clinical experience with muscle testing seems to validate that some causes for nonpolarized responses appear to result from sources outside the physical body, which then influence how the physical body operates energetically. We conjecture that the reason for the locked response is that the patient's energy field is being disrupted by an energy influence originating outside the body. We call these disturbances in the energy field *energy disrupters*.

Energy disrupters can be organic or nonorganic substances or subtle energy sources that interact in a noncoherent fashion with the subtle energy of the patient in idiosyncratic ways. Energy disrupters may include such things as perfumes, dyes, laundry products, foods, cat dander, and electromagnetic fields emitted from appliances, computers, and other electronic devices. Some substances may be overtly toxic to the individual and are defined as allergy causing agents that produce physical symptom like sneezing, rashes, watery eyes, and respiratory distress, or cause other physical symptoms, such as dizziness or physical weakness. Energy disrupters can be instrumental in effecting psychological symptoms such as depression, anxiety, impulsive behavior, and states of psychological reversal, and they also appear to cause nonpolarized responses to muscle testing. It has been repeatedly observed by the authors that reversed polarity in muscle testing can be a direct result of proximity to an energy disrupting substance, especially when the energy disrupter is a substance that is reportedly addictive to the patient. Gallo (2000) wrote:

> When a substance results in an energy toxic effect, the energy system evidences an imbalance such that generally effective therapeutic methods are blocked or impaired in their ability to alleviate the psychological problem. The energy toxin causes a recurrent reversal and neurologic disorganization, blocking other efforts to balance the energy system and remove the subtle energy codes within the thought field (perturbations). (p. 195)

Callahan (1995) initially described one form of energy disrupter as *energy toxins*. In observing their effects on his work with patients he stated, "the discovery of the role of energy toxins in the treatment of complex psychological problems is a major original contribution to the field of psychotherapy. From experience we know that an energy toxin is, by far, the most likely reason for the return of a successfully treated problem." Callahan also points to the presence of energy toxins as the reason why some psychological reversals do not correct. Although we agree with Callahan that energy disrupters (or energy toxins) can contribute to the existence and return of a psychological problem, we do not agree about their frequency. We have found clinically that the diagnosis and treatment of unknown blocks, as well as the ability to correct nonpolarized muscle responses via diagnosis and treatment of meridians, have sharply reduced the frequency of incidents, which in the past we would have attributed to the deleterious effects of energy disrupters. However, when these newer methods fail to successfully correct the muscle-response pattern or to sustain treatment results, then it becomes necessary to look for outside influences (i.e., energy disrupters) that can disrupt the personal energy field.

Physician Robert Becker (1990) was the first person to research the link between illness and electromagnetic fields. He reported that every organism produces electromagnetic fields, which expand beyond the body's physical space. His research, which was mainly centered on electromagnetic energy, indicated that when the fields from two different organisms interact, one could have a negative effect on the other. Chiropractor, nurse, and acupuncturist Devi Nambudripad, who developed the Nambudripad allergy elimination technique (1993), hypothesized that that when a person's energy tries to block adverse energies, that person's energy field can weaken, causing the energy pathway of the body to create blocks. Her work with allergies focused on the adverse interaction of the human energy field with the energy signatures of both organic and non-organic substances. She posited that allergies result from two energy fields repulsing each other: the human energy field and the allergen.

> The repulsion of energies can happen between two living organisms, (e.g., between two humans, such as father and son; two siblings, husband and wife; two friends, animal and human being, etc.). It can also occur between one living organism and one non-living organism. For example, between a human being and fabrics or food; between one living organism and energies of other substances (i.e., food, a cat, other

human beings like husband, mother, child, co-workers, etc., fabrics, furniture, fumes, trees, pollens, chemicals, work materials, radiation from the television, microwave, radio, sun, etc.) at the same time. (Nambudripad, 1993, p. 9)

Nambudripad believes that if you put the allergen in contact with the body during an energy treatment, the body becomes a powerful charger and is strong enough to change the adverse charge of the allergen to match the body's frequency. Other researchers, including pediatrician Doris Rapp (1989) and neurophysiologist Carla Hannaford (1995) have noted the link between the adverse reactions to foods, chemicals, electromagnetic fields, and common allergenic substances to changes in thought, perception, and behavior in children.

In our own work we have seen many examples of how energy disrupters can adversely affect the muscle-testing responses of our patients. In Chapter 4 we described how Diepold observed that a patient's deltoid muscle "locked-up" (i.e., nonpolarized strong/strong response) when the patient was wearing a new, unlaundered t-shirt. When the patient, a male athlete, removed the t-shirt and put on a well-worn and washed shirt, the lock-up phenomenon disappeared and Diepold was able to resume muscle testing. Of interest was the observation that the locked-up muscle response occurred not only when the patient wore the t-shirt, but also when he held his hand at his side and just touched a part of the shirt. Diepold hypothesized that this shirt represented a type of "contact" energy disrupter, in contrast to an energy disrupter that could be ingested or inhaled. Since manufacturers commonly treat clothing with formaldehyde and other chemicals, it was suspected that this was the culprit.

Energy disrupters can have varying effects on different people. What is disruptive energetically to one person may not be to another, nor may the reactions be the same. The duration of an energy disruption can be brief or long-lasting. For example, one patient reported feeling dizzy and nauseous for several hours after exposure to a space heater that was used without affect on other family members. When fluorescent lighting is used during our workshops, we often observe that the nonpolarized or reversed muscle responses of some trainees change immediately when they move out from under the light source, while other trainees are completely unaffected either way.

Energy disrupters can also adversely affect the behavior and psychological health of an individual. In a case treated by Britt, a patient who had previously been easy to muscle-test, and who responded extremely well to EvTFT, arrived for a session uncharacteristically depressed and unable to explain her psychological distress. When muscle-tested, Britt found the patient to be "locked-up" with a strong/strong response, a phenomenon that had not occurred over the previous year of treatment. Extensive inquiry regarding changes in the patient's contact with possible energy disrupters (e.g., deodorants, cosmetics, dry cleaning fluid, new foods added to the diet, contact with plants and flowers) revealed no changes. When asked if *anything* was new in her work or home environment, she remembered that her landlord installed new carpets in the hallways that week. Through muscle-testing, it was revealed that the culprit was the new carpeting and most probably it was the epoxies used to hold it down that adversely affected her.

When clinicians inquire about possible energy disrupters that could be affecting the patient, the following are some areas to consider: all inhaled or ingested substances, including medications and nutriceuticals; environmental changes, including new construction and newly installed electromagnetic equipment; use of new substances, such as laundry agents and body care items; recent hair treatments; contact with known allergens; trips to shopping centers, including hardware stores that carry many toxic materials and malls that have new construction; trips to food markets, specifically the laundry aisles; heavy metal toxicity, such as mercury and lead; fluorescent lighting; and objects that may distort light coming into the retina, such as new eyeglasses. Anything and everything is suspect when searching for the source of the changed response.

In the last 80-plus years, tens of thousands of new substances have been introduced into our environment, all of which emit their own energy signatures and interact in some way with the human energy field. In addition, natural substances and foods that we commonly eat have been genetically altered from their original states. Finally, in the last one hundred years, the introduction of electrically-powered devices into our environment has created the single greatest energetic change in the history of the human species (Becker, 1985). The massive shifts away from natural energies in the last century are here to stay and clearly new methods are needed to counteract adverse reactions.

Identification of Energy Disrupters and the EvTFT Diagnostic and Treatment Protocol

The following protocol for treating the effect of energy disrupters was developed by The BDB Group; the protocol for testing for the effect of energy disrupters[4] was developed by Roger Callahan (1995). Our goal in using this protocol is to clear the patient's energy field of blocks created by specific energy disrupters to performing EvTFT diagnosis and treatment. Based on clinical experience, we believe that energy disrupters can and do create nonpolarized or reversed responses to muscle testing, which impedes the diagnostic process.

We want to be clear that we are not directly attempting to cure allergies or allergic reactions in the medical sense. However, field-shifting an individual's energetic response to an environmental energy disrupter in the direction of coherent functioning may have a positive influence on physical and psychological health.

In utilizing these protocols, the actual physical presence of a substance is not necessary but it can be useful to have it at hand. When the substance is available, the patient can hold the substance (e.g., a bottle of deodorant) or place it next to his or her central abdomen while being muscle-tested. The indicator muscle will respond weak if the substance is an energy disrupter. When the substance is unavailable, the therapist (or patient) can do any of the following when muscle-testing for the effect it has on the patient:

- write the name of the suspected energy disrupter on a piece of paper and have the patient hold it;
- work with an image, picture, or other representation of the suspected energy disrupter; or
- have the patient verbally state the name of the item to be tested.

For example, one patient was allergic to cats and when shown a picture of a cat, her indicator muscle responded weak. The diagnosis then proceeded using the picture as the thought field in lieu of having an actual cat or a cat dander sample present. It is posited that the energetic signature of the energy disrupter is present in each form and representation.

When testing for possible energy disrupters, all suspected substances that are not physically present during the testing must have been previously in the patient's energy field. In other words, we do not recommend testing a substance as a possible energy disrupter if the patient has not had prior contact with that substance unless you are testing the physical substance directly.

The muscle-testing procedure is used to assist in the identification of energy disrupters that may foster a polarity reversal. This is a two-step procedure:

1. Have the patient state the name of the suspected energy disrupter (e.g., wheat, sugar, cat dander, electromagnetic field), and add, "I want to be healthy," and check the muscle response. If the muscle response is weak, the substance is an energy disrupter for that person and it adversely affects the patient's health/energy field, creating

reversed polarity. If the muscle response is strong when repeating the statement, proceed to step two;

2. Have the patient state the name of the suspected energy disrupter once more and add, "I want to be sick" and muscle-test. If the muscle response is weak the substance is not considered to be an energy disrupter. However, if the substance is an energy disrupter, then the muscle response will test strong to this second statement.

Callahan believes a strong muscle response to this second test question suggests that the substance is problematic for both the patient and the therapist. We are reminded, however, of the work of clinical kinesiologists Susan Levy and Carol Lehr who wrote "muscle tests may change with time, based upon current body balance, the season of the year, or what may be occurring in the individual system" (1996, p. 165), suggesting other factors may be involved.

The Treatment of Energy Disrupters

The protocol for the diagnosis and treatment of the possible psychological and polarity effects of energy disrupters is nearly identical to the basic EvTFT diagnostic and treatment protocol. Any of the three diagnostic methods can be used with the following modifications:

- Tuning in to the energy disrupter. As in all EvTFT protocols, attunement to the thought field is required. When working with energy disrupters, the suspected or identified energy disrupter becomes the thought field. Attunement can be established by thinking about the substance, being or imagining being in physical contact with the substance, or viewing a symbolic representation of the energy disrupter. Use your clinical judgment to determine if physical contact with the substance is appropriate.

- It is not necessary to have a SUD or SUE level from the patient regarding the energy disrupter. You will be working without the benefit of this verbal feedback from the patient, as is the case with the diagnosis of unknown blocks. Instead, rely solely on the muscle response of the patient as the diagnoses proceed.

- Conduct the EvTFT diagnosis and treatment session as you would for the diagnosis and treatment of an unknown block using the energy disrupter as the identified problem. (The patient's indicator muscle may show varying degrees of weakness or strength at the beginning of the protocol and get progressively stronger as the treatment moves forward.) After having diagnosed and treated all holons and belief related blocks, the indicator muscle will remain strong when the patient directly contacts the substance or attunes the energy disrupter.

- When the above treatment is complete, invite the patient to have direct contact with the identified energy disrupter or its representation (e.g., the name written on paper) for 10 to 15 minutes. For example, have the patient hold it or put it in a pocket. After this exposure, muscle-test again to check your work; it should be strong to the substance.

  Our rationale for this treatment segment is based on re-introduction of the identified substance after the patient's body energy has been field-shifted. The body energy is now re-acquainted with the substance in a desensitizing mode while in the healthier, field-shifted state.

- Remember to check if additional follow-up home treatment is necessary.

- As may be relevant, after the patient's energy field is cleared, you can return to diagnosing the original psychological problem you were working on before the effects of the energy disruption became evident.

WAYS TO MUSCLE-TEST
AND DIAGNOSE ONESELF

In addition to becoming proficient in the practice of muscle-testing patients, it can be advantageous for the clinician to learn how to muscle test himself or herself. Skillful self-testers can utilize the EvTFT diagnostic protocols to diagnose and treat themselves if desired or they can use themselves for surrogate testing of patients. It takes a good deal of practice to become adept at self-testing and to be confident in the results, but after competence is achieved and the self-testing has proven to be a reliable indicator, it can become a valuable therapeutic tool.

Self Muscle-Testing

There are many ways to muscle-test oneself. In experimenting with muscle testing, it becomes apparent that any muscle in the body can be used effectively. Most self-testers, however, find their hand and finger muscles to be the most convenient and least distracting. Although we have refined our own methods of self-testing over the years, we have also witnessed many creative adaptations our colleagues and students have devised for themselves. The following two methods are those most often employed by the authors, and we offer them as a starting place for readers to begin their own self-testing skill development.

1. Press the pads of the thumb and index finger of your nondominant hand tightly together, forming an O-ring shape as shown in Figure 12.1. Now press the pads of the thumb and index finger of your dominant hand together and flatten the fingers together in the shape of a duckbill. Insert the duckbill fingers inside the O-ring fingers as far as they will comfortably go (as shown in Figure 12.2).

2. Clear your mind and hold the O-ring fingers together. Use the two fingers of your dominant hand (duckbill) to try to pry open the O-ring fingers of your nondominant hand. Usually, you will be unable to pry the fingers apart: This will give you a baseline strong response.

3. While you are muscle-testing your fingers in this way, test for polar-

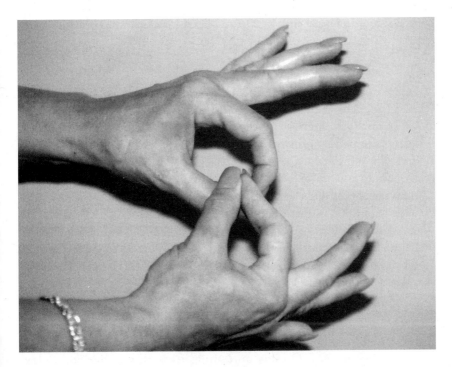

Figure 12.1 Muscle-testing oneself ("O-ring/duckbill" method)

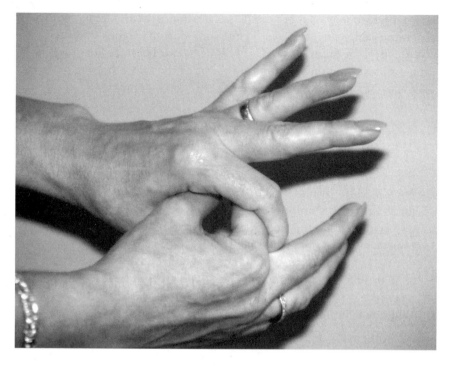

Figure 12.2 Muscle-testing oneself ("O-ring/duckbill" method with fingers inserted)

ized responses to yes/no and true/false statements as you do in the basic protocol. The fingers should remain strongly together for truthful statements and positive thoughts, and weaken and come apart to false statements or disturbing thoughts. This will establish a strong/weak baseline response set.

4. If you are unable to pry the fingers open under any circumstances, then try combining the thumb and the ring finger to form the O-ring with your nondominant hand. The fingers are progressively easier to separate as you move towards the pinky finger of your nondominant hand. If you are still unsuccessful, you may need to treat yourself for neurologic disorganization to obtain a polarized muscle response.

A second method of digital self muscle testing is as follows:

1. Press together the fingertips of your thumb and index finger of your nondominant hand forming an O-ring. Link the thumb and index finger of your dominant hand inside the O-ring at the pads of the

fingers creating another O-ring. This should resemble a chain (see Figure 12.3).

2. Clear your mind and hold the O-ring fingers together. Use the two fingers of your dominant hand to pull open the O-ring fingers of your nondominant hand. Usually, you will be unable to pry the fingers apart: This will give you a baseline strong response.

3. While you are muscle-testing your fingers in this way, test for polarized responses to yes/no and true/false statements as you do in the basic protocol. The fingers should remain strongly together for truthful statements and positive thoughts, and weaken and come apart to false statements or disturbing thoughts. This will establish a strong/weak baseline response set.

4. If you are unable to pry the fingers open under any circumstances, try combining the thumb and the ring finger to form the O-ring with your nondominant hand. The fingers are progressively easier to separate as you move towards the pinky finger of your nondominant hand. If you are still unsuccessful, you may need to treat yourself for neurologic disorganization to obtain a polarized muscle response.

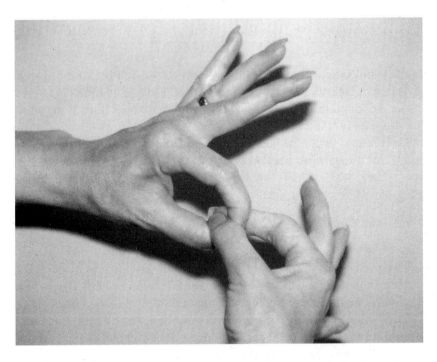

Figure 12.3 Muscle-testing oneself (double "O-ring" chain)

Self Diagnosis

Callahan introduced the successful use of algorithms with patients as self-treatment without the benefit of individual diagnosis. Because of our observations that individualized diagnosis is a more precise and powerful treatment instrument, we reasoned that self-diagnosis would be more accurate when we sought to alleviate some of our own issues. Mindful of the adage that "the physician who treats himself has a fool for a patient," we have discovered that there are many instances in which self-diagnosis and the use of self muscle testing have been an appropriate method of self-healing. Such instances have included diagnosis and treatment of jet lag, anxiety, panic, small *t* trauma, peak performance issues, simple phobia, emotional upset, and allergic-type reactions. Self-diagnosis is also an excellent way for a therapist to practice and sharpen diagnostic skills. When the choice is made to self diagnose, we recommend using the basic EvTFT diagnostic and treatment protocol, and the thought directed diagnosis method. Remember that all the standard checks for polarity and evaluations for belief related blocks and psychological reversal apply.

USE OF SURROGATES FOR DIAGNOSIS AND TREATMENT

On occasions when a patient cannot be muscle-tested because of physical or psychological reasons, the therapist can use a technique discovered by George Goodheart (1987) known as *surrogate testing*. This is an effective alternate method of obtaining the diagnostic information needed for EvTFT treatment, in which the therapist physically muscle-tests another person (the surrogate) on behalf of the patient, instead of directly testing the patient. Occasions when surrogate testing would be appropriate include the following:

- The patient is an infant or a small child who cannot understand or be an active participant in the diagnosis and treatment process.
- The patient is very weak or has a physical disability (e.g., paralysis, neck/shoulder/hand pain, arthritis, confinement to bed) that would prohibit testing and possibly self-treatment.
- The patient would like to receive the benefits of EvTFT but his or her present mental state makes him or her fearful of being touched or being proximate to the therapist.

- The therapist is getting undifferentiated muscle responses and all attempts at correction have failed.
- A known patient is on the telephone and unable to be physically present due to crisis, illness, or physical distance.

Under the above list of circumstances, the therapist can use a designated surrogate to stand in for the patient. For example, a parent or consistent caregiver can be used as a surrogate for a child just as family members or friends can be surrogates for adolescents or adult patients. If the therapist is proficient at self-testing, then he or she can use himself or herself as a surrogate for the patient using the self-testing methods with the thought directed diagnosis method.[5] There have also been occasions when we have been consultants on a case and have invited the primary therapist to be the surrogate for the patient.[6] In actuality, anyone can be a surrogate as long as the patient has given permission for the other person to do so. For example, in our advanced workshops and consultation groups, we often have students who have never before met practice the surrogate model on each other, and they experience overwhelmingly successful results.

Before initiating any form of surrogate testing, the ethical issues must be clearly understood and honored. We strongly recommend that surrogate treatment be reserved for patients who want to be treated in this fashion and who have given their permission to the surrogate to stand in for them. We caution against other use of surrogacy, no matter how well intentioned the therapist. We take the position that we never use surrogacy without permission from the patient. Although parents can provide permission to use surrogates for treatment of their minor children, the child's consent can also be acquired via muscle testing of the surrogate, which is described in the steps that follows.

Use of a surrogate for muscle testing or treatment follows the identical protocols described in Chapter 10, with some modifications. First, it is helpful if an energetic link can be established between the surrogate and the patient, which is easily accomplished by getting both parties to agree to the procedure.[7] This can be readily accomplished by asking the patient if he or she agrees to let the other person serve as a surrogate (i.e., to be muscle tested or treated in his or her stead). A simple "yes" reply will suffice. Then ask the surrogate if he or she is willing to serve as a surrogate for the patient. Again, a simple "yes" response is sufficient.

We offer the following protocol to establish this time-limited energetic contract, which we have used repeatedly with success:

1. With Mary as the patient and John as the surrogate, muscle-test John
    after he says, "My name is John," and then after he says, "My name
    is Mary." John should muscle-test strong to "My name is John" and
    weak to "My name is Mary."
2. Ask Mary if she agrees to permit John to be her surrogate. If she
    answers "yes," then ask John if he agrees to be a surrogate. If John
    answers affirmatively, then proceed with the rest of the protocol. If
    either party is unwilling, then the process should be halted. If for
    some reason the subject cannot give a response to the question (i.e.,
    the subject is a small child named Mary), then the therapist can
    muscle-test the surrogate after saying, "It is okay with Mary if I act
    as her surrogate" and then to, "It is not okay with Mary if I act as her
    surrogate." In order to continue, the muscle response must confirm
    acceptance of John serving as a surrogate.
3. If desired, you could now muscle-test John (the surrogate) once
    again after he says, "My name is John" and after he says, "My name
    is Mary." He should now give a strong muscle response to, "My
    name is Mary." Although this is interesting to do for a training dem-
    onstration, it is not necessary during a therapy session.
4. The energetic contract is now established. Proceed with EvTFT
    diagnosis and treatment exactly as if the surrogate were the patient,
    following the protocol described in Chapter 10. Any of the three
    EvTFT diagnostic methods can be used. Remember that the entire
    protocol is utilized, including having John tune into Mary's problem
    while being muscle-tested, providing the SUD or SUE level if ap-
    propriate, and when necessary, performing the TAB treatment pro-
    cedure on the indicated acupoints as revealed through the diagnostic
    process. The diagnosis and treatment procedures continue until the
    SUD or SUE level is 0.
5. At the conclusion of the session, invite John to free himself from
    being Mary's surrogate, and invite Mary to end the surrogate ar-
    rangement. Now muscle-test John after he says, "I am no longer
    Mary's surrogate" and to, "My name is Mary." John should now
    muscle-test strong to no longer being a surrogate for Mary, and weak
    to his name as Mary.

As noted above, the surrogate can TAB on the treatment points when
the patient is unable to do so. However, we prefer to involve the patient
as much as possible. We therefore ask the patient who is capable of
doing the TAB to treat himself or herself on the corresponding treatment points and to participate in the correction of any belief related
blocks that might appear as the diagnosis progresses. Depending on the

situation, we might also have the patient determine a SUD or SUE level and verify at the end of the diagnostic protocol that a level of 0 has indeed been achieved. We find that including the patient in these ways is not only empowering, but removes the aspect of having something done "to them" (that is not under their control) instead of "by them."

Chapter 13

THE ALGORITHM APPROACH

> . . . There is, it seems to us,
> At best, only a limited value
> In the knowledge derived from experience.
> The knowledge imposes a pattern, and falsifies,
> For the pattern is new in every moment
> And every moment is a new and shocking
> Valuation of all we have been.
>
> —T. S. Eliot, *East Coker*

An *algorithm* is a preset series of thought field therapy treatment points that can be used to treat a specified psychological trauma and negative emotions. Roger Callahan introduced the concept of using a select set of treatment points in his *five minute phobia cure* (1985) for anxiety and phobia problems, and he continues to advocate this method for various forms of self-treatment (Callahan, 2001). Callahan defines algorithm use in the Callahan Techniques™ as "a recipe or formula for treatment of a particular problem discovered by TFT diagnosis which has been tested on many people and has been found to have a high success rate" (Callahan & Callahan, 1996, p. 98). He stated the algorithm treatments to be "75 to 80 percent" effective (Callahan, 2001, p. 11).

It is interesting that the word *algorithm*, which is defined as "a set of rules for solving a problem in a finite number of steps" (*Webster*'s, 1996, p. 52), has in itself a history of Eastern to Western transitions. Muhammed ibn Musa al-Khwarizmi, a ninth-century Persian mathematician, having studied arithmetical sources from India, wrote a work entitled *Al-jabrwal mugabalah*. A variation of the first part of this title produced the English word *algebra*, and the name of the town from which the author came formed the word *algorithm*.[1]

Callahan indicates that algorithms were the most frequent treatment sequences derived from a diagnostic method of muscle-testing meridian alarm points (therapy localization) when a particular emotional or psychological problem was diagnosed.[2] Callahan believes that the order in which meridians are treated is critical to treatment outcome. When using this approach, the therapist would obtain a subjective units of distress (SUD) level and invite the patient who presents with a particular issue to touch-and-breathe (TAB) on a set of specified points while he or she is attuned to that issue. For example, the most common algorithm treatment for a simple phobia is to use the eye (ST-1), arm (SP-1), and collarbone (K-27) treatment points followed by the integration sequence and a repetition of the eye, arm, and collarbone treatment points. A reevaluation of the SUD level would then follow this algorithm treatment. Callahan also incorporates treatment of the different forms of psychological reversal[3] into the algorithm format, but without the use of affirmations.[4] Whenever the SUD level is reported to be 2 or greater after completing the first algorithm treatment, the patient then automatically corrects for a process-specific psychological reversal (a mini psychological reversal in Callahan's language), and repeats that same algorithm until the SUD level drops to 0 or 1, or switches to an alternate algorithm to use. Sometimes algorithms are repeated many times until the SUD level is reduced (e.g., Emotional Freedom Techniques).

Although our clinical experience with the diagnostic methods over nearly seven years has not generally concurred with the extent of Callahan's claims as to the universality of the specified treatment sets, it is important to note that algorithms do often work to reduce or eliminate emotional distress. Bender once read that Gregor Mendel had fudged his findings on the inheritance of genetic traits in peas. The 2×2 square that we all learned about in Biology I was the product of careful observation, some guess work, and creative rounding of numbers rather than clear-cut results of research. It is Bender's opinion that the algorithms derived from the experiences of those trained in Callahan's diagnostic procedure, as they diagnosed their patients' psychological problems, are probably a case of similar observation and embellishment. This musing is not meant to detract from the genius of Mendel or from the astute observations and well-meant intentions of those involved in the thought field therapy community. Algorithms do work in many cases, and for some specific situations they may be the treatment of choice. However, we believe that therapists must be selective in the use of algorithms until claims of their universal applicability and effectiveness can be substantiated. We also believe, because of the success we have seen clinically as well as overall patient response, that algorithm treatments do no harm and are therefore potentially valuable for patient self-treatment between sessions.

ALGORITHMS OR DIAGNOSIS

Using the algorithm approach instead of a diagnostic method may initially appear to be a much simpler approach for the beginning EvTFT therapist. Muscle-testing is not required, alarm points do not have to be memorized, and the guesswork and intuition is removed from the equation. There are, however, serious trade-offs that relate to clinical effectiveness with the algorithm approach. One could liken this situation to using a word processor as a typewriter: When you take the time to learn all you can do with the word processor, it is frustrating to go back to the limitations of a simple typewriter. The overwhelming clinical indications are that the algorithm treatments have nowhere near the range or precision that the diagnosis methods have in assisting patients. In teaching the algorithms Callahan acknowledges "these are simple recipes that frequently work for associated emotions or problems. Complex problems must be diagnosed and an appropriate sequence determined" (Callahan, 1996, unnumbered manual).

However, there are times when the use of algorithms can be an appropriate and effective treatment choice. For example, algorithm treatments are useful when patients call and could benefit from an intervention via the telephone, but no previous diagnosed patterns are applicable or available. There might also be times with newer patients when muscle testing and touching would be clinically premature or therapeutically risky. Such instances might include sessions with patients who have been assaulted or violated and who are untrusting or fearful of being touched. (The option of using a surrogate form of diagnosis in lieu of touching the patient is described in Chapter 12.) These patients can then be taught specific algorithms to help them self-soothe; this can be especially helpful for patients who evidence difficulty with affect tolerance. The algorithm approach also provides therapists a tool when working in emergency room situations or critical incident debriefing for the immediate aftermath of a trauma. For example, if a patient presents at the initial session with a high degree of anxiety, the use of a trauma or anxiety algorithm can provide immediate and substantial relief. In subsequent sessions the therapist could continue the history and assessment process and then begin using the EvTFT diagnosis methods and protocols to further reduce the symptoms and complete the healing from the presenting issue.

Algorithms are also useful when working with groups. For example, in working with a gathering of people who are learning stress management you might want to demonstrate and teach a variety of algorithms for stress reduction and relaxation techniques. Algorithms also work well in group therapy settings, including family therapy. For instance, if you see a family whose members cannot seem to get beyond their immediate emotional distress, which is blocking initial efforts to work at the beginning of a session, it can be useful to have them all do an algorithm treatment sequence. The algorithm chosen would be based on your understanding of the situation or emotion that is compromising their ability to communicate with one another in your office.

Allied health professionals who routinely work with phobias (e.g., dentists, hospital staff using magnetic resonance imaging technology) can be taught to use the phobia algorithm treatments in their milieu. We also advocate that algorithms can be a useful form of first aid for people in almost any setting (e.g., schools, the work place, emergency rooms, in traffic). For instance, algorithm treatments can be used as a first attempt to quell anxiety and panic attacks or to help deal with an instance of inappropriate anger. People do not need professional therapists to self-administer algorithm treatments. We often say that the worst that can happen to an individual when using an algorithm is that nothing will happen. Lambrou and Pratt explore the many uses of algorithms as a self-help technique in *Instant Emotional Healing* (2000), as do Callahan in *Tapping the Healer Within* (2001) and Gallo and Vincenzi in *Energy Tapping* (2000). The Emotional Freedom Technique (EFT) engineered and popularized by Gary Craig (Craig & Fowlie, 1997) is a universal algorithm approach derived from Callahan's treatment points. Our general view is that algorithms can be very useful in the short term with less involved issues. However, the use of EvTFT diagnostic methods will prove more versatile, effective, and even quicker once you become adept at it than the algorithm approach in most cases involving any degree of complexity.

We recommend that therapists familiarize themselves with the various algorithms and even memorizing several of them for the instances in which they might be utilized. The trauma and anxiety algorithms can be particularly useful, as is the comprehensive algorithm. For instance, Britt, while visiting her child's school, witnessed a six-year-old become extremely upset after having an accident. The teacher, knowing about Britt's work with EvTFT, asked for assistance to help the child. Britt used the trauma algorithm and within a minute the child resumed laughing and playing. In a similar situation several years ago, Diepold witnessed a little league ball player catch a bad hop in the face, bringing blood, tears, and fear of resuming his position at shortstop the next inning. He was not seriously hurt; more shocked and afraid that the ball might hit him again. Since Diepold was assisting with the team, he asked the boy's parents if he could try something that might be helpful to their son to settle him down and even resume his play. They agreed and watched as the trauma algorithm was used regarding the incident. Within a few minutes the boy regained his composure and was again ready, willing, and able to play his position.

USING ALGORITHMS AS A GUIDE
WITH DIAGNOSIS

The beginning EvTFT clinician may use the algorithms as a guide when selecting alarm points to test while doing a diagnostic protocol. These algorithmic guidelines can serve as initial "training wheels" for therapists not yet comfortable with the intuitive process of diagnosis. This is what we refer to as "thinking algorithmically" when doing diagnosis. For example, if the targeted thought field is a known trauma, the clinician might muscle-test the bladder alarm point first, because it is the first point of the trauma algorithm. (The bladder meridian is frequently involved in instances of traumatic experience.) While the bladder meridian may or may not turn out to be the initial treatment point, it is often in the mix when trauma is involved.

As noted in Chapter 3, practitioners of traditional Chinese medicine do not use a system of one-to-one correspondence of emotions to meridians yet the use of some of the algorithms seems to contradict this. We continue to suggest that the direct correlations of an algorithmic treatment to emotions such as anger, shame, and guilt only *seem* to exist. We caution the reader that what truly exists in the meridian-emotion connection is considerably idiosyncratic to the individual and their experience. What is *anger* to one person may be experienced as *rage* or *frustration* by another. The intensity and felt location of the emotions are also quite different, which further suggests the emotion-meridian correlations are more consistent within a person than between or among persons.

THE ALGORITHM METHOD
OF TREATMENT

We advocate that muscle testing be utilized when possible to enhance the accuracy and effectiveness of algorithm treatments. For those times when muscle testing is not feasible, we offer the following set of guidelines. In the absence of muscle testing, it is necessary to assume that the patient has blocks (i.e., psychological reversals, belief related blocks) that require correction. Assuming that appropriate assessment and history-taking have been done, here is the algorithm method:

1. Ask the patient to do one of the polarity correction procedures (e.g., BEC, NOTx).
2. Have the patient perform the correction for a generalized psychological reversal, using the NLR area for correction.
3. Have the patient tune into the problem and get an initial SUD rating.
4. Have the patient perform the correction for an issue specific psychological reversal, using the small intestine treatment spot (SI-3, the karate chop side of the hand).
5. Have the patient touch-and-breathe (TAB) on the appropriate algorithm points for the problem. This is followed by the integration sequence and a repeat treatment of the algorithm points.
6. Ask the patient to re-rate the SUD level.
7. If the SUD has dropped to a 0 or 1, have the patient do the eye-roll treatment.
8. If the SUD level has dropped two or more points but not all the way to 0 or 1, have the patient do the correction for a process-specific psychological reversal, using the small intestine treatment point (SI-3) as the correction site. Then have the patient repeat the same algorithm (step 5 above) and have them re-rate the SUD level. Keep repeating until the SUD level has dropped to 0 or 1, or use an alternate algorithm. The patient then completes the treatment by doing an eye-roll.
9. If the SUD level does not drop or drops only one point at a time, have the patient do the simplified collarbone breathing or the neurologic organizer treatment to correct for the possibility of neurologic disorganization (relating to disruptions in polarity and left and right brain hemisphere interaction). Upon completion, repeat the algorithm treatment procedure. Another alternative for addressing the failure of the SUD level to drop is to have the patient correct for a belief related block (i.e., future, safety, deservedness). When muscle testing is not being used, the clinician must inquire of the patient or make an educated guess as to which belief related block could be present. After doing the correction for the belief related block, the patient should repeat the algorithm treatment sequence.

You can also use the algorithms with muscle testing. To do this, use any of the protocols for the three diagnostic methods found in Chapter 10, and substitute the appropriate algorithm in place of the steps for diagnosing the treatment points. If you are using this method, you will be repeating the same algorithm, or an alternate, over and over until the SUD level drops to 1 or 0. Whenever the SUD level fails to drop to 1 or 0 using algorithms, it is time to consider using the diagnostic method. Another way to combine algorithms with muscle testing and diagnoses is to muscle test the patient to the thought field *after* he or she has completed the first treatment of the algorithm points. If the patient's muscle response is strong, then proceed to the integration sequence. If, however, the muscle response is weak to the thought field, then begin to diagnose the next treatment point(s) to add to the algorithm points and complete the process following the basic diagnostic protocol.

The Algorithm Treatments

Table 13.1 presents a sample of the algorithm treatments we initially learned from Fred Gallo, and then from Roger Callahan, when we began our study of thought field therapy. These and other algorithms can be found in Callahan (2001). The formulations we present have been slightly modified from the originals to reflect the terminology used in this text. The two most notable changes are the substitution of integration sequence (ISq) for Callahan's nine gamut sequence (9G) and the change of the treatment point location for the bladder meridian from the inner tip of the eyebrow (eb or BL-2) to the inner eye (ie or BL-1). The sequencing of treatment points remains the same. The alternative algorithms are indicated where there is more than one algorithm sequence listed for the designated problem or emotion. The idea is that when treatment success is not forthcoming with the initial algorithm the patient has an option to try the alternate algorithm sequences.

The choice of which algorithm to employ is based on the presenting problem of the patient, which is the thought field. However, many algorithms are emotion-focused, which we believe can be a major drawback. The algorithm might neutralize the upsetting emotion, but there could be other emotions not being addressed because the cause of the negative emotion is not being targeted. In most instances the emotional upset resonates as symptoms that result from a past or anticipated event or a belief. As with the selection of a thought field for diagnosis, when using algorithms the thought field should be the event or cause of the upset and not the upset itself. By treating the cause many other possible emotional responses can be treated. The therapist can use the emotional information offered by the patient and string together two or three algorithms (e.g., anger, grief, guilt) while focusing on the source event as the thought field. Again, our preference is to do diagnosis.

Table 13.1
The Algorithm Treatments

PROBLEM OR EMOTION	TREATMENT SEQUENCE
Simple Phobias	e, a, c → ISq → TxSq → ER (*most Simple Phobias*) a, e, c → ISq → TxSq → ER (*spiders, claustrophobia, flight turbulence*)
Common Anxiety	e, a, c → ISq → TxSq → ER
Addictive Urge Anxiety	e, a, c → ISq → TxSq → ER c, e, c → ISq → TxSq → ER a, e, c → ISq → TxSq → ER
Trauma, PTSD, "Love Pain"	ie, e, a, c → ISq → TxSq → ER ie, c → ISq → TxSq → ER (*simple trauma*) ie, e, a, c, lf, c → ISq → TxSq → ER (*with anger*) ie, e, a, c, if, c → ISq → TxSq → ER (*with guilt*) ie, e, a, c, lf, c, if, c → ISq → TxSq → ER (*w/both*)
Anger	lf , c → ISq → TxSq → ER
Rage	oe, c → ISq → TxSq → ER
Guilt	if, c → ISq → TxSq → ER
Pain Management, Depression	bh (extended TAB) → ISq → TxSq → ER
Embarrassment	un, c → ISq → TxSq → ER un, a, c → ISq → TxSq → ER
Shame	ul, c → ISq → TxSq → ER ul, a, c → ISq → TxSq → ER
Relaxation Procedure	ER → ISq → ER
Negativistic Behavior	fix psychological reversal
Reversal of Concepts, Words, or Behaviors	fix psychological reversal
Clumsiness or Awkwardness	SCB or NOTx
Inhalant-Type Allergy	mf, a, c → ISq → TxSq → ER
Nasal Congestion, Stuffiness	un, c → ISq → TxSq → ER
Panic/Complex Anxiety	ie, e, a, c, → ISq → TxSq → ER e, a , ie, c, lf → ISq → TxSq → ER ie, a, e, → ISq → TxSq → ER e, ie, a, lf → ISq → TxSq → ER c, e, a → ISq → TxSq → ER
Grief	t, c → ISq → TxSq → ER
Jet Lag (Going East)	e, c → ISq → TxSq → ER
Jet Lag (Going West)	a, c → ISq → TxSq → ER
OCD	c, e, c → ISq → TxSq → ER a, e, c, → ISq → TxSq → ER e, a, c → ISq → TxSq → ER

The Comprehensive Algorithms

The comprehensive algorithm was first proposed by Roger Callahan as a "when all else fails" approach to self-help. The Callahan Techniques™ algorithm consists of having the patient treat (e.g., TAB) 13 of the 14 treatment points[5] while tuned into the thought field, then doing the integration sequence, and then repeating treatment of all 13 points. This is sometimes referred to as "running the system."

This all-purpose one-algorithm-fits-all method was used by Gary Craig, one of the early students of the Callahan Techniques™, in his emotional freedom technique (Craig & Fowlie, 1997); it is commonly known as the EFT algorithm. There was no predetermined order to the EFT sequence other than treatment of the acupuncture points proceeded downward from top to bottom of the body. Craig is of the belief that order of the treatment is not critical because his treatment is repeated over and over in "rounds" until the SUD level reaches zero. The initial or basic EFT treatment sequence uses all 14 treatment points: ie, oe, e, un, ul, c, a, r, t, if, mf, lf, sh, bh (Craig, 2000). Craig later reduced the number of treatment points to the first seven of the fourteen, and calls this the EFT "shortcut sequence." Craig also discontinued the use of Callahan's nine gamut treatment as he further developed his EFT approach. Lambrou and Pratt, in their variation of the comprehensive sequence, use all 14 treatment points in a particular order and intersperse repeat treatment of the kidney meridian three additional times and the stomach meridian one additional time: ie, oe, un, ul, e, c, a, c, e, r, lf, c, if, c, mf, t, sh, bh (2000).

The comprehensive algorithm can be used as a last resort if none of the other algorithms work. We do find that using a comprehensive algorithm is usually a cumbersome way to achieve an end more elegantly (and often more quickly) attained by the use of the diagnostic method. However, it certainly has proved useful to teach patients a one-size-fits-all prescription to help them through difficult times away from the therapist's office. The hypothesis is that if the patient keeps treating the points over and over again, the right combination or sequence of meridians will be treated, and has been found to be true a remarkable number of times. We are reminded of the 1983 movie *WarGames*, in which the rogue computer was looking for a ten-digit access code to launch a nuclear offensive. It accomplished this by running the possible sequences repeatedly until the code was discovered.

Chapter 14

THE INTEGRATION OF EvTFT INTO PSYCHOTHERAPY

Evolving Thought Field Therapy challenges
our previous beliefs about the nature and treatment of psychological problems.
—John H. Diepold, Jr.

This chapter is intended as a guide for psychotherapists who wish to incorporate Evolving Thought Field Therapy (EvTFT) into their clinical practices. We will discuss avenues and opportunities for integrating EvTFT into everyday practice, and briefly describe a diagnostic spectrum of clinical case examples. The clinical vignettes that follow include case examples on trauma, posttraumatic stress disorder, anxiety disorders, phobia, dissociative disorders, depression and suicidal ideation, anger/rage, unhealthy attractions, shame, embarrassment, nail biting, pain management, obsessive compulsive disorders, and peak performance issues. We will also discuss working with children, using surrogates, and family therapy interventions.

INTEGRATING EvTFT INTO CLINICAL PRACTICE

EvTFT is a powerful, versatile, and effective psychotherapy that can greatly enhance treatment effects when appropriately incorporated into a clinical psychotherapy practice, regardless of the practitioner's orientation. We do not envision EvTFT as a panacea or a one-trick psychotherapeutic pony. We adamantly encourage a strong commitment to ethical practices and procedures, which permeate our beliefs and teaching, when integrating EvTFT into the therapeutic repertoire. Accordingly, the following advisory appears at the beginning of our workshop training manual:

Clinical Ethics Reminder

All Contact and Thought Directed Diagnostic and treatment procedures in this manual are for use by licensed and/or certified mental health professionals only.

The BDB Group strongly recommends, in accordance with appropriate clinical practice, that you take a complete psychosocial history, and have an understanding of the problem(s) within the context of the individual and their environment. Effective psychotherapy requires a trusting relationship between therapist and patient. The BDB Group recommends that an appropriate therapeutic relationship exists before initiating Contact and/or Thought Directed Diagnoses and treatment.

The BDB Group strongly recommends that the population (adults, adolescents, children), and types of mental health issues (e.g., anxiety, dissociation, eating disorders), with which you work remain within your area of training and expertise.

The BDB Group also recommends that you take the time to adequately inform and/or prepare your patient with information about EvTFT and energy psychotherapy procedures. To the best of our knowledge, there have been no reported ill effects from using EvTFT when the appropriate precautions and procedures are used.

The BDB Group adheres to the American Psychological Association's *Ethical Principles Of Psychologists and Code of Conduct*. The BDB Group *requires* that all clinical information shared during the course of this training (via practicum experiences and live demonstrations) be honored as *confidential* in accordance with APA guidelines. (Britt, Diepold, & Bender, 1998)

As with all psychotherapy, establishing and maintaining rapport with the patient is critical to initiating treatment. In fact, we believe the energy that resonates between patient and therapist accounts for the phenomenon we describe as *rapport*. There are many ways in which rapport can be established and many methods to acquire clinical assessment information that exceed the scope of this chapter. We therefore encourage therapists to use the style and methods that they have previously learned and employ them in setting the stage for therapeutic intervention when considering the use of EvTFT. Decisions regarding when and with what issues to use EvTFT will come with clinical experience. The more the therapist understands the concepts and the versatility of EvTFT the more knowledgeable and creative they and their patients will become in its application.

As part of our case formulation we assess whether EvTFT is appropriate for the patient based on the referral information, personal and problem history, and standardized clinical assessment tools. As appropriate, we discuss the option of using EvTFT with the patient and determine when and where the use of this treatment would be most efficacious. Often, new patients are unfamiliar with EvTFT, so time is needed to verbally explain, demonstrate, and provide reference literature and websites for their knowledge.

Because EvTFT is an excellent modality to provide rapid, effective relief from disturbing affect, we often find it beneficial to use EvTFT as a first-line intervention. This is especially true in cases where the patient is experiencing acute distress requiring immediate intervention (e.g., flashbacks, panic anxiety, abreaction). As the treatment issues manifest during the course of therapy the therapist can apply EvTFT when target incidents or beliefs are identified (i.e., events reported by the patient that trigger disturbing affect and/or self-defeating cognitions and behavior). It is our hope that the case examples will demonstrate the versatility and the quick relief patients can experience at any point in their course of psychotherapy.

The Callahan Techniques™, which is one of the roots of EvTFT, had developed a reputation of being an effective short-term treatment methodology (e.g., Figley & Carbonell, 1995). However, we have also observed that EvTFT is easily incorporated into longer-term individual treatment models, such as psychodynamic and cognitive behavioral models, as well as the newer coaching models. When working on an issue, the therapist and patient can target specific events, behavior and symptom patterns, beliefs, and even characterological trait issues. They can then interweave the EvTFT diagnostic protocol into the existing therapy model, thereby greatly enhancing the process.

We have observed that therapists can glean a great deal of traditional diagnostic information from the EvTFT causal diagnostic process. For instance, the nature of the various PRs and belief related blocks (safety, deservedness, future) could spark insights for the patient or the therapist. As an illustration, Britt observed during one session that a patient was surprised to find that the *deservedness* belief related block kept turning up. Further exploration of this phenomenon was addressed during the *talk therapy* segment of the session, which prompted the patient to acknowledge the previously repressed perception that he was an adult child of an alcoholic and as as child had experienced a great deal of emotional abuse. This insight provided the springboard for future sessions in which the patient was able to progress with the help of a combination of EvTFT and insight-oriented treatment.

EvTFT WITH CHILDREN
AND ADOLESCENTS

EvTFT is an appropriate and valuable treatment choice when working with children and adolescents. As previously noted in Chapter 4, before beginning treatment with a child it is always necessary to discuss the EvTFT treatment procedures with the parent(s). It is prudent to make sure that the parent(s) are absolutely clear about the limited physical contact on the arm or fingers that occurs during EvTFT diagnosis. Demonstrating the process of muscle testing on the parents can be useful in providing an experiential understanding to supplement the verbal description of how meridian-based psychotherapy works. Depending upon the age of the child and the focus of treatment, it is advisable to have the parent stay in the room while using EvTFT on the child, at least for the initial session.

Although the EvTFT diagnostic and treatment protocol remains essentially the same when working with children, we recommend minor adjustments to accommodate the developmental stage of the child. Instead of having the child say, "I *deeply accept* myself even though I have this problem . . . ," the child could say something like, "I *really like* myself even though I have this problem. . . ." Often children will suggest their own language changes, making it a more personal fit for them. Making the evaluative procedure a more visual experience usually makes the subjective units of distress (SUD) and subjective units of enjoyment (SUE) rating scales more meaningful to a child. In this regard we like to draw a progressive series of simple faces, ranging from a smiley face indicating a 0 or no upset to a very unhappy face indicating an upset level of 10. Keeping children attuned to the thought field can sometimes be a creative effort. Reminding them often to tune in, having them draw a picture, or having a toy or object represent the thought field are some ways this can be accomplished.

EvTFT is adaptable to most play therapies. For example, for children with whom verbalization or attention span can be an issue, the therapist can have the child draw a picture of a particular fear or upset he or she is experiencing and then have the child focus on the picture during the diagnostic protocol. Dolls, puppets, and other toys can also be used to creatively facilitate the process so that EvTFT becomes a smooth-flowing and integral part of the overall treatment. To illustrate, in one case when Diepold was working with a five-year-old child, a wizard puppet was used to give instructions to both the therapist and the patient about muscle testing and treatment points. The playful power of the wizard minimized any difficulty with compliance, and created a comfortable format for future treatment interventions. Children can easily be shown how to do home treatment when necessary and are often eager to do it. Home treatment also has the added effect of empowering children by providing a tool to master their anxieties.

Adolescents tend to enjoy and appreciate the EvTFT model as well. They usually find it intriguing and it is rare to encounter resistance to the protocol. Teens can be secretive for various reasons (e.g., distrust of adults, desire to set boundaries, fear of embarrassment or punishment), so they usually do not mind participating in a model where they do not have to talk much if they choose not to. When a teen does not wish to reveal specifically what he or she wants to work on or is disturbed about, the therapist can still use EvTFT diagnostic methods because *the patient* knows the issue and it is not necessary for the therapist to know what the patient is attuning. It is, however, important that the patient remain with the same thought field until diagnosis and treatment are completed. Following the usual procedural steps of the protocol, and using the SUD or SUE scale as a guide, successful treatment is readily accomplished. After the issue has been cleared of emotional resonance, teens are often willing to talk about the problem, perhaps because they experience it as less problematic now that it is no longer emotionally upsetting for them. The judicious therapist will constantly attend to the ebb and flow of the therapeutic relationship with teens and intermix talk therapy and other techniques with the EvTFT approach. For the most part, the language of EvTFT can remain the same for adolescents as with adults, with the therapist making adjustments as deemed appropriate.

THE USE OF EvTFT IN MARRIAGE AND FAMILY THERAPY

Family therapists are well aware that dynamics in a family can emotionally intensify during treatment sessions, and strong negative feelings (e.g., anger) can block even the most well planned intervention. EvTFT can prove helpful in removing some of these blocks during conjoint sessions and, if necessary, in follow-up individual sessions. For example, most marriage therapists have faced the experience of going out to their waiting room to greet a couple only to find angry-looking adversaries, sitting at opposite ends of the room, waiting to have their fight adjudicated. It can sometimes be prudent for the therapist to invite one of the marital pair into the treatment room and explain that the session will be far more effective if the anger levels diminish to a point where communication becomes possible. Upon securing the agreement of the party to work on the anger-causing issue, the therapist can use EvTFT to reduce or eliminate the angry feelings so that work can progress.[1] After the work is done, invite the other party into the treatment room and offer them the same opportunity.

Similar methods can be applied in family therapy sessions where the parties find it difficult to work cooperatively because of a variety of impediments to treatment, including negative emotions, pattern repetition, and unknown blocks. In family sessions, where anxiety with one or all parties is prevalent, it may be useful to do either an EvTFT diagnosis and treatment with the most anxious person or to use an anxiety algorithm as a family exercise to lower the anxiety level. In cases where a parent and an adolescent are locked into a mutual dance of anger and frustration with neither party being able to back off their positions, consider using EvTFT to reduce the tension and facilitate resolution of the problem. With the other people present in the room, the therapist can use the diagnostic protocol with parent and child in turn (using clinical judgment to determine who should go first) to alleviate those feelings that are blocking the process. Following this, the family session can proceed.

There are times when participants in conjoint sessions feel blocked, not by anger, guilt, or other so-called negative emotions, but by what they describe as an unknown entity. For instance, Britt observed in a marital session focused on sex, that the wife reported that whenever the sex topic was broached, a "wall" would come down, prohibiting her from thinking, feeling, or even communicating about it. The diagnostic protocol for unknown blocks was utilized and the particular block was neutralized. After the EvTFT intervention, the woman was able to name the issue and openly discuss it.

CASE CONSULTATION WITH EvTFT

The authors are often approached by other therapists to do one or more EvTFT consultation-treatment sessions with their patients. These cases can be equally rewarding for the patient and therapist, as several of the case histories discussed later in this chapter will illustrate. When doing this type of treatment consultation we follow the stringent guidelines:

1. Get a clearly defined picture from both the referring therapist and the patient of what work needs to be done. Contract with the patient for the approximate number of sessions the work will take;

2. Obtain a release from the patient so that you can work closely and report back to the referring/treating therapist;

3. Inform the patient that this is a short-term consultation and that there is no plan for him or her to become a regular patient. This approach tends to focus the work, short-circuit the possibilities of splitting, and helps maintain good relations with the referring therapist;

4. Invite the therapist to observe or take part in at least the first session. We find many therapists are interested in doing this both out of concern for their patient's comfort and out of curiosity of what we do with EvTFT. We welcome the therapist's presence because it can serve as a bridge to establishing therapeutic rapport between the patient and us. Because of the short-term nature of this interaction, the usual pattern of history gathering, assessment, and relationship building is truncated, so having the therapist present can help the patient feel safer. Safety is especially important if the patient has been diagnosed with post-traumatic stress disorder, a dissociative disorder, or has a history of abuse. The presence of an additional therapist also gives us the option of doing EvTFT using a surrogate;

5. Work closely with and report back regularly to the referring therapist, and ask him or her for feedback as to how the patient is progressing;

6. Follow-up your work with the referring therapist at regular intervals whenever appropriate.

TYPICAL TREATMENT APPLICATIONS AND CASE EXAMPLES

EvTFT methods are highly versatile and applicable to a wide range of treatment issues. Once the knowledge and techniques of EvTFT are mastered the diagnosis and treatment aspects flow with relatively quick and lasting therapeutic results. We emphasize that EvTFT is not a stand-alone psychotherapy, but a powerful psychotherapeutic intervention. A skilled EvTFT practitioner integrates these potent methods with his or her prior training and orientation in psychotherapy. Listening to our patients helps us determine what issues need to be addressed. When the time is right to do the work, EvTFT enables the patient to resolve his or her emotional distress quickly and easily.

In all of the case examples that follow the authors used one of the EvTFT diagnostic methods and the touch-and-breathe (TAB) treatment approach for the described issues. The cases range from single-treatment examples, to sample sessions of ongoing psychotherapy addressing a specific issue, and to longer-span of treatments in which EvTFT was used at various times. In each sample case, the identifying patient information was changed to safeguard identities. To further protect the identities of the patients being described, the primary therapist is not identified except for previously published cases. Thus, the first person pronouns used (I, we, our, etc.) may refer to any of the three authors.

Case 1: A Referral for Depression

This first example involves a 48-year-old medical receptionist who was referred for reactive depression resulting primarily from the death of her husband of 25 years. He died two months after his diagnosis of pancreatic cancer, and she was understandably traumatized. Eighteen months had passed since his death and she described her situation as "I'm stuck in limbo and having a hard time moving on." She had not touched her husband's personal belongings since his death; his wallet remained on the bureau and his ashes were kept in the house.

She was seen for a total of eight sessions in which only two sessions employed EvTFT. The first treatment issue targeted the death of her husband ("He's not here"). When asked to report her level of upset on a the 0 to 10 point SUD scale, she immediately said "20, 30, 40," emphasizing her high level of distress from just thinking about her husband's death. She was found to have an issue-specific PR to overcoming this problem; the PR was successfully corrected on the side of the hand (SI-3). Four meridians were diagnosed using thought directed diagnosis and treated using TAB in a single holon. When asked to re-rate her distress level she smiled and said, "That's different, it's zero." This Ev-TFT intervention was then completed with the ground to sky eye-roll treatment. When she returned for a psychotherapy session two weeks later she exclaimed, "I cleared my husband's stuff out," and she had made plans to bury his ashes in a grave. A six-month follow-up found that she continued to be upset-free regarding her issues about his death. She remained depression-free and was again living in a more rewarding fashion. Although "depression" had never been the focus of treatment, her symptoms of depression abated.

Case 2: A Family Tragedy

This case involved a 12-year-old boy who, when he was 4 years old, witnessed the drowning of a younger brother in the family pool. The deceased brother had a twin brother who was also involved in the pool mishap and became wheel-chair bound, severely mentally handicapped, and unable to speak as a result. This younger brother continued to reside with the family. The patient was brought in for therapy because he was struggling in fifth grade and had told his teachers he believed he was responsible for his brother's drowning eight years ago. While gathering intake information, I learned that for the past eight years, this 12-year-old patient had been experiencing repeated flashbacks, a series of four nightmares of the accident, and other odd dreams related to his brothers. Often "tingling, nausea, chills, and shakes" accompanied his flashbacks. The presence of his surviving handicapped brother served to trigger the flashbacks, "especially when he's sick."

At the second session his recall of the accident was the target of treatment. His mother remained in the room during the first treatment session so she could observe this form of therapy and ask questions if desired.[2] When thinking of the accident her son reported a SUD level of 8 and described seeing his brothers falling into the pool. After diagnosis and treatment of the first holon, the boy reported a SUD level of 2. A second holon of three meridians was then diagnosed and treated. When asked to re-rate the SUD level, he said "zero" then instantly reported "seeing" a new memory of watching CPR performed on the brother that died. The SUD level for this new memory (a new thought field) was 5.5. Six meridians were then diagnosed and treated in this initial holon. When asked to re-rate the SUD level, he said "about one." However, the ground to sky eye-roll did not reduce the SUD level to 0. A second holon with three meridians was then diagnosed and treated. He then reported a SUD level of 0. However, yet another memory popped into his mind. This memory was of when he taught his little brother to climb the small fence around the pool. To this new memory he gave a SUD level of 9.5. Four meridians were diagnosed and treated as he attuned to this thought field. He then reported a SUD level of 0 with no additional intruding memories. A ground to sky eye-roll treatment completed the EvTFT session. At this time the 12-year-old stated that he was able to see and think about all three connected flashback images without any distress.

The following week the boy reported that he had been free of flashbacks, even when he was in the company of the surviving twin. The above work with the 12 year old transpired within one 50-minute session. The flashbacks and dreams never returned, and he was much relieved. When I asked his mother what she thought about this form of therapy she said, "I never imagined when I brought him for therapy that it would be like this, but it sure works." The boy, however, remained in therapy for approximately one year to address other accident-related, personal, family, and school-related issues.

Case 3: Delusional Disorder

This case was referred for consultation by a marriage and family therapist who was seeing the client and her family for a multitude of chronic problems. At the time of the referral, the patient, a 43-year-old woman, had been experiencing what she called an "eye problem" for a period of about eighteen months. The problem was that she was experiencing the delusion that people were constantly staring at her breasts. Her profession required her to be out in public and to interact face-to-face with large numbers of people each day, and thus the delusion was a source of constant disturbance. Neither her therapist nor her consulting psychiatrist was able to diminish or eradicate the delusion, even with an array of antipsychotic, anti-anxiety, and antidepressive medications. The delusion was hampering her ability to do her job and was also having an impact on her personal life. It served to exacerbate an already serious generalized anxiety disorder and to further the deterioration of her marriage. There did not appear to be any precipitants to the problem, nor was there a personal or family history of delusional thinking.

The woman was seen for a total of three sessions. The first session was used to take a history and to make a preliminary assessment. The following two sessions were EvTFT diagnostic and treatment sessions that specifically addressed the problem. The first thought field to be treated was her perception that people were staring at her breasts. The standard EvTFT protocol using the thought directed diagnosis model was used. There were no immediate blocks present, nor was there a polarity issue; five holons were diagnosed, each time lowering the SUD level. At a SUD level of 4, a safety belief related block manifested itself and was cleared using the governing vessel as the correction point. Another single-point holon was then diagnosed, and the SUD level dropped to 1. The eye-roll treatment did not lower the SUD to 0, and at this point, a process-specific belief related block for safety was uncovered and corrected on the small intestine treatment point. Another single-point holon was diagnosed, and the SUD level dropped to 0. The treatment was completed using the eye-roll. No homework was needed.

Two weeks later the client reported that the delusion had not manifested itself since the last session. However, she was concerned that even though no one was staring at her, they might do so, and therefore she continued to experience anxiety. We then decided to treat the thought field that although people were not looking at her breasts, they *might* decide to do so. The initial SUD level was 7, and once again, there were no immediate blocks or polarity issues. Seven holons were diagnosed with a pattern of single-point drops in SUD level. After two one-point drops, the patient was evaluated to see if neurologic disorganization was present and if a simplified collarbone breathing exercise was necessary, but it was not. One safety belief related block was uncovered and treated.

After this diagnostic segment, the client no longer felt anxious that someone might be looking at her, but she expressed concern that this anxiety might return in the future and that she would be wondering when someone might start looking at her. This constituted the last thought field. The pattern of her not having any immediate reversals or polarity issues remained constant, as did the pattern of one-point drops.

Follow-up reports from the referring therapist at six months, one year, and two years indicated that the patient remained free of this delusion and did not experience any other delusions.

Case 4: MRI Refusal

As part of a coordinated effort between the departments of psychiatry and radiology at the University of Medicine and Dentistry of New Jersey-Newark, there is a variety of ongoing research in addition to patient-care utilization of the scanning devices. Studies have ranged from imaging the physical aspects of unexplained illnesses, especially chronic fatigue syndrome and fibromyalgia, to studying the effects of touching specific acupuncture points.

On one occasion while I was present at the scanning facility, a situation occurred in which, despite the usual coaxing and assurance, a patient was unable to enter and stay within the scanning device long enough to complete the necessary imaging. Within moments of being put into the device, the patient asked to be brought back out. He was a large man and very apologetic about his inability to stay in the scanner. On urging from colleagues who knew I did work with phobic responses, I went in and spoke with the man. When asked what he was thinking, the man said, "My wife had cancer. One of the last memories I have of her is her having to take an MRI. I hate this thing." I asked him, "Are you willing to try something to help you go into the scanner or would you prefer to stop now?" The man assured me he wanted to accomplish what he had come there to do.

Thinking it might be a grief-related problem I instructed the man to tune into the memory of his wife in the scanner and to touch his thumb treatment point (demonstrating the procedure to him), take one full respiration, and then touch his other thumb and take one full respiration. In doing this, the patient treated the lung meridian treatment point (LU-11) bilaterally. He then performed the integration sequence and repeated the bilateral treatment of the lung meridian. Seated on the edge of the tube slide, the man looked around and said, "Ok. I don't know what you did but I'm ready to go back in there." He did go back in and stayed in for the entire time the procedure required. The members of the technical staff expressed interest in the particulars of the phobic response resolution, citing the refusal as a common scanner problem. Their interest was not simply related to the high cost of scans and the value of the time and personnel required for the operation; they were interested in the soothing effect the treatment provided to the patient.

Case 5: Suicidal Ideation

This case example involves a 38-year-old mother of two daughters who was referred for management of trauma, pain, and depression resulting from a car accident that involved her children. As the course of therapy progressed, she reported a longstanding history of suicidal ideation (with no actual attempts) that was exacerbated with the recent life stressors. The origin of her suicidal thinking was connected to her strong desire to escape from the abandonment she felt when her mother died at an early age; this desire was jolted when the woman realized that she could have died in the car crash, leaving her daughters behind. The woman said she never felt the love and approval she needed (her father was also now dead) and she deluded herself in thinking she could get love and approval from her parents if she joined them in death. Because depression with suicidal ideation is a classic area of concern for both patient and therapist, this issue was addressed using the elaters protocol[3] to diagnose and treat the positive thoughts and emotions that appeared to influence the woman's self-sabotaging patterns.

When the woman was asked to explain why she engaged in thoughts about suicide she said it was a way "to get away" and "to be with my parents . . . to finally get their approval and love." When asked how much she enjoyed the feelings she experienced when she thought about suicide she reported a SUE level of 5, even though she knew it was not good for her and her family. There was no issue-specific PR to resolving the suicidal ideation. Four meridians were diagnosed and treated in the initial holon while she was attuned to her positive thoughts and feelings connected to suicide. When asked to re-rate her SUE level she stated "three." Although there was no process-specific PR, there were two belief related blocks that were diagnosed and treated; these pertained to issues of safety and future (e.g., "I will always have this feeling of enjoyment about dying because I had it a long time . . ."). After re-treatment of the initial holon she reported a SUE level of 1. A ground to sky eye-roll treatment reduced the SUE level to 0. However, with a slight smile she said, "I feel better, but how do I know it will last?" (This statement is an example of what Callahan and Callahan [1996] called the *apex problem*.) The following week she reported no suicidal ideation at all since doing the treatment, which marked the first time she had felt relief "in years." Six weeks later she continued to be free of suicidal ideation. She did, however, remain in therapy to address other issues influencing her depression.

Case 6: Ongoing Case with Posttraumatic Stress Disorder and Severe Family of Origin Issues

This patient self-referred for EvTFT after she had tried a number of different traditional psychotherapies, none of which were helpful in resolving her posttraumatic stress disorder (PTSD). Nine years previous to the therapy, she was on an early morning run and was abducted, dragged into the nearby woods, and brutally attacked. She was sexually assaulted and her back was broken during her struggle with the attacker. The attacker outweighed the woman by at least 100 pounds; over a foot shorter than her assailant, she managed to escape by means of sharp intelligence, previous military training, and pure courage. The patient also had a history of related and unrelated medical trauma and issues of severe dysfunction in her family of origin. Her symptoms included disabling flashbacks during which she relived various parts of the assault; a multitude of severe anxiety producing triggers; unpleasant and disturbing physical symptoms; and rage and depressive episodes. Her rage was directed not only at her attacker but also at the legal and health care systems, especially insurance companies. She scored a 35 on the dissociative experiences scale.

The client was seen for a total of 21 sessions over a period of six months. EvTFT was the primary modality used to treat all phases of the presenting problem, with traditional psychotherapy and family therapy being employed when deemed necessary for clinical effectiveness.

The first EvTFT targets were her flashbacks: She had nine particularly severe ones, all concerned with the attack. Each flashback was treated separately. Often additional thought fields would come up while doing the EvTFT diagnostics and they would have to be diagnosed and treated as well. For example she would sometimes have a memory of another aspect of the attack—e.g., an olfactory flashback—that needed to be addressed first.

Disturbing bodily sensations often appeared when working with this client. Sometimes they spontaneously cleared during the diagnostic and treatment process of the initial thought field and sometimes they needed to be treated separately. Muscle testing became an important tool in the determination of when and how to treat these powerful sensations when they arose. When a sensation manifested itself during treatment, the patient was muscle-tested in order to ascertain whether the sensation should be addressed as it came up or after the flashback sequence was treated. One particular thought field elicited a strong body sensation that needed to be treated even after a verbal 0 SUD level was achieved for the flashback. Although the SUD level for that remaining body sensation was 6, it was completely eliminated and reduced to a 0 with one holon.

After successfully treating the flashbacks, work began on eliminating the triggers that would cause a variety of negative reactions in the patient, including severe anxiety, dread, and depression. These included smells and seeing strangers wearing items of clothing similar to what the attacker wore. In contrast to the treatment patterns for the flashbacks, the treatment patterns for the triggers were far less complex. They would involve one to three holons with a minimum of blocks.

A constant feature of the therapy was treatment of the many physical sensations that the woman experienced as a result of the attack, her hospital stay, and her long physical recovery. She would experience physical symptoms like "buzzing" in her shoulders, spine, and feet, as well as "twitching" in her head and neck, all of which had not responded to treatment by the physicians and allied health professionals with whom she was working. These physical sensations were all successfully treated to some degree using EvTFT: Some were completely eliminated and some were greatly lessened in intensity. All of these sensations lost their ability to trigger anxiety, depression, or flashbacks.

Having dealt with the trauma over a period of two months and about ten sessions, the attention turned to other areas of distress in her life. These included anger related to ongoing situations in her life over which she felt she had no control, such as her continuing fights with insurance companies over her treatment, her situation with her family of origin, and her quest to be a competitive runner. Although much of her anger was appropriate and served as a motivating force for positive actions, some aspects of her anger disrupted her life, and these were specifically targeted and either alleviated or brought under control with the EvTFT protocol. Following this segment of the treatment, the woman was able to think more clearly and was empowered to act in ways more helpful to her cause. Having resolved the presenting issue of the trauma, the woman was then able to concentrate on her family of origin. Family therapy techniques, including intensive genogram work, were interspersed with EvTFT, which was used to eliminate negative shame-based beliefs about herself and to reduce the powerful effect of early painful memories. From this work, the woman was able to take positive action regarding her family. The last segment of treatment for this patient was peak performance work regarding her efforts to be a competitive runner, after which she was discharged.

Follow-up after three years has indicated that the major work done with EvTFT has not diminished in its effectiveness. The client is free of flashbacks and other trauma symptoms. Because of the severe bodily damage inflicted upon her during the attack and because she is an athlete, ongoing physical issues remain, however they no longer act as triggers for the trauma.

Case 7: Stress Related Trauma and Eating Disorder

This case involves a 47-year-old wife and mother who sought treatment because she had not been able to eat during the previous two weeks. She reported having lost ten pounds already and being able to "eat a little bit only after 6:00 P.M." She had no idea why she found herself suddenly unable to eat.

Prior to the onset of the eating problem she reported two traumatic experiences and described the past year as "the year from hell." The stressful year pertained to her husband, who had experienced multiple health problems with the possibility of prostate cancer looming. However, two weeks before our session she related a story of having witnessed a car hit a tree and flip over on its roof. She left her car and went over to inform the people in the overturned car that help had been called. When she arrived at the car she saw the driver upside-down against the roof. She said she held his hand and talked with him until the ambulance came. When she arrived home her daughter told her that her mother-in-law had fallen and broken her shoulder. The following day her daughter told her that she had a sore toe, so they went to the podiatrist's office for treatment. After the podiatrist numbed her daughter's swollen toe in order drain it, the doctor left the room. No sooner had the doctor left the room than the daughter "passed out and wet herself," and fell against her mother's shoulder. The mother screamed because she thought her daughter had died. Although she was told her daughter had only fainted, the mother was convinced that "it was more than a faint . . . I haven't been able to eat since." She also reported frequent flashbacks about the way her daughter's head fell on her shoulder.

This articulate woman was a prior patient who quickly supplemented her background information. Although upset and acutely depressed, she was highly motivated. The targeted thought field was the incident in the podiatrist's office where she thought her daughter had died and about which she was having flashbacks. She reported a SUD level of 9 when attuned to this memory. There was no generalized or issue-specific PR. Using thought directed diagnosis, only one meridian was diagnosed and treated using TAB in this initial holon. The SUD level decreased to 8. As there was no process-specific PR, diagnosis yielded another single meridian in this second holon, which was treated. Now a SUD level of 5 was reported. Again there was no process-specific PR and diagnosis was resumed. This time five meridians were treated in a third holon. The SUD level was now reported to be 0, and was confirmed via a muscle test. A ground to sky eye-roll treatment completed the EvTFT interventions. When the treatment was finished, she said, "It was terrible, and I'm glad it's over. I think I can see and eat food without pulling away from it."[4]

This was the only session with this patient regarding her eating disorder. She looked and sounded so much better immediately following treatment that I asked her to call in a couple days to inform me of her status and to reschedule based on her report. She called to say she had been eating again without difficulty and was doing well. She also called several months later to say she had continued to eat well, and that her husband is also doing well. She was both grateful and surprised about her change and her relief after a single treatment session.

Case 8: Fear and Inability to Swallow Pills or Medication

This case involves a single-session consultation regarding a fear of pill taking with a 45-year-old woman who would soon have major surgery requiring post-operative pain medication. This fear and inability to swallow medication was evident in childhood and had persisted despite her many efforts to resolve the difficulty. Medication was often broken apart or ground up and mixed with food (e.g., applesauce) to help the swallowing process, however this was only occasionally successful. Her physician had recently referred her to a local therapist for hypnosis and relaxation work, which she said was helpful, but she was still having difficulty swallowing pills. Time was running out, so she sought this consultation.

A history of her problem revealed that when she was "young" she had tried to swallow pills when ill and recalled "trying to swallow and it wouldn't move." She said the pills would get caught in her throat "a lot of times" and that this problem had continued over the years. When asked to think about swallowing a pill and having it get caught in her throat she reported a SUD level of 8. Muscle-test responses were initially weak to all statements, but the responses corrected after she drank a small glass of water. There was no generalized or issue-specific PR regarding this problem. Thought directed diagnosis revealed a sequence of eight meridians in this first holon, which were treated by TAB. The patient now reported a SUD level of 5. After a process-specific PR was diagnosed and treated at the side of the hand (SI-3), re-treatment of the first holon was completed. The SUD level was then reported to be 2. Diagnosis of a second holon yielded four meridians, which were immediately treated with TAB. The SUD level was now reported to be 1 when she thought about swallowing a pill and it getting caught. The ground to sky eye-roll treatment was completed, but she reported no change in her SUD level. However, a muscle-tested SUD revealed a distress level of 0 to the swallowing problem. The fact that she was still reporting distress (i.e., SUD 1) suggested that there was something interfering that was adjacent to this thought field.

Upon inquiry she stated that she started to think that she was "afraid to throw up." This related thought field relinquished its emotional upset after two holons were diagnosed and treated. Upon completion, she stated that another thought came to mind that pertained to the pill "hitting my throat." This thought field cleared after diagnosis and treatment of the stomach meridian. Now she reported a third related thought field that came to her mind involving the sensation of the pill in her throat. Diagnosis yielded a single holon of three meridians for this thought field. Now she claimed to be free of distress when she attuned the original thought field regarding swallowing a pill and having it get caught. She was also free from emotional distress from the other related thought fields. The entire treatment was then completed with the ground to sky eye-roll. Her verbal report of being free of distress now matched her nonverbal report.

I therefore invited the woman to take her current medication with some water instead of breaking it or mixing it with food, and she was able to do so successfully without distress or difficulty. She went on to have successful reconstructive back surgery and was able to take her pain medication without swallowing problems. Several years have passed since that treatment, and she continues to be free of swallowing difficulties.

Case 9: Posttraumatic Stress Disorder
with Ongoing Stressors

The client, a 49-year-old man, was referred by his treating psychologist for what appeared to be intractable symptoms of PTSD, which proved crippling enough that he was unable to work. The therapist reported that in addition to the trauma symptoms, the patient also had an axis II diagnosis and problems with rage, impulse control, and depression. He was taking a host of antidepressant and anti-anxiety medications. The constellation of PTSD symptoms included chronic anxiety, flashbacks, a variety of triggers, avoidant behaviors, and shaking and crying when confronted. The man had been traumatized for a number of years by his wife's ex-husband who stalked the couple. The ex-husband would call dozens of times a day, both at home and at work; he would also be verbally abusive and at times physically confrontational. Ultimately, a permanent restraining order was obtained against him, but the trauma still remained in the form of flashbacks and severe reactions to triggers, such as a ringing phone, encounters with men who resembled the ex-husband, and any kind of confrontation.

The patient was seen for a total of six sessions; the first two were mainly concerned with history and assessment. In the second session, he was asked for a SUD rating of his overall level of anxiety as he was sitting and talking. He rated it a "five" and was then taught the simplified collarbone breathing (SCB) treatment. After doing that treatment, he was asked to re-rate his SUD level and was surprised to find himself much calmer; he noted that the SUD had gone down to "one." He was instructed to do SCB several times a day, especially when he grew anxious. In the following session he reported that it was very useful for him.

In the third session, EvTFT was used to desensitize him to both hearing a ringing phone and answering the phone. He worked on several aspects of the phone trauma: memories of when the perpetrator would call, instances of people yelling at him on the phone at work, and hearing a ringing phone at home. In all but one diagnostic protocol, the client did not exhibit any signs of a polarity reversal, nor were generalized PRs present. Most treatments contained an average of three short holons with either an issue-specific PR or a safety belief related block. Each time, the SUD level went down to a 0 and no homework was indicated. The future performance imagery index was used with him imagining answering the phone comfortably and without anxiety.

The man came to the fourth session very angry about occurrences in his home situation that were unrelated to the trauma. Before continuing with the trauma work, it was necessary to diffuse that anger and EvTFT was selected as the treatment of choice. This was the only time a generalized PR was evident. The anger was quickly resolved, with the SUD level dropping from 8 to 0 with two blocks and one holon. The remainder of the session was focused on the traumatic incidents related to his wife's ex-husband. The patient was diagnosed and treated with EvTFT for the three worst incidents: a physical confrontation in which the police were called, the memory of being threatened, and the experience of being harangued at his place of work. All three treatments involved safety belief related blocks. The first involved two holons and the other two consisted of one holon. The SUD levels were progressively lower for each incident treated.

In the fifth session the man reported having seen a person who closely resembled the perpetrator, but the patient reported that he was not triggered. He also had not been bothered by phones in any way, nor was he troubled by flashbacks. The man again described being overwhelmed and depressed by his home situation and consequently the session was spent in doing EvTFT work on this since it was clear that he could not concentrate on the trauma issue. This work was done in combination with the future performance imagery index in which he was asked to imagine himself at home and remaining calm. He was able to accomplish this and left feeling calmer and more optimistic about his home life.

The sixth and last session was concerned with clearing the remaining triggers, including the man's reactions when he heard or saw the ex-husband's name. The SUD levels for the triggers were all very low (in the 3 to 4 range) compared with the much higher ratings in the earlier sessions. All triggers cleared easily with only one or two holons and no reversals in each treatment. We decided that the trauma work was completed and he was referred back to his primary therapist for ongoing treatment. The man noted that he felt "smarter" and more empowered by the treatment session. In a follow-up consultation, his psychologist confirmed that the PTSD symptoms appeared to have been resolved and that the client was much more stable.

Case 10: Stroke Victim
with Obsessive-Compulsive Disorder

A 65-year-old woman was seen for a one-time consultation for treatment of an obsessive compulsive behavior that was creating a problem for both her and her family. She had suffered a stroke that had left her severely compromised physically and cognitively; she was several years into her rehabilitation. The woman was making great strides physically, but an old behavior that had minimally bothered her before the stroke seemed to be growing in strength. She had a compulsion to count sides of squares, and when she had counted four sides, she would obsess over whether or not she had truly counted four sides. Therefore, she found it necessary to go around and around a square making sure she had counted four sides and all squares had to be counted.

The woman came early for her appointment, and when she finally entered my office she illustrated the extent of the problem by asking if I knew how many squares were on the thermostat in the waiting area? It occurred to me that the stroke or all the medications she was taking may have compromised her polarity, so I first checked polarity by muscle testing. The patient showed a nonpolarized response: strong/strong. The first treatment offered was a brief energy correction, which did not correct the locked response. Next I tried the collarbone breathing treatment, which also was not successful in weakening the palm-up response. In an attempt to get a weakening of the palm-up response, I decided to diagnose the system disruption. Using the thought directed diagnosis method, when I thought "pericardium," (i.e., the circulation-sex meridian) the muscle weakened for the palm-up position. The patient then treated the middle finger (CS-9) bilaterally, did the integration sequence, and again treated the middle finger bilaterally. She then showed the appropriate strength to palm-down over the scalp and weakness to palm toward the ceiling.

I then asked the patient if she noticed anything. The patient responded, "No." I asked her to describe what she was *not* noticing. The patient responded, "Nothing. The pictures on your wall are just pictures; the ceiling tile is just ceiling tile; books are just books. Everything is as it should be." When her husband was called into the room from the waiting area, she pointed to his glasses and said "See, they're only glasses. I would go around and around his square glasses; now I can see just glasses. I can look at his face and see glasses." No further sessions were necessary for this problem.

Case 11: Chronic Nail Biting

This client, a successful middle-aged business executive, was treated twice for a chronic decades-old nail biting habit in which he bit his nails down to or below the quick. The first time he was treated, the elater protocol had not yet been developed so a standard perturbation EvTFT protocol was used. The second time, eighteen months later, the elater protocol was used. The first treatment unfolded as follows: Starting with a SUD of 10 regarding his disturbance over biting his nails, there was a polarity reversal, an issue-specific PR, a future belief related block, a process-specific PR, and two holons. The SUD level then went down to 0. There was no homework needed. In a follow-up phone session, he reported being symptom free.

The client requested another session eighteen months later. He had been symptom free for over a year when his mother died and he gradually resumed the old nail biting habit after experiencing this loss. This time, the elater protocol was used. The treatment was swift and simple. It is interesting to note that in both instances the initial pattern was the same: a reversal of polarity and an issue-specific PR. A one-year follow-up indicated that the problem did not return.

Case 12: Fear of Heights and Elevators

This case involves a 40-year-old woman who was already in treatment for several months for multiple traumatic experiences. She also suffered physical injuries from the traumatic events, which affected her comfort and her ability to navigate stairways where she worked as a teacher's aide. She specifically reported an inability to use the building elevator because of a longstanding fear of elevators. As I probed for more historical and related information she related that she also experienced intense fear about escalators, heights, and bridges. She had never driven over a bridge in all her years of driving and could only do so as a passenger if she put her head between her knees. She described her fears as extremely distressing, and now they were exacerbating her adjustment difficulty because of her physical injuries. To obtain a baseline measure of her reported distress, I walked her out to the office-building elevator and observed that she was unable to even approach a closed elevator door without obvious panic-like anxiety. She was also unable to look at the ground from my office window, which was only two floors up.

Because of her physical injuries, I used myself as a surrogate to do the diagnosis. The woman, however, did the TAB treatments on herself. Through our discussion we determined that her fear of heights seemed to be the common denominator of her related fears. Accordingly, her fear of heights was the targeted thought field, to which she reported a SUD level of 10. There was no generalized or issue-specific PR. Three meridians were diagnosed and treated with TAB in this first holon. She then reported a SUD level of 8. A process-specific PR was diagnosed and treated, and repeat treatment of the initial holon followed. She then reported a SUD level of 5. Three meridians were then diagnosed and treated in this second holon. A SUD level of 1 was then reported. The ground to sky eye-roll treatment was performed, and the SUD level was now 0. The patient also reported a future performance imagery index rating of 7 (the clearest). Her affect was noticeably different as she excitedly walked over to my office window to look down at the ground. She joyfully exclaimed, "I'm looking at the ground . . . I can see the ground . . ." in tones of surprise and disbelief. She then rode the office-building elevator up and down with excitement and joy.

The following week she reported that she rode the elevator at work, went to the mall with her daughters and took the escalators, and drove over a bridge and back for the first time "without my head between my knees!" A one-year follow-up found that she continued to be free of those life-long phobias.

Case 13: Flashback Trauma: Dissociation/DID

The patient was a 38 year-old woman who was referred with a diagnosis of major depression, chronic pain, and dissociative identity disorder (DID). At the time of this session she had been in therapy with me for nearly four years. The primary life interference was recurrent flashbacks to childhood sexual and psychological abuse, which she recalled came from both of her parents.

There were approximately 30 identified adult, adolescent, and child resources[5] at the time of this case example. Over the previous eight months, however, she had become increasingly aware of probable cult experiences whose memories were most likely influenced by her daughter's age (4 years old), which was the approximate age when she became subject to her described cult experiences.

During the session prior to the one that is being presented, the woman commented, "There's a new somebody inside," and she provided a name and an age. She also reported that two resources already knew about "her." At the next session five days later one of the resources reported that he was trying to keep the woman asleep "because she is having body memories [pain] and she does not know why . . . It feels to her like when she had [her daughter], but it is coming from [the new resource]." It was reported that this new resource had both the memory and the physical experiences of some types of cult trauma. When I asked what brought this resource out at this time I was informed that my patient and her fiancée were discussing how to expand their family. This woman had had a hysterectomy at a very young age and was reportedly feeling "guilty" that she could not have another child. This apparently triggered other associations and memories, which included her experience of "major guilt" about an abortion while in high school and no recall of how she became pregnant. The abortion was described as "therapeutic" and was recommended by her physician because the woman had undergone an x-ray of the hips for a sports injury without knowledge of the pregnancy. This new resource was reported to have memories of "all the deliveries she had to go through . . . and that is what [the patient] is feeling." The new resource was reportedly in severe pain and being kept "in a room" (away from my patient's conscious awareness) by another resource who was looking after her. I was informed that the resource with the memories and severe pain was in no condition to do therapy, but the one looking after her said he would be willing to serve as a surrogate to help her. The EvTFT intervention was then conducted using this helping resource as a surrogate. The entire therapy session lasted nearly ninety minutes, which is atypical when using EvTFT, even with this population.

The targeted thought field was identified as "the experience of labor time and time again." The SUD level was 10. Via muscle testing, permission was requested for the helping resource to be a surrogate, and the distressed resource with the pain and memories consented to allow the other to serve as her surrogate. The hand over head polarity check was normal, and there was no generalized PR. However, the muscle test was strong to the thought field. A deservedness belief related block was diagnosed and was successfully treated under the lip (CV-24). The muscle test was, however, still strong to the thought field. A safety belief related block was then diagnosed and successfully treated under the nose (GV-26). The muscle test was now weak to the thought field, so diagnosis of the identified issue could begin. There was no issue-specific PR. Using the thought directed method of diagnosis, three meridians were diagnosed and immediately treated in this initial holon using bilateral TAB. A SUD level of 5 was then reported.

There was no process-specific PR, but the muscle test was again strong to the thought field. When this occurs there is usually a belief related block, an unknown block, or a change or interference with the thought field. There was no belief related or unknown block. However, when I inquired of the patient what was happening that may have been blocking the completion of the work I was informed that "[the patient] is in the way . . . she wants to get [her daughter] for a dress fitting [for the wedding]." After she was assured that she would be leaving shortly she stepped aside and allowed the therapy to continue with the resources. Since the muscle test was now weak to the thought field, four meridians were diagnosed and treated in this second holon. A SUD level of 2 was then reported. There was no process-specific PR, but once again the muscle test was strong to the thought field. This time a process-specific belief related block for safety was diagnosed and successfully treated (bilaterally) at the side if the hand (SI-3). As is protocol after correcting a process-specific PR, the TxSq → ISq → TxSq was again performed for this second holon. The SUD level was now reported to be 0. The EvTFT intervention was then completed with the ground to sky eye-roll treatment.

Feedback from the surrogate resource was, "It was terrible what happened . . . but it doesn't upset her now . . . She is not in any pain, she's breathing normally, and she's sitting up comfortably now." Upon completion of the work, the two resources readily relinquished their surrogate relationship. In the seven months that have transpired since this treatment there have been no further flashbacks, physical discomfort, or emotional distress regarding the targeted thought field.

Case 14: PTSD with Phantom Digit Pain[6]

This case involves a 28-year-old man, a mechanic, whose right index finger was severed in a truck engine fan belt. An orthopedic surgeon had attempted to save the finger, but nine months later, two-thirds of the finger needed to be amputated. When treatment began, this patient was 11 months post-injury and two months post-surgical amputation. He reported recurrent dreams and flashbacks about how the finger was originally injured, and phantom limb (digit) sensations involving "itching, pins and needles, pain where the edge of the finger nail is [was]. It hurts where there's no finger, there's a feeling of pressure, and [sometimes] it's numb, like asleep." He was unable to return to his usual duties as a mechanic because he kept experiencing flashbacks whenever his hand was anywhere near the fan belts. He harbored unresolved anger at both the person who caused the injury by starting the engine and the orthopedic surgeon who reportedly "told my parents and my fiancée that if I were a concert pianist, he would have sent me for microsurgery."

The patient was seen a total of six sessions. The first two sessions involved information gathering, and the last session was a wrap-up. EvTFT was used during the middle three sessions to address four specific thought fields related to his trauma and complaints. He had no prior knowledge of or exposure to EvTFT.

The first thought field pertained to his memory and flashbacks of seeing his finger fall off. When asked to rate his discomfort on a scale from 0 to 10, he reported 15. There were no body polarity problems and no general or issue-specific PRs. Using the thought directed diagnosis method, the patient then treated five meridian treatment points (treatment sequence or TxSq) using TAB as each meridian was diagnosed. Next came the integration sequence (ISq), followed by a repeat of the TxSq. He was then asked to rate his SUD level, and with a puzzled look he said, "one." The ground to sky eye-roll treatment was then completed, whereupon his SUD level was reported to be 0. When asked to comment he said, "I'm relaxed. I'm not mad. I don't know but I just don't feel upset or mad." Of interest was his observation that somewhere during the treatment all of the "pressure" and phantom digit sensations went away. This was the first time he had been completely free of these discomforts since the initial injury. He also reported that he was no longer angry with the man who started the engine.

The second thought field pertained to his hand being near fan belts. When he attuned to this thought field, he rated his SUD level a 10. There was no issue-specific PR. Diagnosis revealed four meridians requiring treatment (TAB) followed by the ISq and a repeat of the TxSq. The SUD level was now at 2. The patient was not found to have a process-specific PR, and thus another perturbation was diagnosed in a second holon. After a single-point treatment, the SUD level was reported to be 0. The ground to sky eye-roll treatment was then performed.

The third thought field involved an image the patient had of the fan belt taking his hand into the pulley whenever he imagined reaching for a fan belt. Interestingly, this thought field preceded the first thought field in terms of actual accident chronology. He reported a SUD level of 10. There was no issue-specific PR. Diagnosis revealed two meridians requiring treatment. After the ISq and repeat of the TxSq, he was unable to state a SUD level. (An inability to report a SUD level, or a tendency to underestimate a SUD level, is most often seen in trauma cases when elements of dissociation and repression are evident.) The patient was then muscle-tested and a SUD level of 6 was determined. (Muscle testing was used to acquire a nonverbal assessment of his SUD level.) There was no process-specific PR. Diagnosis within a second holon resulted in treatment of four meridians. After the ISq and repeat of the TxSq in the second holon were completed, muscle testing indicated that the SUD level was 3. A third holon was subsequently diagnosed, indicating that perturbations now needed to be treated in four meridians. After the ISq and repeat of the TxSq in this third holon, muscle testing indicated a SUD level of 0 to 1. The ground to sky eye-roll treatment then brought the SUD level to 0. An observation of minimal cues prompted me to check for a belief related block. A safety belief related block was then diagnosed and treated.

Three weeks passed before the next session. During this time the patient claimed to be continually and completely free of phantom digit sensations and of dreams or flashbacks of the accident. As a result of the last session he also reported, "I changed a [fan] belt," but added, "I made sure the keys weren't in the truck at least 10 times, but I did it." Accordingly, the fourth thought field treated pertained to his concern about keys being in the ignition. Diagnosis and treatment of three meridians were then completed, followed by the ISq and repeat of the TxSq. Belief-related blocks related to future and safety issues within this thought field were then diagnosed and treated. Re-treatment of the TxSq → ISq → TxSq in the holon was then completed, followed by a ground to sky eye-roll treatment. A SUD level of 0 was reported; the patient commented, "I feel good, relaxed."

When this patient was seen for follow-up six weeks later, all the therapeutic gains had been sustained: He remained free of flashbacks, dreams, phantom digit sensations, and was working on trucks. He was now aware of the nuisance factor of having a third of a finger that sometimes got in the way, was not always helpful, and got caught on things. He dealt with this in a matter-of-fact fashion, and was planning to consult the surgeon about removing the nonfunctional stub. He had successfully resolved the emotional and physical trauma of the injury, and he was most grateful.

Case 15: Compulsive Eating and Treatment of Elaters[7]

This case regarding the treatment of elaters involves a 36-year-old woman who was being treated for repeated childhood trauma issues. During one session she described her uncontrolled, late-night eating pattern of several years as "grazing." She had been overweight for most of her life and an insulin-dependent diabetic since age 25. She frequently ate dark chocolate and popcorn late at night, which negatively affected her blood sugars and her waistline. She reported that she had been unsuccessful in stopping and was fully aware that the behavior was not healthy for her. When asked why she ate this way, she said, "[because] it tastes good." She reported a SUE level of 9 when attuned to her late-night "grazing." Thought directed diagnosis methods revealed ten meridians in need of treatment; these were treated with TAB at the corresponding treatment sites as each meridian was diagnosed. The ISq treatment and a repeat treatment of the TxSq followed. The SUE level was then reported to be 0. The ground to sky eye-roll treatment was used to complete the EvTFT intervention. Upon completion, she laughed and spontaneously stated, "I'm remembering the heartburn I felt at 4 A.M. this morning," which had been blocked from her memory.

A two year follow-up indicated that the "grazing" had ceased since the day of treatment. Such results have become common when treating the elater component of self-defeating behaviors.

Case 16: Uncomfortable Attraction to Another[8]

This case demonstrating the treatment of elaters involves a 50-year-old salesman, who experienced strong feelings of attraction toward his dental hygienist. Although the patient was no longer married, the hygienist *was* married. This patient was in treatment for an obsessive-compulsive disorder and, not surprisingly, he frequently obsessed about his attraction to the hygienist, which often involved fantasy behaviors he did not want to enact. He had a dental appointment scheduled for the upcoming week and was feeling increasingly uncomfortable. A SUE level of 10 was reported when he was asked to think about his attraction to the hygienist. Using the thought directed diagnostic method and the TAB treatment approach, two holons, each with several elaters, were identified and treated. There were no PRs or belief related blocks. The SUE level was then reported to be 0 and the ground to sky eye-roll treatment was used to finish the EvTFT intervention. When asked about his thinking regarding the hygienist, he stated that his experience of enjoyment (attraction) was no longer perceived as problematic since he "knows" he would never act on it. He additionally commented, "I have no more angst" about the upcoming appointment. Two weeks later the patient reported that he had "no problem" with his appointment with the hygienist. He further stated that there had been no obsessing and that "she's a goodlooking woman, and that was the end of it." In this instance it was evident that treatment of the positive emotion causing his distress enabled him to think, feel, and act in a more comfortable and socially acceptable way.

Case 17: Sport Performance Issues: College

This case example involves a consultation session with a 21-year-old woman who was a standout player on her university's field hockey team. She had been seen twice over the previous four years for sports related issues. This time she wanted assistance with her negative attitude about running for conditioning in her sport, as well as a problem she was having in playing her defensive position.

The first thought field pertained to her issues about running. Specifically, she reported that she would become "real tense" when she ran for conditioning and that she would "get all worked up" about the running.

She had no clear idea about when or why she started feeling this way. When she thought about the running a SUD level of 8 was reported. There were no problems with body polarity. There was no generalized or issue-specific PR about the running. Using thought directed diagnosis, two meridians were identified and immediately treated with TAB. The ISq was performed, followed by a repeat of the TxSq. She now reported a SUD level of 4. She then muscle-tested strong/strong for a process-specific PR, which was successfully corrected at the side of her hand (SI-3). As is protocol after correcting a process-specific PR, she repeated treatment of the holon (TxSq → ISq → TxSq), after which she reported a SUD level of 0. The ground to sky eye-roll was then completed. When asked how she was doing, she said with a smile, "I feel like I want to go running." The future performance imagery index (FPII) rating was reported to be 7 (highest on a 1 to 7 scale) regarding how clearly she could imagine herself running and feeling as comfortable and confident as she did at the session.

The second thought field pertained to her concern about getting beat in her defensive position because she was planting her feet. She verbalized that she needed to keep her feet moving to play her position effectively. As she spoke about the problem she recalled "getting beat" in a prior field hockey game in overtime. When she attuned that memory she reported a SUD level of 6 or 7. There was no issue-specific PR. The thought directed diagnosis method identified four meridians that were treated using TAB. The ISq was then performed followed by a repeat of the TxSq. The patient now reported a SUD level of 3. There was no process-specific PR; however, she muscle-tested strong to the thought field. No future, deservedness, or safety belief related blocks were identified. However, an unknown block was diagnosed and subsequently treated. There was no issue-specific PR regarding the unknown block, and a single meridian was diagnosed and treated regarding this unknown block. The ISq was then performed followed by a repeat of the one meridian for this unknown block. Having cleared the unknown block, the TxSq → ISq → TxSq was repeated for the previously diagnosed holon of this thought field. The woman then reported a SUD level of 0 to the memory of getting beat at her position. The ground to sky eye-roll treatment then completed the EvTFT intervention. When asked if there was any change in her thinking she said, "I think I can change what happens when I play now . . . When I make a mistake I don't have to keep repeating it in my head . . . and my feet can keep moving."

After this session the woman went on to a stellar collegiate career in her sport and earned national recognition. After graduation she has continued to play at the national and international levels, and she has not had a recurrence of these issues.

Case 18: Sport Performance Issues: High School

This case involves a high-school wrestler who acknowledged anxiety about performing at the state championships, which were to begin in about one week. He said he was experiencing a great deal of pressure to win a state championship after failing to do so in the previous three seasons. He was a talented and skilled wrestler, but as a freshman he lost in the finals, and as a sophomore and junior he lost in the semifinal rounds. When he thought about competing in the state tournament he kept remembering his earlier losses, which were distracting and upsetting. Aside from these intruding memories he believed he was ready to wrestle and win the state title. It was discussed how some events can be traumatizing and interfering, which would necessitate resolving his issues related to the events. Like many teenagers, he was guarded and minimally expressive about his feelings. However, with the encouragement of his coach, we agreed to address and resolve the interference from his prior losses to enable him to focus solely on the current year's tournament.

The first thought field pertained to his first loss in a high school match during the final match of the state tournament as a freshman. When attuned to this memory he reported a SUD level of 7. Hand over head polarity was normal, and there was no generalized or issue-specific PR. Using thought directed diagnosis, five meridians were identified and immediately treated using TAB. The ISq was then performed followed by a repeat of the TxSq. He then reported a SUD level of 2. There was no process-specific PR. A second holon was diagnosed involving only the gall bladder meridian, which was treated with TAB. The ISq treatment was then performed, followed by a repeat of the TxSq for this holon. He now reported a SUD level of 0. The ground to sky eye-roll treatment was then performed to complete this treatment intervention. As a young man of few words, he simply stated that he was no longer bothered by the memory.

The second thought field involved his loss in the semifinal round of the state tournament when he was a sophomore. He reported a SUD level of 5 to this memory. As before, there were no difficulties with hand over head polarity, and no generalized or issue-specific PR. Thought directed diagnosis revealed two meridians to be treated in this single holon. The ISq was then performed, followed by a repeat of the TxSq.

He now reported a SUD level of 1 to the memory. Completion of the eye-roll treatment brought the SUD level to 0.

The third and final thought field pertained to the loss he suffered the previous year as a junior in the semifinal round. To this memory he reported a SUD level rating of 8. Again, there were no problems regarding body polarity, and no generalized or issue-specific PR. Using thought directed diagnosis, two meridians were identified and treated with TAB as they were diagnosed. The ISq was then performed, followed by a repeat of the TxSq. The patient then reported a SUD level of 3. There was no process-specific PR. Another holon was diagnosed involving a single meridian, which was treated by TAB. The ISq was then performed followed by a repeat of the TxSq for this holon. He now reported a SUD level of 0. As in each of the preceding thought fields, all SUD level reports of 0 were confirmed by a muscle test. The eye-roll treatment completed the EvTFT intervention.

The young man now denied experiencing any upset about any of the prior matches he had lost. He also reported that he could now focus more clearly on the upcoming tournament. Using the future performance imagery index, he reported his ability to clearly imagine himself performing in the state tournament to the best of his ability as a 7 (highest on the 1 to 7 point scale). This talented wrestler then went on to win the state title, and in doing so defeated a returning state champion in the finals.

Case 19: Foul Smells and Gagging

This case example involves a single treatment session with a first-year medical student who, like many medical students, had concerns about tolerating the foul smells in anatomy lab. Although she was psychologically handling the strong odor of formaldehyde and the stench coming from the cadavers, she found that the smells could trigger the gagging reflex and all that could follow. She reported spending about 10 hours per week in the lab. The lab had been four weeks in progress with 12 more weeks to go.

The first thought field pertained to what she described as "the rotting body smell." When she recalled this smell, she reported a SUD level rating of 6. The hand over head polarity check was found to be nonpolarized; she tested strong to all statements and tests. She was in lab the day before and exposed to formaldehyde, which may account for the disruption in polarity (see Rochlitz, 1997). She then performed the neurologic organizing treatment, which restored proper polarity when retested. There was no generalized or issue-specific PR. Using thought directed diagnosis, the stomach meridian was diagnosed as the single meridian in this holon and it was immediately treated using TAB. The ISq was then performed followed by a repeat of the TxSq. She now reported a SUD level of 3. There was no process-specific PR. A second holon was then diagnosed involving the kidney meridian and the governing vessel, which were also treated using TAB. The ISq was then performed followed by a repeat of the TxSq for this holon. She now reported a SUD level of 0. The eye-roll treatment then completed this treatment intervention.

The future performance imagery index was then used to assess how clearly she could imagine herself tolerating the rotting body smell without distress. She reported a rating of 6 on the 1 to 7 point scale. Since the goal was to enable the patient to imagine herself in the future with a rating of 7, she performed the treatment steps involved in this procedure to improve her clarity. Specifically, she was directed to touch under her arm (SP-21) and take three respirations, more if she wanted, while imagining herself in the lab and tolerating the rotting body smell. She then repeated this procedure while touching at her inner eye (BL-1). The ISq was then performed, followed by a repeat treatment under the opposite arm and then the opposite inner eye. She now reported a rating of 6.5. When asked if she knew what the source of interference might be she said, "I'm not one hundred percent convinced about not gagging."

The concern about gagging in the presence of the obnoxious lab smells became the second thought field. She did not evidence an issue-specific PR to this thought field. Using thought directed diagnosis, the stomach meridian was identified as the only meridian in this holon and it was therefore treated using TAB. The ISq was then performed, followed by a repeat of the TxSq. There was no process-specific PR, and she again tested weak to the gagging related thought field. The spleen meridian was then diagnosed and treated as the single meridian in this second holon. The ISq was then performed, followed by a repeat treatment of the spleen meridian. There was no process-specific PR, and she now tested strong to the thought field and was without distress. No belief related blocks or a recurrent PR were evident. The eye-roll treatment completed this segment of the EvTFT intervention. She then re-rated her clarity in imagining herself in lab a 7 while tolerating the smells and feeling comfortable in her throat.

Over the remaining 12 weeks of lab that followed treatment, she reported only one instance of a minor gag response. Aside from that one occasion, the rotting body smells were more comfortably tolerated, and the gag reflex became a non-issue.

Case 20: Treating Negative Beliefs in a Cluster

This case example involves a 58-year-old man who had been in treatment for nearly 18 months for personal and relationship issues. He was already familiar with EvTFT because this approach had been frequently used to facilitate the substantial changes and progress he had experienced in many areas of his life during the prior months of treatment. This therapy excerpt pertains to an area underlying his characterological issues that was seemingly connected to the many discouraging comments he recalls his mother having directed to him throughout his lifetime. He stated that the discouraging comments blocked him from realizing his potential in many areas of his life because the comments endlessly "ring" through his head. At the close of the session in which these issues were introduced, he was asked to list three to five of the most discouraging comments and to bring the list with him to the next session.

At the next session he provided his list of five haunting statements: (1) You can't do that because . . . ; (2) We can't afford for you to go to college; (3) Why can't you be like your sister?; (4) You always start things and never finish them; and (5) Don't do (this or that). The patient then reported a SUD level rating of 9 for each of the first four statements, and 10 for the last statement. I then asked the patient to cluster the five comments together and to imagine placing them into a container of his choosing.[9] The thought field then became "the container," without the need for him to focus on any particular comment (now clustered within the container). In this way all five thought fields were being addressed simultaneously. No SUD level rating was required for this modified thought field because diagnosis progressed solely according to the response of the muscle testing while following the EvTFT protocol.

The patient showed the desired polarized responses when muscle-tested, and there was no evidence of a generalized or issue-specific PR regarding "these problems."[10] Thought directed diagnosis identified four meridians involved in the first holon, which were treated with TAB. The ISq was then performed followed by a repeat of the TxSq. There was no process-specific PR and the patient again muscle-tested weak to the thought field. A second holon involving three meridians was diagnosed and treated. The ISq was then performed, followed by a repeat of the TxSq for this holon. There was no process-specific PR, and now he muscle-tested strong to the thought field. No belief related blocks or a recurrent PR were evident. The eye-roll treatment then completed this EvTFT intervention. I then asked the patient to remove the five comments from the container and to rerate the SUD level for each. The SUD level for each comment was reported to be 0.

At the following session the man stated, "For the first time in a lot of years I feel good . . . and excited about things . . . a whole new positive outlook on things . . . I don't feel like I'm just getting through the day, or life now." He attributed these changes to being free of the limiting beliefs. He also reported that he had made arrangements to finish the necessary course work for his doctoral degree, as well as plans to follow through with his desire to become a deacon in his church. A one-month follow-up revealed that he was still making progress toward achieving his goals and was feeling much freer and happy with life.

Case 21: Ethnic Prejudice

This case example involves a 35-year-old woman who was in psychotherapy for panic attacks and childhood sexual abuse. She was employed as a sales representative in a department store and had contact with a large number of customers. During the course of a session she began discussing her thoughts and feelings about prejudice regarding Mexican and Puerto Rican customers. She stated that she did not like them to come to her counter and that she would become instantly "angry and irritated" when they did. She further reported that she did not like "how they act," and that she had the same feelings about both men and women. The patient said she had no idea why she felt this way, and she initially stated that she was unaware of any traumatic experiences with people of these nationalities. Within minutes of her reporting this, however, she recalled an incident while babysitting at age 15 when the father of the children, "who was one of them," tried to get into the bed with her. She said nothing happened because she immediately left the bed and the house without another word ever being said. She denied any emotional upset regarding that isolated incident.

Upon further exploration the patient said she was not aware of having prejudice toward any other race or nationality, however her husband had told her that she also showed prejudice toward Koreans and people from India. She did, however, acknowledge that she had dislike for these groups. I stated that EvTFT might be helpful in addressing her feelings of prejudice[11] if she wanted to do so. Since she encountered people of these nationalities regularly on her job, she agreed to try it. A SUD level rating of 10 was attributed to her thought field regarding Mexicans and Puerto Ricans, and a 7 to each thought field involving Indians and Koreans.

The first thought field to be treated was the one involving the Mexicans and Puerto Ricans because it evoked the highest SUD rating, and because it was the most pronounced in her experience.[12] There was no problem with body polarity and there was no generalized PR. However, an issue-specific PR was diagnosed and successfully treated at the side of the hand (SI-3). Contact directed diagnosis-patient was used to identify three meridians, which were treated. The SUD level was then reported to be 9. Diagnosis of the second holon revealed two meridians to be treated. The patient reported no change in SUD level after this treatment. A test for neurologic disorganization indicated that the collarbone breathing treatment was needed. However, because the session time had expired, the patient was quickly guided through the collarbone breathing treatment and asked to repeat of the last holon after the session.

At the next session the woman reported that she had not noticed any Mexican or Puerto Rican customers in the store since the last session, although she said she would ordinarily notice them. She did, however, notice an Indian man whom she waited on "all the time." When I inquired about a SUD level for the Mexican and Puerto Rican thought field she stated it was "zero" with a puzzled look on her face. When I asked her to assess her level of upset regarding Indians she stated a SUD level of 4. An issue-specific PR was evident with this thought field; it failed to correct at the side of the hand (SI-3), but it did successfully correct at the neurolymphatic reflex area. Diagnosis yielded three meridians which were treated. The SUD level was then reported to be 3. There was no process-specific PR. Two meridians were then diagnosed and treated in this second holon.

At this point the woman said she "didn't know" her SUD level, but she muscle-tested to a SUD level of 2. There was no process-specific PR, and once again she muscle-tested weak to the thought field. Two meridians were then diagnosed and treated in this third holon. The muscle-tested SUD was then rated at 1. Because the eye-roll treatment did not reduce the SUD level to 0, a fourth holon involving a single meridian was diagnosed and treated, which reduced the muscle-tested SUD level to 0. The eye-roll treatment was then performed to complete the intervention. At this point the patient reported a SUD level of 0 for every thought field pertaining to Mexicans, Puerto Ricans, Indians, and Koreans, which came as a surprise to her. Follow-up inquires regarding her experience of prejudice at three months and nine months indicated that she had "no problems."[13]

Case 22: The Parent of a Son with ADHD

The number of children diagnosed with attention deficit hyperactivity disorder (ADHD) has been steadily increasing, and most of the care and treatment emphasis is directed toward the afflicted child. Parents, however, are also affected by their children's behaviors, which can be exasperating. This session example involves a 42 year-old mother whose 12-year-old son was diagnosed with ADHD. Like many parents of ADHD children, she followed all of her physician's recommendations, including medicating her son, which was reported to be helpful. However there were many times when the medication wore off or did not control the boy's impulsive and oppositional activities. She was frustrated and intermittently negative about her son, and also upset with herself for thinking and feeling that way. I offered to use EvTFT as a way to assist her, and she accepted.

The targeted thought field was the woman's son and his behavior. When she attuned to this thought field she reported a SUD level rating of 10. Her hand over head polarity check was fine and there was no generalized PR. However, there was an issue-specific PR that was diagnosed and successfully treated at the side of the hand (SI-3). Using thought directed diagnosis, three meridians were identified and treated with TAB. The ISq was then performed followed by a repeat of the TxSq. The SUD level was then 4. There was no process-specific PR. Diagnosis revealed only the spleen meridian needed treatment in this second holon, followed by ISq and a repeat of the TxSq. She then reported a SUD level of 0. However, upon checking, the muscle-tested SUD level was "greater then 0." When queried, she said there was a slight "something," but very low. The eye-roll treatment did not reduce the muscle-tested SUD level. However, she muscle-tested weak again to the thought field, and a third holon was diagnosed with the gall bladder meridian in need of treatment. After completion of the ISq and repeat treatment of the gall bladder meridian, she stated that she felt "calmer." The muscle-tested SUD level was now 0, and the eye-roll treatment was performed. When I asked if there was any change in her thinking she said, "I can laugh at him now," which she was unable to do previously.

Because being with her son was an ongoing activity, I then used the Future Performance Imagery Index (FPII) to assess her perception in the future. I asked her to rate (on a 1 to 7 scale) how clearly she could imagine herself with him (and he acting as he does) and feeling as comfortable as she does now. She reported an FPII rating of 7, the highest level. Therefore, no further interventions were engaged. The next time I saw her she said, "It's great. You gave my son back to me . . . When he started his stuff . . . I was able to roll with it, and laugh, . . . and I even had a rubber band fight with him (laughing)." A two-month follow-up indicated that she was continuing to deal more effectively and lovingly with her son. She also muscle-tested strong to the treated thought field, which suggests the continued absence of perturbations.

Case 23: Complex PTSD with Dissociative Disorder Not Otherwise Specified

This case involves a 38-year old woman from a fundamentalist religious background who had a history of ongoing childhood sexual abuse. Her presenting problems included debilitating flashbacks, suicidal ideation, body memories, constant episodes of dissociation, deep fears of abandonment, and sleep disturbance. She lived in a continual state of terror as she went back and forth between dissociative memories, switching into dissociated ego states when triggered by internal or external cues. Three years previously, she had recalled being a victim of incest over a period of more than ten years, making her childhood and adolescent home "a house of horror." Following the initial recall, she entered into traditional psychotherapy, which yielded some relief, especially in the attachment area of her pathology. She was also heavily medicated with antidepressants, antipsychotics, tranquillizers, and mood stabilizers. However, the therapy and medication were not enough to stave off the constant onslaught of flashbacks and other symptoms. An intelligent, well-read woman, she had read about thought field therapy among other newer treatments for trauma, and felt that it might help her.

As is necessary with survivors of abuse, the treatment is first concerned with stabilization and safety. Among the first stabilizing techniques she was taught was simplified collarbone breathing. This helped to "ground" her by lowering her anxiety level. She was also taught the neurologic organizing treatment procedures and several other grounding techniques, all of which she incorporated into her daily life with some success. Although EvTFT treatment with trauma progresses rapidly, it needs to be titrated in accordance with the pace set by the patient.

The EvTFT work, which went on for over two years of weekly sessions, centered on the scores of triggers and flashbacks that made the woman's everyday life unbearable. There were a myriad of objects, odors, sounds, emotions, events, sights, and bodily sensations that would put her into states of terror and dissociation. During the first several months of treatment, most treatment sequences included reversed polarity on the hand over head check and generalized and issue-specific PRs. The PRs were always cleared at the neurolymphatic reflex area site for this patient. The reversed polarity was usually corrected with simplified collarbone breathing. As the treatment progressed, there were fewer incidences of generalized PR and since she incorporated simplified collarbone breathing into her everyday routine, her hand over head polarity check was reversed only occasionally. Sometimes the work would center on abandonment issues because her husband was often required to go on business trips and this was disturbing for her. However, she was far less disturbed by these trips as time went by. As with most survivors, issues of shame and guilt were also present. These were also diagnosed and ameliorated using EvTFT.

Almost all of the EvTFT therapy was done using the thought directed diagnosis method. However, there were times when the woman was experiencing too much terror to be muscle-tested. At these times, I would rely upon previous treatment patterns or the trauma algorithm. After two or three repetitions of a prior pattern or algorithm, the SUD level would be reduced enough so that she could be muscle-tested and proceed with the EvTFT diagnosis, which would always result in a SUD level of 0.

It was remarkably apparent from this patient's affect and facial expressions when she was being influenced by a child ego state. As the SUD levels dropped, she reported that her ability to self soothe was operant. Often, she would experience the physical sense of energy leaving her body, "whooshing out" through her feet. When this happened, there was a clear difference in her physical demeanor and her subjective sense of reality from one minute to the next. As soon as she said, "it's gone," her face would become composed and peaceful, and she would assert that she was no longer disturbed by a thought field that minutes ago had proved painful and debilitating.

Once the triggers and events that would precipitate dissociative states and suicidal ideation were diagnosed, treated, and resolved using EvTFT, they showed no evidence of returning. Many aspects of this woman's life that were stolen from her were restored in these treatment sessions.

Case 24: Emergency Treatment Using Algorithms

A serious event occurred in my practice one day when a young woman was brought in by her parents, who requested an emergency visit. The parents had received a phone call from their daughter's roommate (in another city) and were informed that their usually very healthy daughter had become nearly catatonic. No one knew what had happened to put her in such a state, and it was requested that they come get their daughter immediately. The parents sought help in that city's hospital emergency room and were advised to hospitalize her. Being reluctant to do this so far from home, they brought her home to New Jersey, where she was seen by a psychiatrist in a local hospital emergency room, who also advised hospitalization. The emergency room social worker knew about EvTFT and suggested that they see a practitioner before hospitalizing her, and accordingly the patient was lead to me.

The patient arrived with her parents at the office. She appeared to be frozen in a state of terror. I attempted to communicate with her but the patient was unable to speak; she could however follow directions and was compliant. After having made the office space as safe as possible, I explained the procedures that would be used. The woman was first led through the brief energy correction and then prompted to do the corrections for a generalized PR and for an issue-specific PR while I said the affirmations for her. She then was led through the extended trauma algorithm (ie, e, a, c, lf, c, if, c → ISq → TxSq). This clearly yielded some relief because color began to return to her face and she was visibly more relaxed. She repeated the trauma algorithm three more times until it seemed that she had reached a plateau, but she seemed a good deal better. After a half-hour the patient uttered her first words since her roommate had found her: "I was raped." When asked if she felt strong enough to do further work on the trauma at that time, she shook her head indicating "no," but said, "Later, now I need to go home." The patient wanted to go back to the city where she lived and was referred to a trauma specialist there. As she stood up, she almost smiled and she said, "Thank you." These were all the words she spoke in the session. In a follow-up call, the parents said that she was not hospitalized and was proceeding with psychotherapeutic treatment for the trauma.

Case 25: Expanding the Energy Psychology Paradigm: Successful Treatment of Enuresis "at a Distance"[14]

This brief review describes a case study of an 11-year-old boy who had been enuretic on a nightly basis since the age of five. According to the boy's mother, the onset followed a beating by the boy's father. Apparently, the son awakened the father when he got up to use the toilet, and was subsequently beaten. Nightly bed-wetting had resulted over the ensuing six years despite several attempts by professionals to resolve the problematic occurrences. The father and mother had been divorced for the past two and a half years. The son and his sister, and two half-sisters, lived with the mother. The father had no contact with his children since the divorce.

The boy's mother was in therapy with me and, thereby, was familiar with the therapeutic effects derived with EvTFT methods. The son was in treatment with another psychologist who practiced more traditional psychodynamic therapy. During one of her therapy sessions, the mother began sharing her concerns about her son's ongoing problem and asked if I could help him. Mindful that the son already had a therapist, I did not want to disrupt the therapeutic relationship that had been established between them. Nevertheless, the mother's concern and frustration about her son's reported anguish and shame around the bed-wetting could not be ignored. I offered to try an EvTFT intervention using the mother as a surrogate for her son, which would not require the boy to be present in my office and thereby possibly disturbing the rapport he had with his own therapist. The mother spoke with the son's therapist about her intention to consult with her own therapist about her son's bed-wetting and the therapist voiced no objection. She also spoke with her son about talking with her therapist about his problem, giving no further specifics about her intention. The boy did not ask for any details nor did she offer any.

Muscle-testing procedures verified that mother was willing to serve as her son's surrogate and that the son gave permission for his mother to serve as his surrogate. While this may appear to be a "leap of energetic faith," the important part is that permission to proceed was acquired at the nonverbal energetic level. Treatment efforts would have immediately ceased if either party denied permission as assessed via muscle testing. In like fashion, confirmation to release each other in the surrogate role was verified when treatment was completed.

The first thought field the mother attuned was the beating her son experienced at age five when he went to the toilet and awakened his father. There was no generalized PR or issue-specific PR. While the mother thought about the beating incident thought directed diagnosis revealed perturbations in two meridians, which were immediately treated with TAB. The ISq was then performed, followed by a repeat of the TxSq. The muscle response assessing a process-specific PR was strong/strong, but attempted treatment to correct this block was unsuccessful at the two usual treatment sites (side of hand and neurolymphatic reflex area). Another hand over head polarity check indicated a strong/strong nonpolarized condition, which was restored with the neurologic organizing treatment after the brief energy correction failed to restore her polarity. A recheck for a process-specific PR, however, was again strong/strong, and this time I diagnosed two meridians in need of treatment to clear it. After the process-specific PR was cleared, retreatment of the TxSq → ISq → TxSq followed, per protocol. The mother then muscle-tested weak to the thought field, and a second holon was diagnosed and treated involving just the heart meridian. The ISq was then performed, followed by a repeat of the heart meridian. There was no process-specific PR. A third holon was diagnosed and treated with the governing vessel (GV-26). The ISq was then performed, followed by a repeat treatment at GV-26. Muscle tests then showed that the mother held strong to the thought field and that there was no process-specific PR, belief related blocks, unknown blocks, or a recurrent PR. The woman's hand over head polarity check was normal and she muscle-tested strong to a SUD level of 0.

At the following session the mother reported that there was no change in her son's problem. At this point, I wondered if there were additional issues that needed to be addressed or if this form of surrogate work simply did not work. In addition, it is interesting to note that the mother never said a word to her son about the surrogate work she had done.

Three weeks after the initial treatment of the thought field related to the beating, another attempt was made using mother as the surrogate. This time the targeted thought field was the bed-wetting problem directly. Permission was again obtained, and there was no generalized or issue-specific PR. Again, using thought directed diagnosis while the mother thought about the bed-wetting, four meridians were diagnosed requiring treatment. The ISq was then performed followed by a repeat of this TxSq. There was no process-specific PR. Three meridians were then diagnosed and treated in this second holon. The ISq was then performed, followed by a repeat of the TxSq for this holon. There was no process-specific PR at this point and, the mother again muscle-tested weak to the thought field. A third holon was diagnosed and treated involving the gall bladder and spleen meridians. The ISq was then performed followed by a repeat treatment of these two meridians. A process-specific PR was diagnosed and successfully treated at the side of the hand (SI-3) followed by a repeat of the TxSq → ISq → TxSq for the third holon. The mother then muscle-tested strong to the thought field. A deservedness belief related block was diagnosed and successfully treated using the central vessel (CV-24). After a repeat of TxSq → ISq → TxSq, the mother muscle-tested weak again to the thought field. A fourth holon was diagnosed and treated that involved only the stomach meridian. The ISq was then performed, followed by a repeat treatment at ST-1. There was no process-specific PR and the mother tested strong to the thought field. There were no other belief related or unknown blocks. The eye-roll treatment then completed the work on this thought field. Upon completion, the mother described a "spacey" feeling, along with an increase of energy, tingling in her hands and feet, cognitive clarity, and a lack of inhibition. I therefore had the mother complete the neurologic organizer treatment to stabilize and ground her. Upon performing this procedure, the mother's reported sensations subsided.

The following week the mother reported that her son wet himself on two days when he fell asleep on the couch. However, he did not wet in the bed. During the other five days, he was reported to be completely dry in bed and on the couch. The mother said that her son had never been dry for five days in a row before. A third thought field was identified and treated, which pertained to any remaining problems connected to wetting or staying dry in any situation or location. Permission was again obtained, and thought directed diagnosis and treatment was completed while the mother was attuned to this thought field. Assessment of an issue-specific PR yielded a strong/strong response, which was successfully corrected at the neurolymphatic reflex area after it failed to correct at the side of the hand (SI-3). Muscle testing of individual meridian alarm points revealed that only the gall bladder meridian required treatment in this holon. The ISq was then performed, followed by a repeat treatment of the gall bladder meridian. There was no process-specific PR and the mother muscle-tested weak to the thought field. A second holon was then diagnosed involving the stomach meridian, which was treated with TAB. The ISq was then performed followed by a repeat treatment of the stomach meridian. Muscle testing was then strong/strong for a process-specific PR, which was successfully corrected at the side of the hand (SI-3). After correction, a repeat of TxSq → ISq → TxSq for this holon was completed. The mother then muscle-tested strong to the thought field and did not evidence belief related or unknown blocks or a recurrent PR. The eye-roll treatment then finished the EvTFT intervention. Upon completion of treatment, the mother stated "I feel a release of independence for my son."

At the next session the mother reported that her son had been dry for 12 continuous days. At the time of this writing, 16 months had elapsed post-treatment, and the boy had maintained a dry bed for nearly 12 months before he had another problem. (The occasional "accidents" were described to be stress related, and never lasted for more than a few days.) As might be expected, the mother observed that her son became more cheerful in the morning and was seemingly gaining self-confidence. I find it intriguing that the mother never spoke to her son about the surrogate work she did for him regarding his problem, and her son never spoke to her about the sudden elimination of his problem.

Perhaps the cessation of the bed-wetting problem, which directly followed the surrogate treatments, was entirely coincidental. However, the fact that a six-year problem that had not responded to other interventions progressively abated suggests that the surrogate treatments may have been instrumental. If so, this outcome is very challenging to explain. It was a single-blind situation; the boy did not know a new form of treatment had been introduced. Current hypotheses about the mechanisms that are involved in the use of EvTFT specifically, and energy psychology methods in general, do not adequately explain such results from an "at a distance" surrogate treatment model. Although Chapter 15 offers a conceptual frame that successful outcomes using meridian-based psychotherapy result from attainment of frequency resonance coherence between and among meridians as they resonate with the thought field, an expanded paradigm is clearly needed to account for the intriguing type of outcome described in this case study and, incidentally, also reported with some frequency by other practitioners of EvTFT and other energy-based psychotherapy methods.

Chapter 15

UNDERSTANDING THE EFFECTIVENESS OF EvTFT[1]

Whether inner or outer self, wave superposition
forms all. And, collectively, although appearing
separate, we are not. Our wave constituents flow
and ebb, join, flicker, disperse and reunite.
Patches of order form, radiant power densities
escalate and incandescence flowers. First in
one and next in all—then we are one!

—William A. Tiller,
Science and Human Transformation

This chapter will expand the hypothetical underpinnings of why and
how Evolving Thought Field Therapy (EvTFT) and other meridian-based psychotherapeutic methods achieve their rapid and robust
effects. The concept of *frequency resonance coherence* (FRC) will be presented as a possible explanation, and meridian activity and the function
of chi will be elaborated. We will also address the controversial issue of
treatment sequence in algorithm and diagnostic approaches using the
FRC metaphor to describe the process and explain the results. Further
extensions of FRC will be presented using hypothetical models of dynamical energy systems to better comprehend the far-reaching scope of
our synergistic mind-body-energy relationship. Lastly, this chapter will
explore the interface of EvTFT with consciousness and spirit and illustrate how thought fields serve as a bridge to the vast resources of a
timeless unconscious.

HYPOTHESIS MUST
PRECEDE THEORY

The field of energy psychology is in its infancy and answers to why and
how meridian-based thought field therapies work continue to be sought
by both current users and their critics. Theory development would appear to be the reasonable next step toward understanding the effective-

ness of EvTFT and other meridian-based psychotherapies. However, we are most likely decades away from any unifying theory. *Webster's* (1966) defines *theory* as "originally, a mental viewing" or "contemplation" about the way to do something or about how something works. The definition also incorporates "a formulation of apparent relationships or underlying principles of certain observed phenomena *which has been verified to some degree*" (italics added). It is this later aspect of verification that distinguishes theory from hypothesis. Accordingly, *theory* "implies considerable evidence in support of a formulated general principle explaining the operation of certain phenomena." In contrast, *hypothesis* "implies an inadequacy of evidence in support of an explanation that is tentatively inferred, often as a basis for further experimentation."

All too frequently it seems that the terms *theory* and *hypothesis* are used interchangeably. Perhaps in our case, regarding the exploration of energy psychology and thought field therapies specifically, we have used the term *theory* prematurely to describe or conjecture about what is happening. Despite the use of the term *theory* as found in the available writings, publications, and presentations on meridian-based psychotherapy, it appears that we are most likely at the hypothesis stage of development in our fledgling discipline. We are very much in need of "considerable evidence" before the term *theory* can be used appropriately. The terms *model, model building* or even *metaphors* are more fitting as we endeavor to formulate hypotheses, construct preliminary representations, and develop insights about the nature and mechanisms of meridian-based psychotherapy and EvTFT.

This chapter contains no absolutes. However, we do offer speculation based on available information and clinical experience. It is our hope and intention that the hypothesis development, metaphors, and model building presented in this chapter will serve to inspire other interested professionals to think more deeply and differently about the phenomena of why and how meridian-based psychotherapies operate. Additionally, we hope that the presented ideas will excite therapists to experimentally test and expand the presented material and work toward securing the much-needed "considerable evidence."

THE ISSUE
OF TREATMENT SEQUENCE

The issue regarding the sequential order in which meridian acupoints are treated remains a controversial and often debated topic. Is the sequence of treatment points obtained via individual diagnosis truly indicative of a precise natural code, as Callahan posits, or simply an artifact of the linear nature of the diagnostic process? If the nature's code hypothesis were the only true answer, then why and how does Gary Craig's sequence-less emotional freedom technique work? Why can different but effective treatment sequences be diagnosed for the same person by the same or different therapists? In addition, what effect does the therapist have on the patient's energy system by his or her mere physical presence and intention?

Callahan teaches that the muscle-test response of a patient will be different (strong/strong) when the therapist is psychologically reversed, indicating that the energy of the therapist is reflected in the patient. A similar phenomenon has also been observed when the patient and therapist share the same issue of treatment.[2] Research at the Institute of HeartMath in Boulder Creek, California, has provided quantifiable data that "when we touch someone else, an exchange of electromagnetic energy—from heart to brain—takes place" (Childre, Martin, & Beech, 1999, p. 160), which also occurs when people just stand close together. But why and how does the neutralization or elimination of problematic emotions occur, and why does it occur so quickly? We speculate that the answers lie in how meridian activity changes as a result of treatment and therapist influence.

FREQUENCY RESONANCE COHERENCE

It has been postulated (Gerber, 1988; Tiller, 1997) that human beings are made up of a complex network of interwoven energy fields that operate within and around the body. The acupuncture meridian system is but one aspect of this complex array, which has interactive influence via subtle energetic forces. The energetic influence of the meridians has been explored by creative Western minds from physicists to medical pioneers with the aid of advanced technology. Nevertheless, our knowledge about meridians and subtle energy is limited to the available technology and the prevailing theoretical constructs. In an effort to discuss what happens during diagnosis and treatment with EvTFT and other meridian-based psychotherapies, the creative concepts presented here will be couched using familiar terminology.

Diepold (2002) hypothesized that successful treatment using meridian-based psychotherapies results from attainment of *frequency resonance coherence* (FRC) between and among the meridians as they resonate with the attuned thought field. When there is emotional upset resulting from perturbations[3] in the thought field, there is a disruption in frequency resonance coherence. A bodily experience of distress often accompanies unpleasant emotions or feelings precisely because of the resulting *inco*herence. When elaters are driving unwanted behavior, there is additional resonant discord between the feeling state and the behavioral state. The following explanatory metaphor is offered.

For the non-physicist, an operational definition of terms and some background information would be helpful. Since EvTFT falls under the broad umbrella of energy psychology, let's begin with energy. *Energy* is defined in physics as simply the ability to do work. The forms of energy include heat, chemical energy, and mass, with light, sound, and electricity serving as forms of energy transmission (although they each have intrinsic energy contents of their own). Quantum theory holds that energy is emitted and absorbed in a micro-bundle called a *quantum*. These quanta reportedly behave like particles of matter under some conditions and like waveforms under others. The term *wavicle* has been proposed by some to convey this duality: electrons and photons are neither waves nor particles, per se, because of their rapid ability to respond to a condition in either form. A further extension of quantum theory, referred to as *quantum field theory*, deals with the interactions between particles that produce electromagnetic forces from the exchange of photons. A wave of electromagnetic energy results from the transfer of electrical energy via vibration or oscillatory movement.

Frequency, in classical physics, refers to the number of oscillations, or vibrations, in cycles per second or cycles per centimeter. The energy of a wave is proportional to the square of the amplitude of the wave. A wavelength is the distance the energy travels, at the speed of the wave, during one full oscillation. For example, when the frequency is higher, the wavelength is shorter, and vice versa. *Resonance* refers to the natural vibratory reinforcement that occurs in a body (or energy system) when it is exposed to a vibration of about the same frequency from another body (or energy system). The result is an enhanced absorption and emission of energy involving simultaneous adjustments in the two systems. Resonance is a form of synchronized dynamic interaction (Schwartz & Russek, 1997). *Coherence* is the quality of harmonious cohesion and integration. In physics, waves are considered coherent when they have the same frequency and phase or when they have a fixed ratio of frequencies and the same phase. *Incoherence* would indicate a lack of correlation between, or synchronization of, wave phases. In other words, being and feeling "out of sync" is exemplary of incoherence.

The electrical resistance of the 12 bilateral pairs of organ-specific meridians used in EvTFT has a direct and measurable relationship to the status of their corresponding internal organs (Voll, 1978). A single unilateral meridian is energetically connected to its twin and simultaneously connected to all of the other meridian pairs, forming an interconnected and synergistic vibratory loop of the 12 meridians along with the governing and conception vessels. Stimulation of the peripheral acupoints affects brain activity (Diepold & Goldstein, 2000; Dubrov & Pushkin, 1982), and can restore health, or improve performance on tasks (Tiller, 1997).

It can be reasoned that EvTFT serves as an info-energy modifying treatment, impacting the interface of mind and body through attainment of frequency resonance coherence. As a result of attaining the state of FRC, the attuned thought field is "shifted" in its essence and not merely balanced or re-balanced. The dynamical interactions between and among the meridians with the attuned thought field during EvTFT result in *field-shifting*. By this we mean the intrinsic make-up of the thought field is shifted, usually permanently, because of a resulting FRC due to the elimination of interference previously stirred by perturbations and elaters, which is reflected in meridian activity. Because of their apparent reciprocal relationship, meridians ultimately respond in the service of the thought field and the thought field responds in kind to meridian activity.

Perhaps acupuncture meridians entrain to thought fields in a manner similar to how the brain entrains to the heart.[4] Research at the Institute of HeartMath concludes that the heart produces the most powerful electromagnetic field of any organ in our body; it is nearly "five thousand times greater in strength than the field produced by the brain" (Childre & Martin, 1999, p. 33). Although there is shared information and communication between the heart and brain via nerve impulses, hormones, neurotransmitters, biophysical pressure waves, and electromagnetic field interactions, the heart is the major player. That is not to say that the brain and all its ability to facilitate thought, memory, imagery, calculation, deduction, and so on in its linear and logical manner is diminished in any way. However, by comparison, the heart's feeling-related character is associated with love, intuition, caring, understanding, compassion, and so on, which seem to operate less linearly, and therefore provide broader input for the brain to analyze, recognize, sort, compartmentalize, and transform the input from the sensory network and convert it into perception, cognition, and emotions.

Intentionally using brain activities (e.g., thinking, imagining, remembering) can bring about profound changes in heart functioning, both positive and negative. Again, the HeartMath researchers have found that focusing attention on our hearts or heart issues increases the synchronization between heart and brain. The change in heart information is then fed back to the brain so loudly via the electromagnetic output of the heart that the whole body (and others) can "hear" and respond, as we appear to literally broadcast (and receive) emotional information. In fact, measurements of the heart's electromagnetic field have been detected between eight and ten feet away from the body (Childre & Martin, 1999).

The described inner teamwork of the heart/brain connection may be analogous to the hypothesized relationship between thought fields and meridians and serve as a model. If meridians have a responsive and reciprocal relationship to thought fields (i.e., meridians entrain to the thought field), then treatment of the meridians will result in changes or shifts in the thought field to which the meridians will entrain. The ensuing entrainment to the "shifted" thought field may be contributory to the quick and lasting results that often accompany EvTFT.

The frequency resonance coherence metaphor is based on the assumption that meridians have a frequency range, and that each meridian has its own signature frequency that resonates with the others. Recall in Chapter 3 (about the acupuncture meridians) that Woollerton and McLean (1979) posited that yang is analogous to high frequency waves and yin to lower frequency waves. Since the degree or amount of yin and yang are never absolute, the stage is set for a huge number of high and low frequency combinations that could exist between the meridians and vessels. Accordingly, the amount and type of information received, transmitted, and processed by the meridians and vessels would be enormous.

The 12 bilateral meridians are often described as separate yet they are connected by various divergent meridians and radiant circuits, and they thus share a synergistic relationship among each other and the governing and conception vessels. When there is ample flow of healthy chi, the meridians operate in a coherent manner and provide for optimal physical and emotional well-being. When the chi influence is disrupted and unhealthy, there is illness or emotional distress because the meridians become incoherent and are unable to optimally use the information carried by the chi. Successful EvTFT hypothetically affects chi in a two-fold manner: (1) It restores a balanced or ample flow of chi in the treated meridian, and (2) it modifies the information-bearing signals flowing with, or carried by, the chi so that the information becomes usable and conducive to health as evidenced by a state of FRC. Accordingly, chi can be conceptualized as a carrier wave that flows along or through the meridians and carries information-bearing signals relative to thought fields, as well as other information relative to our living and learning.

Figure 15.1 illustrates the flow of chi in acupuncture meridians as it is typically imagined to operate relative to health and illness. Part a in Figure 15.1 shows a balanced and optimal flow of chi in all 14 predominate yin and yang meridians and vessels, which is thought to correlate with the desired model of health. Part b in Figure 15.1 portrays a hypothetical illness model resulting from less than optimal and an imbalanced flow of chi in the 14 predominate yin and yang meridians and vessels. In the illness model, chi flow can become either too great or restricted along the meridian pathway resulting in differing effects on physical and emotional experience.

Consider the analogy of a farmer who under ideal conditions of soil, sun, and water harvests a bumper crop. Let this be the optimal health model described above. Now imagine that the same farmer experiences a period of drought and the crops are smaller in size and the production is diminished because of the lack of rain. Now imagine that the farmer experiences a period of excessive rain and flooding where the soil is overly saturated and the roots are unable to hold and even rot. Again the farmer's harvest is diminished, but the cause and resulting features are quite different than those resulting from a drought. However, the idea

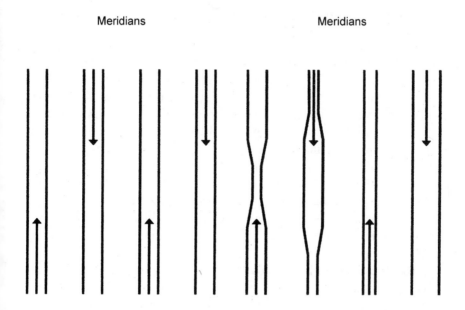

a. Health Model
Based on the Balanced Flow of Chi

b. Illness Model
Based on the Unbalanced Flow of Chi

Figure 15.1 Acupuncture meridian flow in health and illness

that all that is really needed is a balanced amount of rainfall is short sighted. What if the ideal amount of rainfall contained acid rain or some other contaminant from an environmental hazard via irrigation that adversely affected the growth and development of the crop? To put it another way, having the water pipes cleared of clogs so that the water flows freely will not be the final resolve if sewage is still seeping into the line. Clearing what flows in or along with the chi (i.e., information-bearing signals) is equally important, if not more important, than just adjusting the flow. Additionally, it is hypothesized that the changes in chi flow are the result of changes in the information-bearing signals, which are influenced by EvTFT procedures. Meridian-based psychotherapies affect the information-bearing signals (e.g., perturbations and elaters) carried by the chi because of attainment of FRC with the targeted thought field.

Our bodies are constantly transmitting and receiving information-bearing signals of varying frequency and intensity. At the meridian level, I propose that the information-bearing signals are

1. transmitted, received, and amplified at the numerous acupoints, which serve as frequency regulators,
2. converted into electrical signals by the central nervous system, and
3. used to modulate newly received or internally generated chi.

The newly modulated chi is similarly amplified and regulated at the acupoints and converted into electromagnetic wavicles, which then radiate throughout and around the body. Each of the 12 paired meridians and the two vessels are sensitive to their respective frequency and intensity ranges of information-bearing signals. When the waves produced by the information-bearing signals are coherent as they resonate with the thought field, a state of optimal health (emotionally and physically) is evident. Accordingly, the phenomena of emotional distress and psychological reversal can be viewed as interfering information-bearing signals that cause polarity disruption and blocks the meridian system's capacity to restore immediate, complete, and lasting coherence (i.e., healthy change).

Muscle-testing can be considered a *time sample* of the energetic state of coherence in response to a given thought field. When the body energy resonates with the thought field, the muscle holds strong because the meridians are vibrating at optimal frequency, reflecting coherence with the attuned thought field. When there is a lack of or reduction in resonance between the body energy and the thought field, the muscle tests weaker due to an altered and less than optimal meridian frequency, suggesting incoherence. To put it another way, when there is disruptive body energy resonance to the thought field, the overall integrity of the energy system is compromised, as evidenced by the weak muscle response due to incoherence. As Childre and Martin wrote, "Coherence is more than a powerful, harmonious concept, . . . It's the state that makes the difference between a book light and a laser beam. . . . There are high levels of coherent organization and patterning throughout nature. . . . When a system is coherent, virtually no energy is wasted, because all its components are operating in harmony. It follows, then, that when every system in the body is aligned, your personal power is at its peak" (1999, p. 50).

TREATMENT SEQUENCE REVISITED

The treatment sequence obtained via the EvTFT diagnostic procedure (regardless of the method used) is analogous to acquiring a time-based energetic signature of the mind-body-energy interrelationship (i.e., the mind-body interface) relative to the thought field. Much like Alfred Adler's reference to handwriting as a frozen sample of personality, the diagnosed sequence reflects a linear, code-like interpretation of a more complex state of being. Therefore, to think that the resulting treatment sequence is the *only* viable sequence or "code" would be, in our opinion, an erroneous conclusion. We believe this viewpoint is also supported by the work of Bohm and Hiley (1993) regarding their thinking about implicate and explicate order, as previously referenced in Chapters Two and Seven. With specific regard to the diagnostic process, the explicate order (a resulting diagnostic sequence) can only be a representative subset of the implicate order plucked from an unbroken wholeness for our treatment purposes. Because we can only step into the implicate order at some arbitrary place when we begin diagnosis, the perspective from that place may be different than if diagnosis had begun at another arbitrary place. In other words, the resulting diagnosed sequence represents a sample of explicate order, which is a limited expression of a more encompassing implicate order. Therefore, the diagnostically determined sequence can be but one of an unknown number of possible treatment sequences. Elements that contribute to the explicate nature of a treatment sequence include

1. the linear (one by one) approach to diagnosing meridian involvement,
2. the intuitive or knowledge-based source used by the therapist to select a meridian to test,

3. the energetic effect of treatment on the other meridians, and
4. the impact of the therapist's energy field on the patient.

In addition, a host of other intervening variables can affect treatment. For example, time-of-day differences, overall physical and structural health of the patient (and therapist), nutritional fluctuations, presence of environmental or energy toxins, and so on can all affect energy flow and meridian activity.

Figure 15.2 illustrates our concept of the interplay of frequency and coherence between and among meridians and vessels when attuned to a thought field. Although specific values and wave descriptions are unknown, a general direction of impact can be hypothesized: When frequency is coherent to the attuned thought field, the frequency pattern comfortably conforms to a signature threshold or range of resonance that constitutes health and well-being. In contrast, when frequency is incoherent, the resulting energy patterns fall outside the range of resonance to the thought field, thereby deviating from the optimal signature pattern of emotional and physical health. When there is incoherence, the specific meridians that respond to the information-bearing signals of perturbations and elaters are detectable via the EvTFT diagnostic methods.

Figure 15.3 illustrates a hypothetical and linear view of meridians when a person is attuned to a disturbing thought field. In this example it can be seen that meridians 3, 4, 7, 8, 9, and 14 demonstrate incoherence and are therefore diagnosable. With EvTFT methods of diagnosis, any of these six meridians would muscle-test strong when the patient is attuned to the targeted thought field when the alarm point was tested.[5] When an incoherent meridian is identified by the strong muscle response, it is immediately treated with TAB. The remaining eight coherent meridians would muscle-test weak, if they were checked, and thus

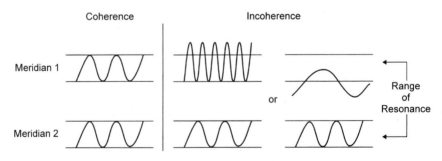

Figure 15.2 Interplay of frequency and coherence between meridians when a person is attuned to a thought field

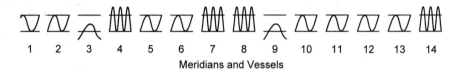

Meridians and Vessels

Figure 15.3 Hypothetical linear view of meridians when a person is attuned to a disturbing thought field: Coherence versus incoherence

not require treatment at this time. Accordingly, the treatment sequence could begin with *any* one of the incoherent meridians because the therapist has no way of knowing which or how many meridians are currently in a state of incoherence and therefore involved in maintaining the emotional distress.

It is further hypothesized that the treatment of whichever meridian is diagnosed first will have a synergistic impact on the other meridians, thereby affecting the state of coherence. This hypothesis is based on the concept of closed strings or string loops as characterizing the interconnections between and among the 12 paired major meridians and the two vessels. Additionally, the treatment effect appears consistent with the concept of enhanced activation of deltrons from the emotional domain, which ultimately alter information patterns in order to be realized in our physical reality (Tiller, Dibble, & Kohane, 2001).

For the purpose of this example, let's say the therapist diagnosed meridian 7 as the first meridian to be treated. After having the patient TAB on the prescribed acupoint for that meridian to adjust to the information-bearing signals of perturbations or elaters, meridian 7 now demonstrates coherence. However, this single-point treatment of meridian 7 may also have any of the following effects, (as illustrated in Figure 15.4) perhaps a result of enhanced deltron activation.

a. It brought all five of the other incoherent meridians into coherence as well (Figure 15.4a).
b. It brought one or more of the five other incoherent meridians into coherence (4, 8) but not all (3, 9, 14) (Figure 15.4b).
c. It brought one or more of the five other incoherent meridians into coherence (4, 8) and, as a result of the vibrational info-energetic changes, caused one or more additional or different meridians to now evidence incoherence to a degree commensurate with the reduced SUD level (1, 6, 11) (Figure 15.4c).

These three patterns of response generally continue to repeat throughout the diagnosis and treatment process until all meridians estab-

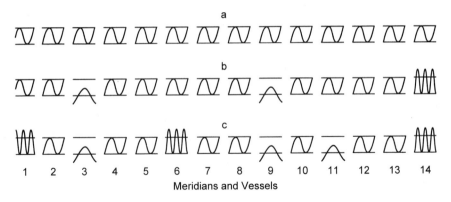

Figure 15.4 Hypothetical changes in coherence and incoherence after treatment of an acupoint

lish coherence in frequency and resonate to the targeted thought field without perturbation or elater influence or interference.

Because there may be more than one meridian in an incoherent state during any part of the diagnostic and treatment phases, the resulting treatment sequences will vary from person to person and therapist to therapist, not just from thought field to thought field. The diagnosed sequence of treatment points (an example of explicate order) can vary based on the synergistic relationship of the 12 meridians and two vessels, *and* on "catching" one of several meridians or vessels that was detectable when a diagnosis was made. Indeed, after observing hundreds of trainees and colleagues over the past several years who were unfamiliar with algorithms, we can confirm that the diagnosed treatment sequences *often* vary from the list of popularized algorithm treatment sequences. Although shorter treatment sequences that involve anxiety tend to be more similar to some algorithms, complex or involved issues can produce lengthy treatment sequences that are dissimilar to algorithms. Other reasons for the variations most likely involve the interaction or contribution of the therapist's energetic influence on the patient by way of physical presence or intentional thought and the built-in variance between how the patient and therapist perceive and emotionally respond to the targeted thought field. In other words, the manner in which the therapist and patient resonate within each other's bio-energy field will influence the treatment sequence obtained via diagnosis, as well as the form and frequency of chosen algorithms.

These conceptualizations constitute a way to explain how diagnostic sequences are determined, and why individually diagnosed treatment sequences, specific algorithms (e.g., Callahan, 2001), or the comprehensive algorithm variation of the emotional freedom techniques (Craig & Fowlie, 1997) can all work successfully. The above hypotheses also explain how a particular meridian, not found to be in need of treatment at an earlier time, can later be diagnosed as needing of treatment (a result of one or more of the other meridians having been treated). Further, the above hypothesis would also account for the ecological safety of EvTFT, and perhaps all meridian-based psychotherapies: Treatment of a meridian (frequency) already in coherence will not impact the other meridians, whereas treatment of incoherent meridians does.

Treatment sequence *does* matter but not in the strict sense that there is only one "code." What matters is that the meridians that need treatment get the treatment. Uncovering this information in the most parsimonious manner remains the challenge. Our preference is for individual diagnosis because of the precision of tailoring the treatment. The specific algorithms, or the one-size-fits-all approach, frequently lack precision and often rely on trial and error, repetition, or eventual default to a diagnostic method. As is the case in the emotional freedom techniques, the more points you treat and the increased number of times you treat them, the greater the likelihood of eventually treating the meridians in need. The popularized TFT algorithms offered by Callahan (2001) or Lambrou and Pratt (2000) also lack precision and have a clinically lower success rate than individually diagnosed treatment sequences. While algorithm methods may serve as beneficial self-help tools for the layman or for some patients to use between therapy sessions, for the therapist who is truly interested in knowing which specific meridians are involved when the patient is attuned to the disturbing thought field, individual diagnosis is the treatment of choice. When the patient begins to demonstrate his or her idiosyncratic treatment patterns in response to similar kinds of thought fields (e.g., anxiety situations or trauma), then these patterns can be used algorithmically *for that individual* and modified as needed.

Superstring theory may help our understanding of how EvTFT and other meridian-based psychotherapies work. This theory builds from string theory, which describes elementary particles as one-dimensional curves (strings). Superstring theory combines string theory and supersymmetry to describe how elementary particles form very short closed strings, or string loops. This theory posits that all of the masses, charges, and other elementary properties result from the vibration of these superstrings at different frequencies.

Diepold hypothesizes that the network of meridians and vessels function as interrelated string loops that rapidly channel vibratory information-bearing signals at different frequencies. Not only would vibratory information "channel through" one meridian to another, but the meridians also interact with one another via the space *between* the meridians and vessels in a manner similar to the vacuum-like space between particles in a molecule. If this were so, the resulting emotional change, from using EvTFT, would be rapid and enduring because the change is made at a deeply fundamental level of information exchange. Unsuccessful results could be explained as a result of interference (e.g., psychological reversal, blocking beliefs, and energy toxins), which blocks or negates the treatment-induced changes and therefore impedes the capacity of the meridian system to receive or transmit the information required for change.

DYNAMICAL ENERGY SYSTEMS AND EvTFT

A synergistic view of the mind-body-energy relationship, which we refer to as the *mind-body interface*, is central to EvTFT. Schwartz and Russek (1997) offer an exciting systems theory approach to energy and health, which they call the *dynamical energy systems approach*. This well-articulated model has much to offer the emerging field of energy psychology, and appears consistent with the concept that EvTFT meridian treatments facilitate frequency resonance coherence. Accordingly, Diepold (2002) developed several TFT-related dynamical energy systems models based on the work of Schwartz and Russek. These are presented below with some modification.

Figure 15.5 illustrates the conceptualization of a model reflecting a condition of emotional balance and health. This is the state in which harmonizers are most prominent. This model, like those that follow, has four major ports of information exchange and experience that maintain a dynamical relationship with each other and with *other* information sources, such as morphogenic fields and morphic resonance (Sheldrake, 1988, 1995a, 1995b), energy toxins, and environmental influences (e.g., electric, magnetic, and electromagnetic fields). Port A represents a synchronous and calm thought field influenced by harmonizers. An example of this type of thought field might be watching or remembering a beautiful sunrise or sunset, or the experience of seeing your newly born child for the first time—profound events that language cannot adequately describe. Port B represents the state of coherent, dynamic resonance between and among the meridians when attuned to the thought field in port A, which could be verified by a strong muscle test and indications that no meridians or vessels require treatment. Port C represents an emo-

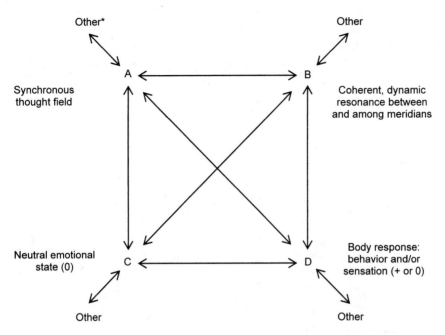

*Morphogenic fields and morphic resonance, energy toxins, and environmental influences

Figure 15.5 An EvTFT-Energy psychology dynamical energy systems model of emotional balance and health (harmonizer effect)

tional state of profound calmness and deep neutrality, which would accompany the sight or recall of the sunrise, sunset, or your new infant. Port *D* pertains to the body response involving behavior and sensation; in other words, the quiet-stillness of the body, the feeling of being awestruck, and the accompanying synchronized rhythms of heart and brain activity. In keeping with the dynamical energy systems approach, ports *A*, *B*, *C*, *D*, and *other* interact with each other recurrently, sharing information through the transfer of info-energy and "literally create[ing] a dynamic memory of their interactions over time through the circulation of their information and energy" (Schwartz & Russek, 1997, p. 50).

Similarly, Figure 15.6 illustrates the psychological and behavioral disturbances resulting from perturbations in the thought field. Such conditions would include anxiety states, depression, trauma, post-traumatic stress disorder, anger, and the like. In this model, port *A* is a perturbed thought field (e.g., experiencing a traumatic flashback or seeing phobic stimuli) with a corresponding state of incoherent, dynamic resonance between and among the meridians, resulting in a dys-synchronous dynamic interaction between and among meridians (port *B*) with the

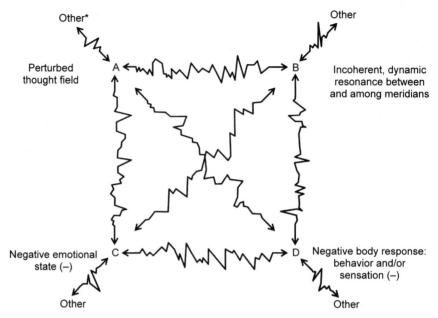

Other*

Other

Perturbed
thought field   A   B   Incoherent, dynamic
                                                                          resonance between
                                                                          and among meridians

Negative emotional   C   D   Negative body response:
state (−)   behavior and/or
                                                  sensation (−)

Other   Other

*Morphogenic fields and morphic resonance, energy toxins, and environmental influences

Figure 15.6 An EvTFT-Energy psychology dynamical energy systems model of psychobehavioral disturbance (perturbation effect)

thought field. Port C reflects the negative emotional state (e.g., fear, anger, guilt, shame), with port D accounting for the unpleasant sensations (e.g., shortness of breath, heart palpitations, sweating) and unwanted behavior (e.g., lashing-out, fleeing, crying, momentary-paralysis).

Figure 15.7 illustrates the psychological and *behavioral disturbances* resulting from the predominance of elaters in the thought field. Port A represents the elated but behaviorally destructive thought field that would involve such events as thinking about having a cigarette, thinking about eating something that is counter to your health goals, misusing a substance, or, for a bulimia patient, thinking about vomiting. Port C is the accompanying initial positive emotional state believed to result from engaging in the event "in order" to experience enjoyment, satisfaction, relief, or escape. However, the associated behavioral responses and sensations (port D) eventually slide into unwanted negative states (e.g., health problems, social isolation, irresponsibility, self-destruction), which in turn create negative emotions (e.g., guilt, shame, embarrassment, depression) because they are not in the best interest of the individual or do not fit his or her overall goals or context. Port B represents the state of incoherent, dynamic resonance between and among the meridians, resulting in dys-synchronous dynamic interaction with the thought field, indicating the need for treatment.

Figure 15.8 illustrates positive and enjoyable emotional experience and *appropriate behavior* in response to elaters in the thought field. This model is the reverse mirror-image of the perturbation-driven model shown in Figure 15.6. Here, port A pertains to an elated thought field, which might include such events as thinking of or being with a loved-one, learning you just passed your licensing exam, talking or thinking about your child's success, or receiving an award. Port C is the accompanying comfortable emotional state (e.g., love, happiness, interest, pride, excitement, and joy). Port B reflects the state of coherent, dynamic resonance between and among the meridians, resulting in a synchronous dynamic interaction with the thought field. Port D represents the pleasant sensations and behavior, reflecting congruence with the individual's (and society's) expectations and health. This model encompasses the positive and healthy emotions (e.g., joy, happiness, excitement, well-

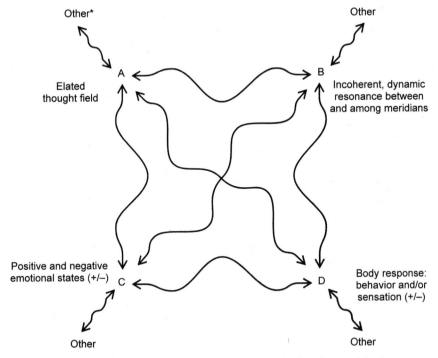

Other*

Other

A

B

Elated
thought field

Incoherent, dynamic
resonance between
and among meridians

Positive and negative
emotional states (+/−)   C

D

Body response:
behavior and/or
sensation (+/−)

Other

Other

*Morphogenic fields and morphic resonance, energy toxins, and environmental influences

Figure 15.7 An EvTFT-Energy psychology dynamical energy systems model of psychobehavioral disturbance (elater effect "in-order")

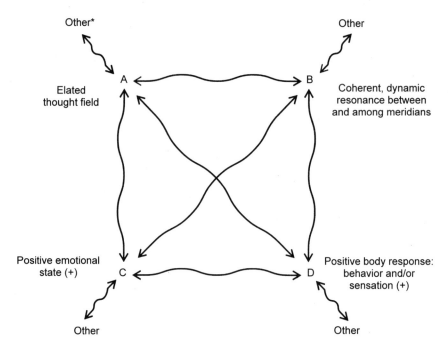

*Morphogenic fields and morphic resonance, energy toxins, and environmental influences

Figure 15.8 An EvTFT-Energy Psychology dynamical systems model of positive emotion and behavior (healthy elater effect)

being) associated with favorable life activities. This is what most individuals strive to experience in daily life.

These dynamical models are offered in an attempt to conceptualize and understand the broad range of influence and effects associated with EvTFT in particular, and with thought field therapies and energy psychology in general. We invite research and other creative and empirical efforts to evaluate and further develop these dynamical energy systems models.

EvTFT AND THE RELATIONSHIP TO CONSCIOUSNESS AND SPIRIT

This section will explore the interface of EvTFT and other thought field psychotherapies with consciousness and spirit. In particular, the section will address conjecture about how the thought field serves as an interfacing bridge or entry into the vast resources of the unconscious mind, which links us to the timeless, collective unconscious articulated by Carl Jung, morphogenic fields and morphic resonance as theorized by Rupert Sheldrake, and ultimately to the spirit and beyond. While the terms conscious and unconscious are familiar to most psychotherapists, the idea and utilization of spirit is less familiar in traditional psychotherapy. Perhaps this is so because the term *spirit* conveys many meanings. However, let's begin with more common ground and the levels of consciousness as traditionally employed in psychotherapy.

Figure 15.9 illustrates a typical two-dimensional view of the mind involving the theorized constructs of the conscious and the unconscious. As can be readily seen, the unconscious area is much greater in size than the conscious area. Diepold remembers an example used in graduate school to exemplify the difference in apparent size and ability of these two mind levels. The students were asked to imagine placing a golf ball on top of the Houston Astrodome. It was then explained by comparison that the golf ball was equivalent to the conscious mind, and the Astrodome equivalent to the unconscious mind. That is a big difference, and as psychologists we have to use the information the patient brings to us with his or her "golf ball" and then locate and treat the related cause somewhere in the "Astrodome" without so much as a floor plan beyond projective psychological testing. However, we believe the concept and utility of thought fields make navigating the known and unknown much easier.

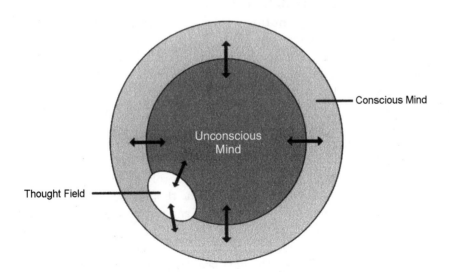

Figure 15.9 Two-dimensional view: Thought field directed energy psychology treatment and the conscious and unconscious minds

The conscious and unconscious minds constantly exchange information as indicated in Figure 15.9 by the double-sided arrows. The information exchange is most likely simultaneous across the many biological, neuro-chemical, cognitive, affective, and info-energetic network systems. We hypothesize that when we attune a thought field multi-level information exchange instantly occurs, bringing conscious and unconscious knowledge and info-energy to the fore regarding the specified thought field. The thought field is an information hub that links conscious and unconscious resources that can be readily accessed and treated with meridian-based diagnosis (e.g., EvTFT, EdxTM, Callahan Techniques™), or in a general generic fashion via algorithms. The resulting changes due to treatment (e.g., field-shifting of info-energy in the thought field, absence of perturbation or elater influence emotionally, cognitive clarity, physiological adaptations) are similarly and instantly communicated from thought field to both conscious and unconscious levels of mind. Accordingly, we think, feel, and act differently and our corporeal structure follows suit in its own way. This is the more obvious and easy part.

So what is really in the "Astrodome"? What is it and where does it come from? How does it work? How does it influence our life now, and how do we influence it? But let's see what happens when we take the flat or front view of the thought field with consciousness, as seen in Figure 15.9, and turn it on its side. Figure 15.10 shows Diepold's interpretation of a four-dimensional view of interactive communications when using thought fields with EvTFT or other energy psychology treatments. In this diagram the unconscious connects to far more than repressed childhood memories and is truly a resource activated in treatment. We now see the richness and the depth of the communication available, which would support the unusually quick and robust results frequently obtained with EvTFT and other energy psychology treatments. The depth and breadth would also account for occasional spontaneous reports by patients about seemingly odd or unusual thoughts, feelings, and images that sometimes accompany resolution of longstanding or complex issues. The rings in Figure 15.10 around the personal unconscious represent different levels or layers of info-energy, beginning with conscious knowledge and thought. The thought field pierces all the interacting levels and layers and transmits and receives info-energy from all areas. The next level involves our physical body energy as reflected in our neurological, biochemical, and electrical activities. We now go beyond the physical body in the next layer and into the electromagnetic, magnetic, and subtle energies that surround us and influence the info-energy we receive and transmit. These outer body energy levels are

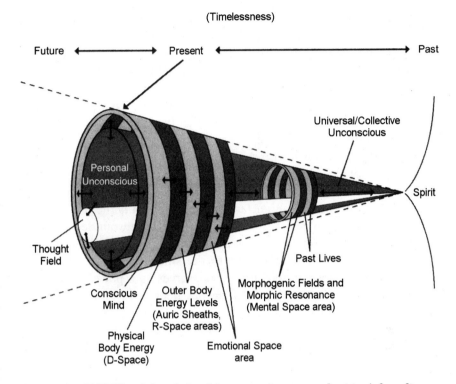

Figure 15.10 EvTFT and the relationship to consciousness and spirit: A four-dimensional view of thought field directed energy psychology treatment

sometimes referred to as *auric sheaths,* or they are delineated in more precise detail as *physical D-space, conjugate physical R-space,* and emotional and mental domains by Tiller (1997) and Tiller, Dibble, and Kohane (2001). The levels or layers of rings are undetermined but they eventually interact with the info-energy from morphogenic fields and morphic resonance (Sheldrake, 1995) and past lives influences (Weiss, 1988, 1992; Newton, 2002) that impact our current life. The universal or collective unconscious melds with the current personal unconscious somewhere in the timelessness beyond Tiller's mental space domain.

Now we are back to the concept and role of spirit, the intangible ingredient of who and what we are. Etymologically the word *spirit* comes from the French *espirit* and the Latin *spiritus,* pertaining to breath, vigor, courage, life, and the soul, as well as from *spirare* meaning to blow or breathe. Spirit is most often used as a noun with a multitude of meanings. *Webster's* (1966) lists 16 definitions and Microsoft Word offers 16 synonyms. The term *spirit,* as relevant to EvTFT and consciousness, would reflect the definitions in *Webstser's* describing *spirit* as "the life principle," which is "regarded as separate from matter," and consisting of "real meaning; true intention." It is neither the intention nor within the scope of this book to infer or discuss *spirit* in a religious sense.

Spirit might be considered the most fundamental aspect of our being, similar to the pure, guiding energy of Shen (Woollerton & McLean, 1979), and therefore it affects our lives in diverse ways that lend to so many definitions. Perhaps it is the spirit that binds the collective unconscious, providing us with the strength, courage, character, fortitude, heart, chutzpah, and will to master life's challenges and strive to overcome adversity without giving up the ghost. The experience of common fears, traumatic events, sorrows, and even the joys of all humankind is contained in the essence of our far-reaching spirit. It is the driving force that guides healers to heal, teachers to teach, and the wounded to mend; it is the force that drives us to seek knowledge. The spirit is our intangible connection to one another and to the simultaneous experience of a timeless past, present, and future that serves as a powerful resource throughout life's journey. While there has been many ways to engage the spirit throughout history, and no doubt many more ways will be devised in the future, it appears at this time that the thought field provides a direct and convenient avenue to the spirit via facilitation of our info-energy system with EvTFT.

EPILOGUE

We are all scientists.
—T. H. Huxley

Throughout this book we have shared our enthusiasm and clinical observations in presenting the background and methods of EvTFT. While it may be customary to bring closure to a book by espousing the accolades of the subject matter, we have chosen to take a different direction. We believe description of the current reality of professional research, and the necessity for same, must be addressed in concert with anecdotal case studies. The current paucity of published research on any of the energy psychology psychotherapy methodologies reflects the current state of affairs and ought to be of interest and concern for clinicians and researchers alike.

History teaches that new concepts and innovative procedures take time to earn their way into the mainstream of any established professional entity. Acceptance of EvTFT and other energy psychology psychotherapy methods will most likely travel the same path. The responsibility to demonstrate the efficacy of meridian-based psychotherapies like EvTFT rests on the shoulders of all who study and use these methods. We recognize that this is no small task and much effort will be needed to accomplish the goal of mainstream utilization based on therapeutic effectiveness. This harsh pill of current reality may be hard to swallow for some who have witnessed the robust effects, but unfortunately it may also serve as reason to criticize these methods. This *is* the reality of where we are.

The idea, desire, and need of researching energy psychology methods are easier said than done. This epilogue will describe the available research and the historical and current trends in conducing research. Controversy not withstanding, we will also offer suggestions about how research could proceed.

RESEARCH: LEVEL
OF SCIENTIFIC DOCUMENTATION

Despite the existence of behavioral kinesiology, life-energy analysis (Diamond), and the Callahan Techniques™ for approximately 25 years, and the more recently evolved forms of meridian-based psychotherapy over the past five to ten years, there is very little in the form of controlled, published research for thought field therapy.

The most frequently cited study on thought field therapy is one by psychologists Carbonell and Figley (1995), which compared treatments for patients diagnosed with trauma using: (1) algorithms; (2) eye movement desensitization and reprocessing; (3) visual kinesthetic dissociation; or (4) traumatic incident reduction. The researchers concluded that while all four therapies were helpful, patients treated with thought field therapy experienced significantly more relief and achieved it more rapidly, than with the other treatments, and that the treatment results appeared to be permanent. While these findings are generally enlightening regarding the quick and lasting results that can be achieved in the treatment of trauma, critics cite design flaws in the procedural aspects of the research (e.g., issues regarding the lack of homogeneity of treatment issues, and the report that some subjects were not considered appropriate for treatment with a particular intervention), which serve to detract from the actual gains realized by subjects treated with algorithms. In a follow-up study using 156 college students, Carbonell and Mappa (cited in Callahan, 2001, p. 43) compared Callahan's phobia algorithm with a placebo treatment[1] for fear of heights (acrophobia). Although both groups showed improvement, the algorithm treatment group evidenced significantly more improvement than the placebo treatment group (Callahan with Trubo, 2001).

Using quantitative electroencephalogram (QEEG), Diepold and Goldstein (2000) found statistically abnormal brain-wave patterns when a patient thought about a traumatic event compared to a neutral (baseline) event. Immediately following EvTFT diagnosis and treatment of the trauma, reassessment of brain-wave patterns revealed an absence of statistical abnormalities when attuned to the traumatic life event. An 18-month follow-up revealed that the patient continued to be free of all negative emotion related to the treated trauma. Lambrou, Pratt, and Chevalier (2001) reported significant pre- and post-physiological, psychological, and behavioral measures involving subjects receiving a single 30-minute algorithm treatment for claustrophobia compared to a control group.

Wells, Polglase, Andrews, Carrington, and Baker (in press) reported significantly greater behavioral and subjective improvement, in laboratory controlled conditions, using the emotional freedom techniques (EFT)[2] algorithm treatment, compared to a group treated by diaphragmatic breathing, with subjects having phobias to small animals.

In *Tapping the Healer Within* (2001), Callahan with Trubo reviewed several single-case and multiple subject studies involving the correlated positive changes in heart function and heart rate variability (the intervals between heartbeats) resulting from treatment using the Callahan Techniques™. Heart rate variability is purported to be a window to the workings of the autonomic nervous system, and thought to be free of placebo effects, which suggests that thought field therapies have the potential to impact both physical and psychological wellbeing. Callahan with Trubo also write about the "science" behind thought field therapy and describe an interesting study on rouleaux as seen under the microscope before and after two treatments with thought field therapy. Still, the research efforts that preceded and followed their book are by no means enough to constitute a "science."

In summary, studies other than those mentioned above consist of case reports, samples with small numbers of participants, and narrow topics using highly specified apparatuses for treatment and evaluation. We emphasize our concern that there has been limited research into meridian-based thought field therapies and that there is a pronounced need for quality research projects that are suitably designed with adequate sample sizes that address the full range of applicability of EvTFT and other meridian-based psychotherapies. Unfortunately, research remains a considerable challenge in light of the history and process of research in general, and research with psychotherapy in particular. The variables to monitor can be as plentiful as the stars, and even if the variables could all be evaluated there is no guarantee that therapists would use the findings as intended. In this regard the interested reader is referred to a letter written by a friend and colleague, psychologist Thomas Tudor, in which he concisely states his case about psychological research and clinical practice (Appendix 6).

SCIENCE, THEORY, AND CLINICAL PRACTICE

In Chapter Two we outlined what we believe to be the historical links for EvTFT to mainstream science. Having done that, we want to discuss what we conceptualize as the next steps for a more rigorous study of EvTFT methods, treatment, and clinical results. You may recall that Lightner Witmer, the father of clinical psychology, espoused a mixture of scientific and clinical practice that would widen the traditional lenses through which psychological investigational studies had been approached.[3] In effect, clinicians could be "scientists," and as a correlate, those in science could put on a clinician's hat, so that there could be perspective and harmony in the questions asked and the ideas exchanged.

It is clear that we need a theory or model of mind and an evenhanded environment for free discussion. Theories of mind in psychology, like theories in physics, have developed in large part on mechanistic considerations. If we take as a model the movement of physics, which enlarged on its classical base, we may glean an exciting template for our next efforts into research design with EvTFT.

Interestingly, some of the problems physicists address when doing research are similar to our own. The limitations of instrumentation, the influence of observation and the fact that the same subject cannot be studied twice (because after study, the subject is not the same by virtue of the study), are problems common to both physics and psychology. The description of what the physicist incurs while studying light allows the social scientists to feel at home, for it reads the same as a study of human variables. It is explained that in studying the wave or particle aspects of light, the physicist is limited to measuring one variable, either momentum or location. "[O]nce an observation has been made on a quantum system, its state will generally change abruptly. . . . It is as though the altered mental state of the experimenter when first aware of the result of the measurement somehow feeds back into the laboratory apparatus. . . . In short, the physical state acts to alter the mental state, and the mental state reacts back on the physical state" (Davies & Brown, 1986, p. 31). For the physicist, as for the psychologist, this raises several questions: If the world is divided into observer and observed, where is the observer positioned? And, where does the measurement begin and end and the observer begin and end?

For physicists the idea of the position of the observer has given rise to multi-dimensions and many-universes interpretations. Issues of multi-dimensions and many-universes are argued by some physicists as preposterous or too metaphysical, while others find them to be the simplest explanation of choice points. We need not concern ourselves as to the merit of those particular arguments, but rather with the fact that we, too, are faced with choices that at first glance may appear preposterous or too metaphysical, and we too are people of science and such discussions are absolutely necessary.

Thought Experiments

If, in this way, we begin to define our knowledge in parallel to another science, we begin to think in different ways. Certainly some of our studies should be *Gedankenexperiment*,[4] experiments in thought.[5] For example, we could ask the questions: What is it we really observe in a thought? How could we know if thought has physical existence? Does thought exist outside the observer? To these points, Rosenthal-Schneider (1980) reacquainted us with some solid psychological ideas, as spoken and written by the greatest scientific minds in physics.[6] They include a return to conceptualizing science and philosophy as interdependent, if not inseparable, notions of differences in systems with and without observers,[7] questions about experience and reality, and as already suggested, experiments in thought. In her introduction, Rosenthal-Schneider indicated that the philosophy and history of science, once regarded as belonging to retired professors, had gained respectability in the second half of the twentieth century, when she wrote her book: "Philosophy and science, identical in antiquity, were for centuries interdependent and often subordinate to religion" (1980, p. 27). She continues that science's break from philosophy meant for centuries that most scientists did not think that scientific philosophy had any relation to scientific practice. There were always a few who recognized the philosophical implications in their theories, but with Albert Einstein and his contemporaries, the understanding that science could not stand without philosophy became institutionalized once again. Rosenthal-Schneider quoted Einstein as having said in 1949, "Epistemology without contact with Science becomes an empty scheme. Science without Epistemology is—in so far as it is thinkable at all—primitive and muddled" (p. 27). Rosenthal-Schneider's interviews and letters reacquaint us with solid psychological ideas, but they do not come from psychologists, they are spoken and written by great physicists.

More recently, we have David Bohm's definition of the thought process that enlarges the scope of what may be the operative field in EvTFT. Bohm wrote, "What is the process of thought? Thought is, in essence, the active response of memory in every phase of life. We include in thought the intellectual, emotional, sensuous, muscular and physical responses of memory. These are all aspects of one indissoluble process. To treat them separately makes for fragmentation and confusion" (1980, p. 50).

Bohm and Hiley wrote that several physicists have suggested that quantum mechanics and consciousness are closely related and that by necessity consciousness will be drawn into the attempts to understand what they call the implicate order of the universe. They state, "[I]t is convenient to introduce the notion that consciousness shows or manifests two sides which may be called the physical and the mental . . . that information is contained in thought, which we feel to be on the mental side, is at the same time a related neurophysiological, chemical and physical activity (which is clearly what is meant by the 'material side' of thought)" (1993, p. 384). Bohm and Hiley go on to say that thought may contain a range of information in levels, that may be viewed from a level beneath or above the present level of the thought. Thus they describe a Janus effect[8] of emerging levels of organization that can in principle could go on forever. When viewed from a higher level, the level beneath or observed is passive in the order of material objects and the higher observing level is active in the order of mental events. "Each of these levels may then be seen from both sides. From the mental side, it is a potentially active information content. But from the material side, it is an actual activity that operates to organize the less subtle levels, and the latter serve as the 'material' on which such operation takes place" (p. 385).

Bohm and Hiley proposed that physical and mental process are essentially the same, and only vary with the perspective. They propose that the experience of "mind" is movement through various levels of subtlety that will "in a natural way ultimately move the body by reaching the level of the quantum potential and the 'dance' of the particles" (p. 386).

Thinking about thinking is not new to psychology; it is in its very roots from the experimental laboratories of Wundt to the more recent studies by Flavell and his students, and now Tiller and his colleagues in their studies on intentional thought (Tiller, Dibble, & Kohane, 2001). We are well equipped to go from constructs of meta-cognition and meta-learning to meta-observation if we choose to do so. Thinking about thinking within an energetic model may be an easier process with professionals working together.

Cooperation Through Dialogue

The issue of developing an atmosphere of cooperation was eloquently addressed by psychologist Kurt Salzinger in his 2002 article, "What If All Psychologists Understood Each Other?" His effort in starting a listserv to open constructive dialogue around a single book has, according to his own report, received great response from the professional community. Perhaps Salzinger could be enjoined to engage the community in discussing an energy psychology book. Certainly in such a context what Huxley called "intellectual honesty" may allow for useful exchanges of ideas.

If an energy psychology book were to be selected, we would recommend *Energy Psychology and Psychotherapy* (2002), edited by Gallo. In the book Gallo gathered contributors who have expertise in other psychotherapeutic specialties, such as hypnosis, EMDR, and biofeedback, and who bring years of experience to their clinical hypotheses and applications. In addition, he has coordinated the effort so that it goes beyond each individual chapter and develops to a meta observation of the possibilities of energy psychology for psychotherapy. In one of these chapters, scientist Mark Furman expressed, as we have, the zeitgeist of this time in psychological history by the very title of his chapter, "Grounding energy psychology in the physical sciences." This book paves the way for serious discussion of energy psychology and in-depth consideration of where we need to go in our research.

A Basic Study

The basic study of a psychotherapeutic method would need to address whether or not the method is effective. The challenge is what parameters should be used to determine the effectiveness of the method. In medicine, the physician is faced with similar dilemas. He or she may have the best medicines *un*available to his patients because of economic constraints (e.g., the insurance company finds them too expensive), or he or she may encounter patient noncompliance because it is laborious or painful to comply with "doctor's orders." Any dentist can tell you that patients do not like pain. Many will suffer with their teeth falling out, rather than go to a dentist. Like the physician and the dentist, we need to measure what is best for our patients, and we too must decide what is the measure of "best." We must decide what works the fastest, inspires the most patient compliance, or is least painful. And like the parallel professions, we need a group of treatments from which to choose. Unfortunately, unlike in medicine where there is a group of similar (yet different) medications, in psychotherapy we are prone to think one therapy fits all and have a low tolerance for variety.

Eddington (1958) asked that we appreciate and develop a new insight revealed to us in a partial truth rather than strive prematurely for only final answers. With this in mind, and despite the fact that there are so many complex issues that drive the possibilities for study in EvTFT, our need to be practical and parsimonious shapes our wish list.

A basic research study could have subjects who cannot for example, enter elevators at all. (Simple phobia may be the least complex of the diagnoses treatable with EvTFT.) Two psychologists, one trained in EvTFT and the other trained in cognitive behavioral therapy (CBT), could spend one hour or less with each subject doing their respective protocols. Each session should be filmed for the observing observer to study, or the observing observer may stay in the therapy room during the session. The therapist should have the subject try to go up and/or down in an elevator after one hour. Success can be adjudged if the patient enters or rides in the elevator, or some number of floors can be counted, or a measure of comfort can also be assessed (e.g., SUD level). The details for success would have to be operationally defined.

The Interdisciplinary Team

Interdisciplinary teams consisting of at least a psychologist or other professional psychotherapist who is trained in EvTFT, a physicist, a neurologist, a biologist, and a philosopher are necessary because of the synergistic possibilities such a combination could offer. Possibilities for such studies could include the use of advanced technology such as neuroimaging, QEEG, and PET scans.

For example, Bender and colleagues (2000) worked with an interdisciplinary team under a grant from the Violence Institute of New Jersey to image the effects of successful treatment with EMDR on subjects diagnosed with post-traumatic stress disorder. It would be of interest and value to do a similar study to image brain effects in treatment with EvTFT on patients with PTSD, or on subjects with a phobia. Comparisons and contrasts could then be viewed from the perspective of each team member's specialty to obtain a more complete and synthesized understanding. At present, The BDB Group is beginning to design and seek funding for basic research projects like those described.

The BDB Group Mission

The mission of The BDB Group is to integrate EvTFT into mainstream psychotherapy and thus facilitate and expand the promise of psychological healing to a more fundamental level than previously believed. In our efforts to accomplish this mission, we continue to train mental health professionals in the EvTFT approach through basic and advanced workshops, and via ongoing support and consultation with interested therapists. Further, we support research interests that will examine the efficacy of the EvTFT procedures. The hypothetical constructs and methaphors offered in Chapter 15, for example, provide fertile ground for research to better understand the intricate workings and widespread effects that EvTFT and energy psychology can have for human development. We view the EvTFT approach as in a continual state of evolution, thus keep an open mind to new ideas, methods, and integrative possibilities as more clinical and research data accumulate.

We remain excited about integrating EvTFT and energy psychology into the every-day practice of psychotherapy, and about bringing the science of mind into the twenty-first century.

A FINAL COMMENT

There is much, much more to be learned and experienced regarding EvTFT and energy psychology. There is much to do experimentally to validate the methods and hypotheses presented in this Handbook. Our purpose and intention is to inspire thought and action regarding EvTFT beyond the usual clinical outcomes and procedural necessities. In this regard we hope your interest has been piqued.

We have shared our experiences, observations, methods, thoughts, and hypotheses pertaining to the hows and whys of EvTFT. We now invite you to use what we have learned to advance this fledgling field of energy psychology and, in the true spirit of psychotherapy, to employ these methods to help those in need.

As we build the EvTFT model, we need to look to what others have noticed in psychotherapy to see if it is possible to use concepts of energy and connectedness as explanations. We would expect that family systems and all psychotherapies that regard the interpersonal relationship as important will benefit from such scrutiny. To paraphrase Bohm and Hiley (1993), consider this our invitation to be free to explore a broader approach to mind and matter, as well as the whole of the psychotherapeutic reality not limited by a particular school of thought. Be good therapists, but be good scientists, and look to each clinical challenge as an opportunity to notice.

AFTERWORD

As I read this fine book by Diepold, Britt, and Bender, I struggled with what I might add that could contribute to such a rich compendium. As I am not a practitioner of this new field, I decided to provide a personal perspective on what I think this general field is all about, where it fits into the rapidly evolving picture of whole person healing, and how some of the practitioner/client information entanglements naturally come about via my higher dimensional physics model.

Based upon my own and my colleague's earlier works (Tiller, 1997; Tiller, Dibble, & Kohane, 2001), the functional capabilities of a human experiencing our world can be usefully expressed in the form of a reaction equation of the type featured in Figure A.1.

In a more pictorial form, Figure A.2 shows the whole person as consisting of three unique parts: (1) the outermost shell of two layers constitutes the personality-self, (2) the middle shell of three layers constitutes the soul-self and (3) the core is the high spirit-self. The outer layer of the personality-self is comprised of electric monopole-constructed substances that travel at velocities less than electromagnetic light, c. The inner layer of the personality-self is comprised of magnetic monopole-constructed substances that all travel faster than c but slower than magnetoelectric light, c^2. This is the body we put on and grow during embryo development and take off during the physical death process. The single lifetime experiences of the personality-self become information modulations of the unique carrier wave frequency of the personality-self and the key information is passed on to the unique, higher frequency, carrier wave of the soul-self during the physical death process. The soul-self grows more and more infrastructure as part of its three layers via the many re-embodiment experiences with different personality-selves. When the soul-spirit has learned all it can from the multiple embodiment experiences in the physical reality classroom, it graduates by being absorbed into our high spirit-self and transfers all its key information to this unique carrier wave frequency.

312

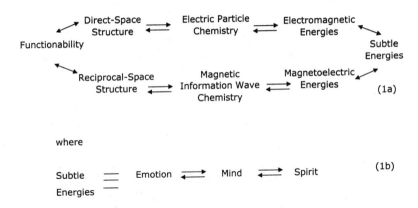

Figure A.1 A reaction equation metaphor connecting a human's ability to function in the world to various structural and energetic aspects of nature.

Returning now to focus on the personality-self, the prime directive is all about growth of personal consciousness and becoming all that one has the potential to become in that particular physical lifetime experience. Some of these experiences lead to traumas that lower the functionability of the personality-self and that is what energy psychologists endeavor to correct via various treatment modalities acting on the acupuncture meridian/chakra system of the individual. Some trauma-structures are built in from the very beginning of a new-life experience. At some time during this personality-self's lifetime, the needed information may have been gained and that particular constraint has the possibility of being removed so the therapist will probably be successful with their treatments because the soul-self will provide positive feedback to support such a change. However, if the necessary information has not yet been gained, the soul-self will provide negative feedback to the therapist's efforts and it will look like an unsuccessful treatment. This is an oversimplification, but it will serve for now.

Our research (Tiller, 1997; Tiller, Dibble, & Kohane, 2001) has shown us that we need to shift our reference frame (RF) for viewing nature from a single 4-space, that we call spacetime, to a particular biconformal base-space (BCBS) RF consisting of two, *reciprocal* 4-spaces, one of which is spacetime. The great advantage of this particular choice is that it yields

1. simultaneous electric particle and magnetic information wave aspects to any measurable quality, so that *any* physical measurement consists of a D-space part *and* an R-space part;

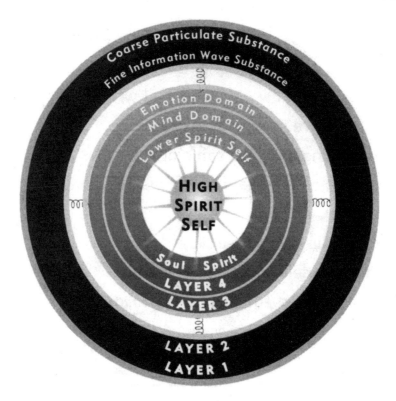

Figure A.2 The whole person, biobodysuit metaphor. Each layer has unique substance and infrastructure. The outer 2 layers constitute temporal physical reality. The middle shell is non-temporal and could be called the soul. The layer infrastructures and the coupling between layers largely determine the state of wellness of the whole person.

2. theoretically predictable connectedness between any point in D-space with any other point in D-space via the mathematical linkage to R-space plus the degree of coupling between the v < c substances of D-space and the v > c substances of R-space;
3. local forces from the D-space aspect and non-local forces from the R-space aspect with the magnitude of the latter depending upon the magnitude of this coupling medium present; and
4. information entanglement between any two seemingly separate parts of a multi-part experimental system in spacetime.

This latter result applies both to spatial separations and temporal separations and this is uniquely relevant to practitioner/client interactions in energy psychology.

To provide the necessary coupler medium, I invented a substance called *deltrons* from the higher dimensional domain of emotion (a 9-space) that is outside of the constraints of Einstein's relativity theory so it can travel at $v < c$ to interact with D-space substance and also at $v > c$ to interact with R-space substance. Thus, the picture we should always hold in mind is that shown in Figure A.3

It is intention from the spirit-self that drives the domain of mind to mobilize the domain of emotion and thus modulate the degree of deltron activation. This process can either weakly or strongly influence substance and events in physical reality (D-space plus R-space aspects). With greater degrees of deltron activation, we witness increases in the magnitude of the R-space contribution to any measurement event.

Our experiments have shown us that larger degrees of deltron coupling present in a given space coincides with a higher electromagnetic (EM) gauge symmetry of the space than the normal U(1) state (towards the SU(2) state, where electric and magnetic monopoles naturally coexist). The SU(2) state is a state having appreciably higher thermodynamic free energy per unit volume than the U(1) state. Because of this, it can deliver useful work to the U(1) state in the form of chemical, electric, and optical processes. These same experiments have also shown us that all humans have the acupuncture meridian/chakra system of their bodies at this higher EM gauge symmetry state. This is the system that pumps chi or prana through the first inner layer of our personality-self (Figure A.2) and enlivens all the processes of the outermost layer. Thus, human bioelectromagnetism is very different from conventional Maxwellian EM.

Turning now to the processes and procedures of energy psychology, it is important to remember that we have electromagnetism for local forces, magnetoelectrism for non-local forces, and deltrons for coupling

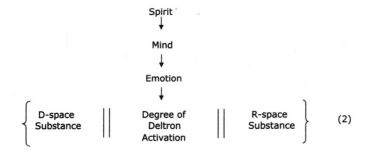

Figure A.3 A Conceptual Process Path Whereby Human Intention, From the Spirit Level of the Soul-Self, Acts on Physical Reality via Modulation of the Coupling Medium Between the Two Layers of the Personality-Self in Figure A.2.

plus modulators of this coupling coming from the higher dimensional aspects of ourselves (i.e., Figure A.3). Thus the very minimum number of parts involved in the practitioner/client system is three:

1. the client's personality-self,
2. the practitioner's personality-self, and
3. the EM gauge symmetry state of the connecting space between them.

The mathematical result of their interaction event will contain terms like (1)(1), (2)(2), (1)(2), (1)(3), and (2)(3). Thus, entanglement of the (1)(2), (1)(3) and (2)(3) types will appear in the results of the treatment events with both spatial and temporal separations involved. Addition of the two soul-selve's connection to the treatment events expands our system to a minimum of five parts with corresponding additional terms connected to and influencing the final result.

Evolving thought field therapy (EvTFT) is implicit in the operational aspects of Figure A.3. Mind is the builder, as many have said, but emotion provides the power for the mind's signal which, in turn, is initiated by the intent from the spirit aspect of self. It is the detailed infrastructure of the acupuncture/meridian–chakra system, which switches are open and which are closed, that determines how well the chi/prana pump is working for a particular individual. We have a variety of mechanisms for altering the switches in this circuitry and various modalities of energy psychology use different procedures for resetting such switches. In this book, the touch and breathe (TAB) procedure is favored. The "science of breath" with focused intent is an ancient and powerful technique coming to us from yogic traditions and acting in us as illustrated in Figure A.3. Repeatedly restoring the proper switch positions in our acupuncture meridian/chakra system is what allows the chi/prana flow to properly nourish all aspects of our personality-selves. Producing a proper lifestyle by the individual is what keeps these switches in their proper position. Sustained and proper intent over time of *all* involved in the treatment events is an important part of the healing process.

William A. Tiller, Ph.D.
Professor *Emeritus*, Stanford University

APPENDICES

Appendix 1

FIELD PHENOMENA: ENERGY DEFINITION OF TRANSFERENCE AND COUNTER TRANSFERENCE

This paper describes some observations outside the expected direction made during evolving thought field therapy (EvTFT) workshops. The variations in the observations could be described in classical terms as transference and counter transference, but an expanded explanation using the concept of *energetic intersubjectivity* is provided. Some parallel discussions and metaphors are drawn from physics to formulate possible hypotheses for EvTFT model building.

The analogy of three baseball umpires discussing their craft—used by Bernstein to explain three theoretical positions for quantum physics—is applicable as well to psychology in the twenty-first century. The first umpire claims, "I call 'em like I see 'em." The second states, "I call 'em the way they are." And the last believes, "They ain't *nothin* till I calls 'em" (1991, p. 96). The first umpire represents the idea that one has only a subjective worldview; the second two represent in a "homey" way the difference between the theories of Einstein and Bohr. Although the three umpires' perspectives are all respresented in various psychological theoretical positions, one could posit that the worldview of psychodynamically-oriented psychologists best fits the subjective claim of the first umpire's statement. One could postulate that the second umpire's statement, which allows for and even commends objectivity, is most consistent with the worldview of behavioral or research psychologists. Unlike the first two umpires' statements, psychologists may have difficulty incorporating the statement of the third umpire into traditional models. Such arguments are reminiscent of those offered by philosophers like George Berkeley and David Hume. Questions such as "Is there an objective reality?" "Does reality exists only with each single observer?" "Is there an ultimate, universal observer?"—all of these were resurrected by physics. But each of these questions is important to psychology as well. The parallel for EvTFT regards what role, if any, the observer/therapist plays in the diagnosis of treatment sequence. In light of the third umpire's conceptualization of a world that exists only because he "calls 'em," what is the nature of interpersonal influences and communications? Can interpersonal influences and communications be described in terms of an expanded model that includes energetic intersubjective fields? Could transference and counter transference be but a subset of the activities occurring in these fields?

During training workshops, The BDB Group provides for extensive practical experiences and participants have opportunities to do EvTFT with immediate feedback. These occasions have become invaluable not only to our participants, but to John, Victoria, and I as well. The title of this book is *Evolving Thought Field Therapy* for this very reason. Each contact with EvTFT has brought us new insights and has raised more questions. As we tell our participants, "You are pioneers in the energy therapies, and it is critical that you not become mechanical or complacent about this clinical work. You must continually use your observations and gathered information to help with the formulation of testable hypotheses."

Extrapolating from the story of the three umpires, one hypothesis is that differences among psychotherapists could result in differences in diagnosed treatment points using EvTFT. It is suggested that such differences in diagnosed treatment sequences could not be accounted for as only an artifact of therapist skill and experience; it is not an aberration or an error. Instead, the possibility exists that the differences result from an energetic interaction that, by the nature of the relationship between the therapist and the patient, must influence diagnosis. Furthermore, it may be possible that, because of difficulties in clearing one's mind, such interactions occur without intention of the therapist. And so it may be that regardless of intention, the thought field of the therapist becomes part of and may even help to create the client's system that is being diagnosed and treated.

It is in the spirit of remaining open to the possible influences that may occur with or without intention—or by the very "what is" of the phenomenon—that I describe our clinical observations and go on to interpret the problems encountered during EvTFT workshops. Both observations and problems have added to our thinking.

Early in my work with thought field therapy workshops, I observed a participant in a practicum group of three muscle-tested strong/strong having stating, "I want to be over this problem/I want to keep this problem." As the facilitator, I informed this practicum group about double reversals; that both participant–client and participant–therapist were possibly reversed. I explained that this could mean that they both were having problems regarding a similar issue.[1] In order to test the hypothesis that both were reversed, I asked if I could muscle test the participant–client before she treated herself.[2] I expected that I would find weak on "I want to be over this problem" and strong on "I want to keep this problem." To my surprise, when I did the muscle testing, the participant–client tested strong for "I want to be over this problem" and weak for "I want to keep the problem." In other words, the participant–client was not reversed for the problem when I tested her. Conjecturing that the reversal in the participant–client may somehow have been "fixed" during the discussion, we had the original participant–therapist muscle test again. The initial therapist again got a strong/strong response. Perplexed, I asked both to rub the NLR area while saying an affirmation ("I deeply and profoundly accept myself with all my problems and limitations."). Yet I found no change in the response for this dyad. They were unable to "fix" the reversal whether by this traditional method, nor by treatment at the side of the hand.

Fortunately, the same training offered a second opportunity to see this same phenomenon occur for another group of three. The participant–client had strong/strong muscle responses when the colleague tested and strong/weak when I tested. This time I had the third group member muscle-test the participant–client and she got results identical to mine. What I then noticed was that the two of us had stood to the side of the participant–client while muscle testing. The original therapist had stood solidly in front. I asked the original participant–therapist to test once more, this time standing to the side of the participant–client and this time he got the anticipated strong/weak response.

At this point, the entire group of participants was asked to experiment, doing the muscle testing in front of one another[3] versus to the side.[4] For most cases, there did not seem to be a difference whether one tested directly in front versus to the side; but, level of felt comfort for the participant–client was clearly in favor of the test from the side. No participant indicated that the position of the therapist to the side engendered discomfort, while a significant number of the participants tested as reversed or non-polarized (strong/strong) with the participant–therapist directly in front of them. It appeared that one factor for the non-polarized or reversed muscle response was related to a clear difference in size between the tester and the subject, when the former was significantly larger in size than the later. This was not necessarily indicative of a double reversal, since the subject was not reversed on the problem. When asked about it, the participant–client related minimal awareness of being uncomfortable with the position of the participant–therapist, but a heightened consciousness when we talked about the circumstances. Interestingly, some participant–therapists when cautioned of this field possibility, kept a position in front of the participant–client and had to be reminded by their now test-wise subjects to stand to the side.

One needs to notice why a skilled therapist would choose to ignore information from their patient.[5] Further, one might wonder about this "field phenomena" and its possible relevance in explaining the traditional notions of transference/counter transference as described by Freud. When Freud suggested that therapists sit away from patients, he was aware that the presence of the therapist influenced the patient. He determined this presence as interference with the progress of treatment. Clearly in psychodynamic parlance, there are occasions in which clients/patients respond to therapists as if the therapists were part of their past or present normal social environment and the therapists responds to clients in kind. This idea that therapist and patient influence one another could be explained in energy terms as tuning into or being connected to each other's bio-field or thought field; and just as psychoanalysts pay careful attention to the experience, we too may gain invaluable information by doing the same.

With this in mind, I have continued to randomly assess participants in EvTFT trainings, to see if my presence created a different response than did the presence of another colleague. In one situation, a participant–client showed a polarity reversal on her name when I tested her and normal polarity when tested by another participant with whom she'd been working. Each time I tested, the participant–client showed strong to a name other than her own (a name of her own selection) and weak to her own, but she responded appropriately strong to her name and weak to the other when the colleague tested. When I was muscle-tested by the colleague, I, too, showed normal polarity. The brief energy correction and collarbone breathing treatment did not correct the problem, nor did attempts to correct with affirmations using the NLR area and the side of hand. I intuited that there might be a problem for the participant with me, and I asked her about that possibility. She agreed it was a possibility. So I had her rub the NLR area and state, "I deeply and profoundly accept myself even though I am having trouble with Sheila." The polarity problem that was previously demonstrated with me muscle-testing her was then resolved. (In hindsight, it could have been possible to treat the problem as an unknown block, but we had not formulated the concept of an unknown block at that time and this guess that resulted in successful correction was an interesting addition to my understanding of energetic exchanges.)

It is critical that we understand that this notion of interpersonal energy interaction carries with it positive as well as negative potential. Victoria, John, and I had occasion to ask Tapas Fleming, developer of TAT (Tapas Acupressure Technique), how she handled polarity reversals. (We were using the term *polarity reversal* in a generic sense because at that time our conceptualization of polarized versus non-polarized responses was less formed.) Tapas said that she did not do anything about reversals because she had never encountered any, and in fact found the idea foreign to her way of thinking. Fortuitously, the next day at a workshop taught by Tapas, Victoria encountered an issue-specific PR when facilitating. Two training participants each checked the participant–client and found the reversal, thus corroborating Victoria's findings. Tapas was then called over so that she could witness an example of the reversal. When Tapas muscle-tested the participant–client there was no reversal, however. Then the members of the group each muscle tested the participant–client once again and now found no reversal. The reversal in this situation had resolved.

It is important to note that, unlike the other related circumstances in which the participant–therapist had negatively influenced the participant–client's polarity, Tapas had seemingly "healed" an issue-specific PR in the client simply through her presence in the participant–client's field. It may be conjectured that some healer's energetic field properly polarizes the field of those in contact with it and that it is this process in itself that imparts the healing potential.

The possibilities for healing and healing at a distance are not foreign. If we allow ourselves once again to borrow from concepts formulated in physics (e.g., the possibilities of action at a distance and speeds faster than light) we can come to a better understanding of the experiences we are describing. Physicists have an edge on psychology in this kind of speculation, in that physicists allow for thought experiments until they have developed an actual apparatus capable of carrying out the experiment. This is a luxury and freedom that we as psychologists have not allowed ourselves.

In the early 1980s Alain Aspect was able to perform an experiment that had been thought about for decades before. The study concerned experimentation on a pair of photons in a way that there could be no communication between them at, or less than, the speed of light. John Bell was later interviewed about Aspect's study (Davies & Brown, 1986). The interviewer summarized Aspect's experiment and suggested to Bell that Aspect's study had challenged Bell's two assumptions. With this in mind, the interviewer asked Bell if only one of his two assumptions could be salvaged, which would he hold onto: an external reality without an observer or no faster-than-light signaling? Bell responded, "I think it's a deep dilemma, and the resolution of it will not be trivial; it will require a substantial change in the way we look at things. . ." (Davies & Brown, 1986, p. 51). In that interview, Bell went on to say that he was convinced that quantum theory was only a temporary expedient and that the founding fathers of the theory prided themselves on giving up the idea of explanation and dealing only with describing the phenomena; they regarded this shift as the price one paid for coming to terms with nature.

These responses are of interest to us because they set an example for keeping an open mind about the possibility of faster than light signaling and, by abstraction, potential explanations for the clinical observations made during EvTFT sessions.

Further conjecture about the energetic basis of transference and counter transference would then require the understanding that we cannot help but act as an influence. No matter how far we stand or sit from our clients, we are bound to them in an energetic relationship. It is therefore most important that we not ignore, and in fact are mindful of, this important connection with them.

Sheila S. Bender, Ph.D.

ADDITIONAL BELIEF RELATED BLOCKS

There are many belief related blocks (BRBs) that can impede successful treatment. The BRBs offered below as examples and are by no means represent a complete list. You and your patient can collaborate on exploring other beliefs, unique to the patient, that may be blocking treatment. All corrections are initially made at the small intestine treatment point on the side of the hand unless otherwise noted. If this correction does not work, repeat the correction using the NLR area. If this does not correct the BRB, then the correction point(s) must be diagnosed. The optional additional statement, "Its cause and all it means and does to me," can be added to any or all of the statements. If this optional statement is used in the test statement, it should be use in the correction statement.

TYPE OF BRB	TEST STATEMENTS	CORRECTIONS
Self Trust	"I am able to trust myself to get over this problem . . . " and, "I am unable to trust myself to get over this problem. . . . "	"I deeply accept myself even if I am unable to trust myself to get over this problem. . . . "
Responsibility	"I am able to take responsibility to get over this problem . . . " and, "I am unable to take responsibility to get over this problem. . . ."	"I deeply accept myself even if I am unable to take responsibility to get over this problem. . . ."
Loneliness	"I will not be lonely if I get over this problem . . . " and, "I will be lonely if I get over this problem. . . ."	"I deeply accept myself even if I will be lonely when I get over this problem. . . ."
Control	"I will be in control if I get over this problem . . ." and, "I will not be in control if I get over this problem. . . ."	"I deeply accept myself even if I will not be in control when I get over this problem. . . . " (Correct using the governing vessel treatment point under the nose.)

TYPE OF BRB	TEST STATEMENTS	CORRECTIONS
Fear of Losing an Important Aspect of Self	"I will keep all important aspects of myself if I get over this problem . . . " and, "I will lose an important aspect of myself if I get over this problem. . . ."	"I deeply accept myself even if I lose an important aspect of myself in getting over this problem. . . ."
Connection	"I will keep my connection with (someone important) if I get over this problem . . ." and, "I will lose my connection with (someone important) if I get over this problem. . . ."	"I deeply accept myself even if I lose my connection with (someone important) if I get over this problem. . . ."
Option	"It is an option for me to get over this problem . . ." and, "It is not an option for me to get over this problem. . . ."	"I deeply accept myself even if it is not an option for me to get over this problem. . . ." (Correct using the governing vessel treatment point under the nose.)
Possibility	"It is possible for me to get over this problem . . ." and, "It is not possible for me to get over this problem. . . ."	"I deeply accept myself even if it is not possible for me to get over this problem. . . ."
Willpower	"I have the willpower to get over this problem . . ." and, "I do not have the willpower to get over this problem. . . ."	"I deeply accept myself even if I do not have the willpower to get over this problem. . . ." (Correct using the governing vessel treatment point under the nose.)
Powerlessness	"I have the power to get over this problem . . ." and, "I am powerless to get over this problem. . . ."	"I deeply accept myself even if I am powerless to get over this problem. . . ." (Correct using the governing vessel treatment point under the nose.)
Intelligence	"I am smart enough to get over this problem . . ." and, "I am not smart enough to get over this problem. . . ."	"I deeply accept myself even if I am not smart enough to get over this problem. . . ."
Deprivation	"I will not be deprived if I get over this problem . . ." and, "I will be deprived if I get over this problem. . . ."	"I deeply accept myself even if I am deprived when I get over this problem. . . ." (Correct using the governing vessel treatment point under the nose.)

THE BDB GROUP FLOWCHARTS

The BDB Group Flowcharts
Phase 1: Evaluating and Preparing the Energy Connection

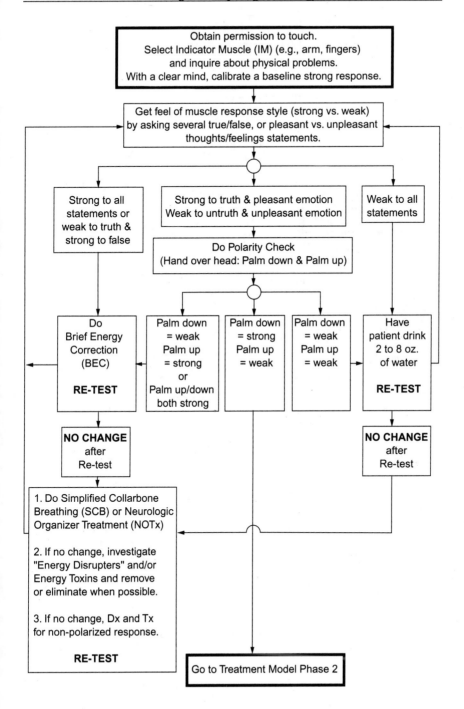

Obtain permission to touch.
Select Indicator Muscle (IM) (e.g., arm, fingers)
and inquire about physical problems.
With a clear mind, calibrate a baseline strong response.

Get feel of muscle response style (strong vs. weak)
by asking several true/false, or pleasant vs. unpleasant
thoughts/feelings statements.

Strong to all
statements or
weak to truth &
strong to false

Strong to truth & pleasant emotion
Weak to untruth & unpleasant emotion

Weak to all
statements

Do Polarity Check
(Hand over head: Palm down & Palm up)

Do
Brief Energy
Correction
(BEC)

RE-TEST

Palm down
= weak
Palm up
= strong
or
Palm up/down
both strong

Palm down
= strong
Palm up
= weak

Palm down
= weak
Palm up
= weak

Have
patient drink
2 to 8 oz.
of water

RE-TEST

NO CHANGE
after
Re-test

NO CHANGE
after
Re-test

1. Do Simplified Collarbone
Breathing (SCB) or Neurologic
Organizer Treatment (NOTx)

2. If no change, investigate
"Energy Disrupters" and/or
Energy Toxins and remove
or eliminate when possible.

3. If no change, Dx and Tx
for non-polarized response.

RE-TEST

Go to Treatment Model Phase 2

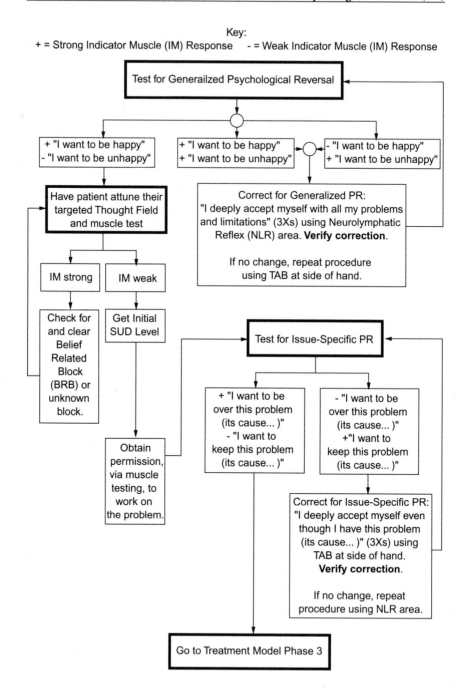

Key:
+ = Strong Indicator Muscle (IM) Response   - = Weak Indicator Muscle (IM) Response

Test for Generailzed Psychological Reversal

+ "I want to be happy"
- "I want to be unhappy"

+ "I want to be happy"
+ "I want to be unhappy"

- "I want to be happy"
+ "I want to be unhappy"

Have patient attune their targeted Thought Field and muscle test

Correct for Generalized PR:
"I deeply accept myself with all my problems and limitations" (3Xs) using Neurolymphatic Reflex (NLR) area. **Verify correction.**

If no change, repeat procedure using TAB at side of hand.

IM strong

IM weak

Check for and clear Belief Related Block (BRB) or unknown block.

Get Initial SUD Level

Test for Issue-Specific PR

+ "I want to be over this problem (its cause...)"
- "I want to keep this problem (its cause...)"

- "I want to be over this problem (its cause...)"
+ "I want to keep this problem (its cause...)"

Obtain permission, via muscle testing, to work on the problem.

Correct for Issue-Specific PR:
"I deeply accept myself even though I have this problem (its cause...)" (3Xs) using TAB at side of hand.
Verify correction.

If no change, repeat procedure using NLR area.

Go to Treatment Model Phase 3

NOTE: Therapist can use CDdx-p, CDdx-t, TDdx, or a combination of these models

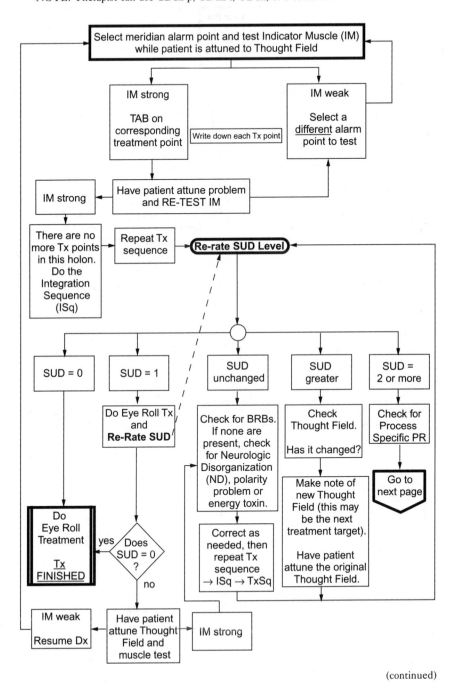

(continued)

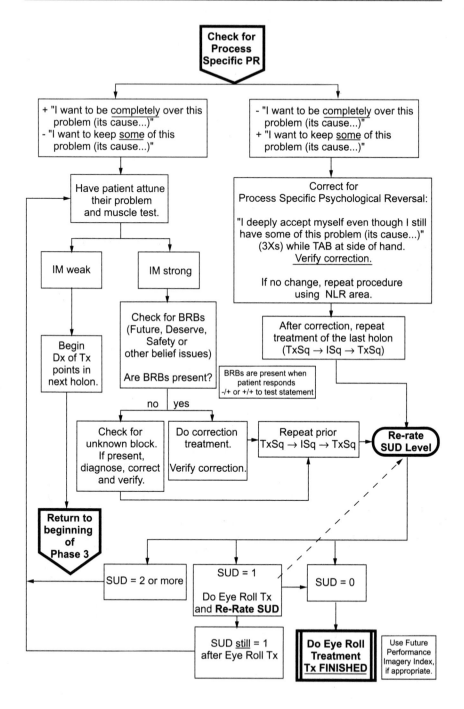

Check for Process Specific PR

+ "I want to be <u>completely</u> over this problem (its cause...)"
- "I want to keep <u>some</u> of this problem (its cause...)"

- "I want to be <u>completely</u> over this problem (its cause...)"
+ "I want to keep <u>some</u> of this problem (its cause...)"

Have patient attune their problem and muscle test.

Correct for Process Specific Psychological Reversal:

"I deeply accept myself even though I still have some of this problem (its cause...)" (3Xs) while TAB at side of hand.
<u>Verify correction.</u>

If no change, repeat procedure using NLR area.

IM weak

IM strong

Begin Dx of Tx points in next holon.

Check for BRBs (Future, Deserve, Safety or other belief issues)

Are BRBs present?

After correction, repeat treatment of the last holon (TxSq → ISq → TxSq)

BRBs are present when patient responds -/+ or +/+ to test statement

no | yes

Check for unknown block. If present, diagnose, correct and verify.

Do correction treatment.

Verify correction.

Repeat prior TxSq → ISq → TxSq

Re-rate SUD Level

Return to beginning of Phase 3

SUD = 2 or more

SUD = 1

Do Eye Roll Tx and **Re-Rate SUD**

SUD = 0

SUD <u>still</u> = 1 after Eye Roll Tx

Do Eye Roll Treatment Tx FINISHED

Use Future Performance Imagery Index, if appropriate.

THE BDB GROUP EvTFT HEALING AT HOME WORKSHEET

Treatment Sequence for   Date:

1. Tune-in to your problem. Rate your level of upset from 0-10.

2. CORRECT (if checked)
Body Energy
- Brief Energy Correction ⇒
- Over Energy Correction
- Simplified Collarbone Breathing
- NOTx

> **BRIEF ENERGY CORRECTION**
> Place fingertips of left hand on your belly button. With right hand:
> - Touch both collarbone points & take one full respiration
> - Touch under your nose (GV) & take one full respiration
> - Touch under your lip (CV) & & take one full respiration
> - Touch base of your spine & take one full respiration
>
> Now, place your right hand on your belly button, and with your left hand repeat the same four steps.

Psychological Reversal
- Generalized Reversal (rub sore spot) ⇒
- Issue-Specific PR (TAB* on side of hand)

- Recurrent Reversal (rub sore spot) ⇒
- Belief Related Blocks ⇒

(Say 3 times)
"I deeply accept myself, with all my problems and limitations."
"I deeply accept myself, even though I have this problem, its cause, and all that it means and does to me."
"I deeply accept myself even though this problem has come back."
"I deeply accept myself, even if
- I will never get over this problem its cause and all it means and does to me" (TAB under nose)
- It's not safe to get over this . . . " (TAB under nose)
- I deserve to keep this problem . . . " (TAB under lip)

(continued)

333

(continued)

3. TREATMENT is done while you are tuned into or thinking about your problem. TAB* one full respiration at each meridian site. Please do in sequence.

☐ Treat bilaterally (if checked)

4. Do the Integration Sequence:
   A. TAB on the collarbone points, while attuned to your problem.
   B. Now do the following in sequence while maintaining contact at the collarbone points:
      1) Eyes open
      2) Eyes closed
      3) Eyes open & look down to your right
      4) Eyes open & look down to your left
      5) Do a 360° circle with your eyes (clockwise)
      6) Do a 360° circle with your eyes (counter clockwise)
      7) Hum a TUNE, out loud for 5 seconds
      8) Count 1 to 5, out loud
      9) Hum a TUNE (again), for 5 seconds

<table>
<tr><td>HEALING AT HOME INSTRUCTIONS</td></tr>
<tr><td>_____</td></tr>
<tr><td>_____</td></tr>
<tr><td>_____</td></tr>
<tr><td>_____</td></tr>
</table>

5. REPEAT entire treatment sequence in step 3 above

6. Re-rate your upset level from 0 to 10.
   A. If upset level now down to 1 or 0, go to Eye Roll treatment (step 7).
   B. If upset level is greater than 1, do the following:
      1) TAB at the side of your hand, saying 3 times, "I deeply accept myself, even if I STILL have SOME of this problem . . . "
      2) NOW REPEAT ALL TREATMENTS in steps 3, 4, and 5.

7. Do EYE ROLL treatment:
   A. TAB on the collarbone points, while attuned to your problem.
   B. While maintaining contact at the collarbone points,
      1) Close your eyes.
      2) Open your eyes.
      3) Lower eyes to the ground.
      4) Slowly roll your eyes upward to the sky, taking 5 to 7 seconds. Treatment is now complete.

* TAB = Touch And Breathe

(continued)

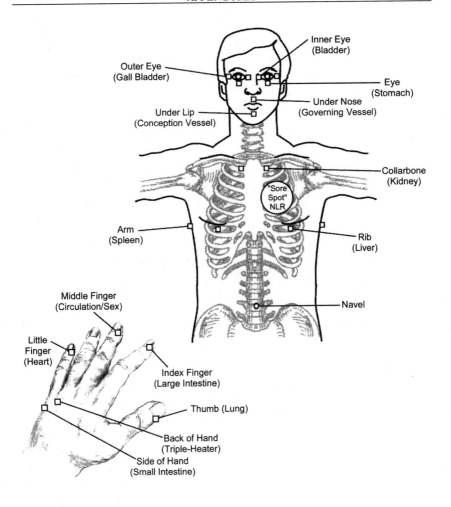

Inner Eye (Bladder)

Outer Eye (Gall Bladder)

Eye (Stomach)

Under Nose (Governing Vessel)

Under Lip (Conception Vessel)

Collarbone (Kidney)

"Sore Spot" NLR

Arm (Spleen)

Rib (Liver)

Navel

Middle Finger (Circulation/Sex)

Little Finger (Heart)

Index Finger (Large Intestine)

Thumb (Lung)

Back of Hand (Triple-Heater)

Side of Hand (Small Intestine)

THE BDB GROUP EvTFT HEALING AT HOME WORKSHEET (ELATERS)

Treatment Sequence for: Date:

1. Tune in your enjoyment of _____, knowing it is not good for you or your body. Rate your current level of enjoyment or benefit from 0 to 10.

2. CORRECT
   Body Energy
   • Brief Energy Correction →
   • Over Energy Correction
   • Simplified Collarbone Breathing
   • NOTx

BRIEF ENERGY CORRECTION
Place fingertips of left hand on your navel. With right hand:
• Touch both collarbone points & take one full respiration
• Touch under your nose (GV) & take one full respiration
• Touch under your lip (CV) & & take one full respiration
• Touch base of your spine & take one full respiration
Now, place fingertips of your right hand on your navel, and with your left hand repeat the same four steps above.

   Psychological Reversal

   • Generalized Reversal (rub sore spot) →

   • Issue-Specific PR (TAB* on side of hand) →

   • Recurrent Reversal →

   • Belief Related Block →

   (Say each statement 3 times when indicated.)

   "I deeply accept myself, with all my problems and limitations."

   "I deeply accept myself, even though I enjoy_____, which I know is not good for me and/or my body."

   "I deeply accept myself even though my enjoyment of _____ has come back."

   "I deeply accept myself, even if
   • It's not safe to be over my enjoyment of . . . (TAB under nose)
   • I don't deserve to be over my enjoyment of . . . (TAB under lip)
   • I never get over my enjoyment of _____, its cause & all it means and does to me" (TAB under nose)

3. TREATMENT is done while attuned to your enjoyment or benefit, knowing that it is not good for you or your body. TAB*, one full respiration, at each meridian site. Please do in sequence.

4. Do the Integration Sequence:
   A. TAB on your collarbone points while attuned to your enjoyment of _____, knowing it is not good for you.
   B. Now do the following in sequence while maintaining contact with the collarbone points:

   1) Eyes open

   2) Eyes closed

   3) Eyes open & look down to your right
   4) Eyes open & look down to your left

   5) Rotate your eyes all the way around one way
   6) Rotate your eyes all the way around the other way
   7) Hum a TUNE out loud for 5 secondsi
   8) Count 1 to 5 out loud
   9) Hum a tune (again) for 5 seconds

5. REPEAT entire treatment sequence in 3 above

```
HEALING AT HOME INSTRUCTIONS

_____
_____
_____
```

6. Re-rate your enjoyment level from 0 to 10.
   A. If enjoyment level now down to 1 or 0, go to Eye Roll treatment (step 7).
   B. If enjoyment level is greater than 1, do the following:
      1) TAB at the side of your hand, saying 3 times, "I deeply accept myself, even if I STILL have SOME of this enjoyment of . . ."
      2) NOW REPEAT ALL TREATMENTS in steps 3, 4, and 5.

7. Do EYE ROLL treatment:
   A. TAB on the collarbone points, while attuned to your enjoyment of . . .
   B. While maintaining contact at the collarbone points,
      1) Close your eyes.
      2) Open your eyes.
      3) Lower eyes to the ground.
      4) Slowly roll your eyes upward to the sky, taking 5 to 7 seconds. Treatment is now complete.

* TAB = Touch And Breathe

(continued)

(continued)

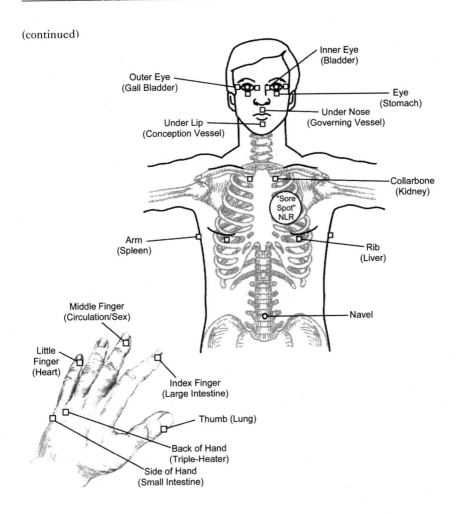

Appendix 6

January 11, 2001
Re: The recent research debate

Hi Everyone,
Here are some politically incorrect thoughts about recent posts concerning psychotherapy research. I know the following thoughts may strike some as intellectually absurd, but somehow I believe they need to be said. And by the way, I was trained in a research-oriented clincal psychology program, so I am quite aware of how one might attack these thoughts; I could do so myself if required.

Having been a psychologist for 30 years, I am totally unimpressed with what anyone might say about the effectiveness of one approach versus another. Positive results tend to get published, negative results don't, so what is published is not a random sample of the research that occurs. I see research as a never-ending series of studies that raises more questions than are answered. Every study ends with the statement "clearly more research is needed in this area." Sounds good, but it only occurs because the real conclusions that can be reached from the study that was done are nil. Somebody publishes a study here, another there; there is no real replication, and therefore no real conclusions can be reached. There are so many variables to consider in any study that anyone can easily criticize and devastate any study done. Heck, I am reading a book entitled *From Placebo to Panacea: Putting Psychiatric Drugs to the Test* (Fisher & Greenberg, 1997). Truth is, even in drug research, it looks like the emperor has no clothes. What could be simpler than giving somebody a pill and assessing the result? Well, how about the attitude of the investigator, the size of the pill, the shape of the pill, the color of the pill? All these have been implicated in how somebody responds to a placebo. If the drug research is really such a mess, and my readings from multiple sources suggest it is, how could we possibly hope that something as complicated as psychotherapy research is going to lead to any universally accepted conclusions? I know, I know, if it is only done right, we can do it. It won't happen, and I would be willing to bet a fair amount of money that in thirty years psychologists and others are going to be arguing about the same old issues, and there will be no body of universally accepted conclusions. Frankly, I see psychotherapy research as irrelevant to what therapists do in the field. Therapists have a huge tendency to pick an approach that matches their personality, practice it, and rationalize it to themselves and others. Really, how many therapists do we know whose approach has been substantially altered by "psychotherapy research?" I've known many therapists over the last 30 years, and I don't see that happening.

So what do I think works in therapy? Listening, compassion, de-shaming people, and Thought Field Therapy. Can I prove it? Nope. But I don't think there has been any double-blind studies done which prove that the sun rises in the East, yet I have a pretty good idea that it does.

And with that I am going on vacation. And surely many readers of the above will say, "Thank God, he sure needs it."

Thomas Tudor, Ph.D.
Cherry Hill, NJ

NOTES

INTRODUCTION

1. A major attribute of thought field therapy is that it either works or does nothing in affecting the disturbance level of the patient. Accordingly, the professional responsibility to do no harm was readily upheld in our learning process.

CHAPTER 1

1. The word *disruptive* refers to any negative or positive emotion that fails to serve a beneficial or healthy purpose. This includes treatment of positive emotions that are instrumental in maintaining unwanted and self-defeating behavior patterns. This is described in Chapter 11 as the treatment of elaters.

2. A more complete discussion of Goodheart and his work follows in Chapter 4.

3. Diamond writes in *Life Energy Analysis: A Way To Cantillation* that the primary cause of psychological suffering stems from hatred for one's mother. Cantillation, which he defines as "a state of spirituality, and the process by which it is sought, and attained, and heightened" (1988, p. 2), is the intended goal of his life-energy analysis.

4. Physics-related definitions of *fields* often refer to a space in which magnetic and/or electromagnetic lines of force are active (e.g., gravity field). See Chapter 2 for history.

5. Callahan wrote, "It is important to state that the two links—acupuncture and applied kinesiology—in my discovery are not at all responsible for my new findings; they are my own, as are any unwitting mistakes" (2001, p. xiv).

6. The number of treatment points varies considerably from patient to patient and from thought field to thought field. While an average could be estimated to be between three and six treatment points, there are some patients and conditions that involve many more.

7. The issues regarding treatment sequence are addressed in detail in Chapter 15.

8. Surrogate testing is described in Chapter 12.

9. The BDB Group (Britt-Diepold-Bender) is the name the authors use when providing workshops on EvTFT.

10. A major attribute of thought field therapy is that it either works or does nothing in effecting the disturbance level of the patient. Accordingly the professional responsibility to do no harm was readily upheld in our learning process.

11. *Thought field therapy basic* is a term we have applied to distinguish the original model from EvTFT.

CHAPTER 2

1. Researchers in many different fields, including sociology and literary criticism, often see themselves as working in or trying to break out of paradigms. In our recounting of the roots of the EvTFT paradigm, we draw largely on the guidelines set by Thomas Kuhn and Charles Coulston Gillispie, who wrote detailed histories of scientific paradigm shifts.

2. Gillispie used by way of illustration the reasons that the labels *anode* and *cathode*, so well thought through and described by Michael Faraday in his time, would not find their way into a modern textbook on electricity. Gillispie wondered how many physicists know why *anode* stands for positive and *cathode* for negative (1960, p. 447).

3. Interestingly, although the words *homicide* and *suicide* have long been in the language, *genocide* was not coined until the 1940s to describe what was happening with Adolf Hitler's regime.

4. For an interesting discussion of this concept, the reader is directed to Arthur Koestler, *The Ghost in the Machine* (1967).

5. Koestler pointed out how the Papez-MacLean theory offers strong evidence for the dissonant functioning of the phylogentically old and new cortex, which provides a basis for the paranoid streak running through human history (1967, p. 296).

6. Nicolaus Copernicus as a young man studied Aristarchos, a Greek astronomer who some 2000 years earlier had maintained that the earth rotated around the sun despite criticism that suggested he be indicted for impiety. Frustrated with the inconsistencies of the astronomy of his day and the fact that even the length of the seasonal year was unexplained, Copernicus wanted to avoid the fate of Aristarchos. For a wonderful sense of Corpernicus's struggle in presenting the paradigm shift to a heliocentric position, see Kuhn (1957).

7. The Eastern story is developed in Chapters 3 and 4.

8. Gillispie wrote admiringly of Faraday "and it is indeed interesting, and to anyone with a sense of the drama of culture across the centuries, it is moving to read Faraday, whose own untutored, self-taught state surely left him the nearest thing to a child of nature, not to say a noble savage, that the history of science can show, coming, after a lifetime spent on doing science with his own hands, to that same dilemma between atoms and the continuum which has given structure to the history of science since its opening in Greece.... For in Faraday it is not geometry, as it had been in Descartes and would be again in Einstein, which encompasses matter and energy in extension. It is imagination: 'To my mind, therefore, the ... nucleus vanishes, and the substance consists of the powers; ... and indeed, what notion can we form of the nucleus independent of its powers?'"(1960, p. 456).

9. In place of the conventional picture of the massy atom, Faraday preferred the atoms of Rugerro (Roger) Boscovich, an eighteenth-century Jesuit philosopher who

was out of the mainstream of science and defined atoms only as centers of force and not as particles of matter in which powers somehow inhere (Gillispie, 1960, p. 455).

10. We are extremely fortunate that there are physicists who are drawn into the construction of a new paradigm for the treatment of mind.

11. The idea of jealousies and other human qualities playing into one's judgment are described anecdotally. One story relates how George Bernard Shaw made fun of Charles Darwin. Shaw's linguistic skills were unsurpassed, and yet history places him in a diminished position because he criticized that which he could not understand due to an insufficient scientific background (Gillispie, 1960).

12. Using one's imagination would seem much simpler for the social scientist than doing mathematics, but social scientists are less likely to accept imagination as possible for research conceptualization than physicists. Thought experiments, a playground for physicists, are not considered acceptable for psychology.

13. See David Bohm and Basil Hiley (1993) for a recent analogy for the concept of fields which suggests that all fields have at every point a potential pair of north and south poles which by necessity overlap. The poles are only abstractions for the purposes of representing what is in actuality an unbroken whole. They go on to relate this to the artificial but necessary distinctions between mind and body. This discussion of implicate order is further discussed in Chapter 7 and the Epilogue.

14. For another interesting historical development that dates back to Socrates, Plato, and Aristotle, the reader is directed to the introduction to the fourth edition of Korzybski's *Science and Sanity* (1980).

15. The reader will find that these points correspond with the points outlined by Kuhn (1996) as being optimal for a paradigm shift.

16. In his book *Gödel, Escher, Bach* Douglas Hofstadter explains how record players are limited to hi fidelity and never reach perfect fidelity. With perfect fidelity, there would be the possibility of the record vibrating at its resonant frequency and thereby shattering. Here is a situation where one might say that perfect is imperfect and imperfect is perfect. In psychology we are frequently faced with situations that have a relative perfection where more is sometimes less and less is more.

17. Thales wrote some 300 years before Aristotle that the primary question was not what do we know, but how do we know it.

18. Konrad Z. Lorenz, Holger Hyden, Wilder Penfield, H. W. Magoun, and Pribram are the contributors.

CHAPTER 3

1. Although the function of blood is fundamental to TCM and is intimately intertwined with chi, it is not overtly relevant to the study of EvTFT. Suffice it to say that blood, according to Jarrett is "a composite of inherited and acquired influences [that] may be viewed as the present embodying the past. Qi, in contrast, may be considered the present creating the future" (1999, p. 300).

2. Walther (1988) noted that therapy localization is most effective when the patient touches the alarm point with the palmer side of the fingers (finger prints) and he speculates that this adds or subtracts "energy" to the system.

3. Treatment location stems from Goodheart's *beginning-and-ending* and *entry-or-exit point* techniques of tapping the beginning and ending points of meridians (Walther, 1988, pp. 211 and 248). This will be further discussed in Chapter 5.

4. All other meridian-based psychotherapies that use a tapping treatment utilize the bladder 2 treatment point (the inside tip of the eyebrow) based upon the Callahan Techniques™. The reason is practical because there is a chance that patients could poke themselves in the eye if they employ tapping on BL-1. The touch-and-breathe treatment eliminates this risk and restores treatment to the preferred point at BL-1.

5. For one of the most enlightening and important conceptualizations of the structure of language and its impact on thinking, the reader is encouraged to read Korzybski's *Science and Sanity* (1980).

6. Woollerton and McLean stated, "The hormones controlled by the pituitary gland include the growth hormone, ACTH, gonadotropic hormones, lactogenic hormones and thyrotropic hormones. The pituitary gland, through the hypothalamus, affects our emotions and the autonomic nervous system. ACTH, or adrenocorticotropic hormone, influences the adrenal glands, which produce epinephrine. This controls blood pressure, pulse, respiration and blood sugar content. It relaxes the bronchial muscles, and it is the trigger for the alarm reaction in an emergency, which releases the reserve of chi stored in the kidneys" (1986, p. 66). It is little wonder that we have observed a more robust effect when treating BL-1, compared to BL-2, for trauma related issues.

CHAPTER 4

1. See the article by Sheila Bender in Appendix 1 regarding transference and counter transference.

2. The reader is referred to Chapter 12 for a further discussion of environmental influences.

3. It has been our clinical observation that these treatments, in and of themselves, can effectively lower anxiety levels. Further, these procedures appear helpful in decreasing levels of chronic rage and instances of unwanted and persistent sexual over-stimulation that can occur with victims of sexual abuse. They may also help increase the ability to concentrate on a task and the level of retention while reading or studying.

4. This is a variation of an exercise commonly known as *Cook's hookup*, developed by Wayne Cook.

CHAPTER 5

1. The core of this chapter originally appeared as Diepold, J. H., Jr., (2000, August). Touch and breathe (TAB): An alternative treatment approach with meridian-based psychotherapies. *Traumatology: The International Journal of Innovations in the Study of Traumatic Process and Methods for Reducing, Preventing, and Eliminating Related Human Suffering*, 6(2), Article 4. Retrieved from http://www.fsu.edu/~trauma/v6i2a4.html

2. Tapping on the bony structure near acupoints possibly causes a piezoelectric

effect, which results when minute amounts of electrical current are generated by stimulating the crystallized calcium in the bone.

3. The *they* in the quote is most likely a reference to chiropractors Goodheart, Walther, and Blaich.

4. Gary Craig, who was an attendee and a presenter at the conference, referred to TAB as *tabbing* (rather than *tapping*), which is how some therapists know this treatment method. The authors are grateful to Gary for the support and exposure he provided for TAB in person and on his EFT Web site.

5. This First Energy Psychology Conference in Europe (2001: An Energy Odyssey) occurred during the first week of July 2001 and was organized by Willem Lammers and the Institute for the Application of the Social Sciences.

6. Eden is the author of *Energy Medicine* (1998) and refers to mudras when she teaches about "radiant circuits" in the body.

7. Gerber described the etheric level as, "The frequency band or octave just beyond the physical octave. Etheric energy or substance vibrates at speeds beyond light velocity and has a magnetic character" (1988, p. 535–536).

CHAPTER 6

1. The ideal intervention for correcting nonpolarized and reversed head-over-head polarity checks is the brief energy correction (BEC) detailed at the end of Chapter 4. If this procedure fails to establish proper polarity, then use another neurologic organizing treatment, such as simplified collarbone breathing or the neurologic organizer treatment.

2. The EvTFT therapist may use the word *problem* to represent the issue being treated. However, the therapist may freely substitute the description of the actual problem (e.g., " I want to be over my fear of bees") using the patient's words when this is judged to be more appropriate and clinically engaging.

3. See Appendix 1 for Sheila Bender's article on energy related transference/counter transference.

CHAPTER 7

1. See Callahan and Callahan's *Thought Field Therapy (TFT) and Trauma: Treatment and Theory* (1996) for an example of "classic" Callahan thinking and terminology explanation. This work contains an extensive Glossary and an annotated bio-energy reference appendix.

2. See the article on energy transference and counter transference in Appendix 1.

CHAPTER 8

1. Like Callahan's choice of the term *majors*, the word *gamut* has a musical reference; it represents the entire series or range of recognized notes in modern music.

2. According to Walther, the six primary EID positions are: (1) eyes down and to the right, (2) eyes directly right, (3) eyes up to the right, (4) eyes up to the left, (5) eyes directly left, and (6) eyes down and to the left (1988, p. 44).

3. See Chapter 13 for information on algorithms.

4. A quick relaxation intervention known as a rapid stress reduction technique sandwiches the ISq between two ERs. While attuned to the identified stressor the patient does the following: eye-roll → integration sequence → eye-roll (ER → ISq → ER).

CHAPTER 9

1. Callahan wrote that meridian diagnosis is a "causal diagnostic procedure because it disgnoses the root cause of the problem, unlike traditional diagnosis in psychology which is diagnosis from categories of symptoms" (1998, p. 14).

2. The number of treatment points varies considerably from patient to patient, from thought field to thought field, and often from therapist to therapist. While an average could be estimated to be between three to six treatment points, there are some patients and conditions that involve many more.

CHAPTER 10

1. With young children, we recommend that the therapist use a progressive series of five to six smiling faces drawn to reflect the 0 to 10-point scale. For example, the first face would be a severely turned down mouth (10), another with a straight/horizontal mouth (5), and the last with a severely up turned mouth (0). The child then points to the face that comes closest to how he or she is feeling.

CHAPTER 11

1. Use of the word *enjoyment* is intended to incorporate any and all positive emotions the individual attaches or derives from the behavior in the identified thought field.

2. Another way to look at the "not being good for the individual" concept is to think of it as "at what cost to me or others."

CHAPTER 12

1. Every meridian site (or NLR area) used to correct psychological reversals in the Callahan Techniques™ thought field therapy is an algorithm approach. That is, each correction site is automatic, depending on the type of psychological reversal, and used because "it works." While there is parsimony in this pragmatic approach, these prescribed correction sites do not always correct the psychological reversal. Bender takes the position that all psychological reversals could be diagnosed for the correc-

tion site and not just those that fail to correct using the prescribed correction sites. Diepold and Britt prefer to diagnose psychological reversals on an as needed basis if the designated correction sites fail.

2. The use of the opposite arm and eye for the re-treatment came about by watching and listening to feedback from patients. Many commented that using the other side was "different" and enhanced the clarity of the imagery even further. These comments were most relevant from patients who previously used this treatment technique without prior regard for bilateral treatment.

3. Instead of using the word *alters* to describe other identity states, we prefer to the word *resources*, which more accurately depicts the defensive and protective functions of the various identity states that are so clearly elaborated with DID patients.

4. Callahan refers to energy disrupters as *energy toxins*. We avoid this term because we can only attest to the disruption in the system and not to the toxicity.

5. For the interested EvTFT diagnostician, a case can be made that both the CDdx-t and the TDdx methods of diagnoses are surrogate models. In this regard the therapist is a functional surrogate for the patient for the process of diagnosis only.

6. The use of the primary therapist as a surrogate for the patient has consistently been at the request of the patients who had dissociative disorder or PTSD diagnoses. All of the patients were abused as children, wanted to avail themselves of EvTFT, and were fearful of being touched by a stranger, but felt safe in the presence of their primary therapists.

7. Although Goodheart (1987) believed that an energetic link is formed and sustained by physical contact, it has not been our experience that this sustained physical contact is necessary in EvTFT. This is not to say that we do not often have a child or infant sit in a parent's lap as the diagnosis on the child is proceeding. Most often this serves the purpose of face-validity. However, because of Goodheart's belief, we also do not use the diagnostic protocol on an adult, for the adult's problem, while a child is being held or is in physical contact with the adult, in case the child's issues should interfere energetically with the adult's.

CHAPTER 13

1. The work of Muhammad ibn Musa al-Khwarizmi was translated into Latin around the twelfth century, bringing the advantages of the Indo-Arabic method of positional counting, including the use of zero, to a western Europe that was still using Latin numerals.

2. Algorithms are a way to structure the many treatment options when diagnostic methods are not used. Remember, if we think of solutions arrived at strictly by chance, the first treatment point has 14 possibilities. The second treatment point can be any of the 13 remaining points. Since a holon can contain the same treatment point non-sequentially, the 3rd treatment point could be any of the other points not selected including the 1st point (13 points). The number of possibilities would be 14×13 to infinity.

3. In Callahan's terminology this would include massive, specific, and mini forms of psychological reversal. In our terminology this would equate to generalized, issue-specific, and process-specific forms of psychological reversal.

4. Callahan used to use affirmation statements when correcting for psychological reversal but discontinued the use to deflect criticism that his interventions were a form of cognitive therapy.

5. Callahan did not include the liver meridian in the comprehensive algorithm.

CHAPTER 14

1. Therapists should be mindful that some people are only willing to relinquish some but not all of their negative emotions under these conditions. Accordingly, a SUD level of 0 is not necessarily desirable or possible at this time. However, a reduction of a few points can make a substantial difference in the session.

2. Having a parent or guardian present to hear a description of the treatment and to witness it at least the first time is a recommended professional protocol with young children and most minors.

3. As described in Chapter 11, when using the elaters protocol, patients are asked to focus on feelings of enjoyment (and sometimes relief and benefit) when they think about their issue, knowing it is not good for them (or their body or their family). In place of a SUD level, a Subjective Units of Enjoyment (SUE) scale is used where 0 equals no feeling of enjoyment (or neutral) and 10 equals the highest feeling of enjoyment. While diagnostic and treatment procedures remain the same with the elaters protocol, the focused thought field attunes to the positive emotions and not the negative emotions. The goal is to reduce the SUE to 0 with regard to the targeted thought field.

4. These are the types of statements and situations that lead to the use of the future performance imagery index (FPII) in non-peak performance cases. A therapist would use the FPII at this time in the treatment to confirm (or enhance) her success in the future.

5. Diepold (1998) used the term *resource*, instead of *alter*, for dissociated identity states. He claimed that these aspects of the traumatized patient emerged as a needed or necessary resource to help the individual cope with the experienced trauma. Diepold also considers the term *resource* to be a more unifying descriptor in treating this population.

6. This case example was originally presented in Diepold (2002).

7. This case example was originally presented in *Thought Field Therapy: Advancements in Theory and Practice* (Diepold, 2002).

8. This case example was originally presented in *Thought Field Therapy: Advancements in Theory and Practice* (Diepold, 2002).

9. The concept of using a container to cluster or bundle thought fields was an adaptation of the "container technique" demonstrated by Fred Gallo during a presentation at the Energy Psychology Conference (November 2002) in Toronto, Canada. Gallo, however, used an algorithm method for treatment, whereas diagnosis was performed in this case example to determine the meridians to treat.

10. Language modifications are required to reflect the multiple thought fields being addressed. For example, in testing for an issue-specific PR, the test statement

would be, "I want to be over *these problems, their* cause, and all that *they* mean and do to me."

11. I had success in treating one previous case involving prejudice, but I am unaware of other therapists who were using thought field therapy for the treatment of prejudice. It is in cases like this that we truly discover how versatile and beneficial EvTFT can be for the betterment of humankind.

12. The cluster technique had not been developed at this time of treatment, but would likely have been used.

13. This case study was included to encourage other psychotherapists to use EvTFT as an effective treatment for prejudice whenever the opportunity arises. Patients, however, are not always ready to let us treat their prejudices because they often view their prejudices as necessary and appropriate. Their reluctance or "resistance" may be interpreted as evidence of PR, which was evident in both of the above treated thought fields. While the origins of prejudice are speculative (e.g., family and cultural influence, traumatic experiences, morphogenic fields), the effects hinder more rewarding humans relations in a shrinking world. Any and all efforts to curtail such unwarranted hindrances with EvTFT are strongly encouraged for humanitarian reasons.

14. There are many fascinating and potentially healing methods that need to be examined, developed, and researched in energy psychology. As we enter into this largely uncharted territory of the mind-body-energy interface, we strongly advocate for responsible and ethical treatment when thinking of using a surrogate format for treatment as described in Chapter 12. We have decided to include this unusual case example to expand the reader's thinking about the possibilities inherent in this therapy approach. In the case that follows, a mother was used as a surrogate for her son after careful consideration of the circumstances.

CHAPTER 15

1. The core of this chapter was introduced by Diepold in a November 11, 2000, plenary presentation in Toronto, and further developed in "Thought field therapy: Advancements in theory and practice" in Gallo (ed.) *Energy Psychology In Psychotherapy* (2002).

2. The BDB Group staff has observed this phenomenon during workshop training practicum.

3. Perturbations are the energetic micro-states hypothesized by Callahan to be the cause of negative emotions.

4. Entrainment of the brain to the electromagnetic field of the heart comes from HeartMath research (Childre & Martin, 1999).

5. In EvTFT, as in several thought field therapies, diagnosis is set up via intention to identify meridians that require treatment when a strong muscle response is obtained. However, a therapist could identify meridians in need of treatment by obtaining a weak muscle response if he or she intended to diagnose in this way. The concept of incoherence remains the determining factor regardless of the intended direction of muscle response to identify meridians.

EPILOGUE

1. The placebo treatment was described as tapping on areas of the body that were unrelated to treatment sites in the Callahan Techniques™.

2. The emotional freedom technique, developed by Gary Craig, is a treatment derived from the Callahan Techniques™. Its methodology involves repeating a single comprehensive algorithm while the patient is attuned to a thought field with the intention of clearing emotional disturbance.

3. See Reisman (1976) for an engaging history of clinical psychology.

4. "An experiment in thought (*Gedankenexperiment*), a word frequently ridiculed by experimental scientists) has usually been of the utmost importance, and may even be regarded as providing the basis of many scientific theories. For Einstein, Laue, and Planck it certainly did" (Rosenthal-Schneider, p. 76).

5. Psychology, like physics, may have different aspects when dealt with on the macro versus the micro level, and we may take our cues to developing research studies from the physicist. For example, as in quantum physics, it may be that we never are able to predict the behavior of a single individual from the behavior of a mob, if our metaphor is the behavior of a single electron in a mass. See Kuhn (1964) for a development of the function for thought experiments.

6. Rosenthal-Schneider (1980), a student of Einstein, von Laue, and Planck, wrote about her discussions with these great men and gave us insight into their characters and thinking.

7. To this point, Eddington (1958) described, there is a difference between the self that experiences and the self that experiences in reference to others. Perhaps we could call this the physicist's recognition of transference/counter transference.

8. In Chapter 7 we described the use of the Janus metaphor for operationally defining the hologram.

APPENDIX 1

1. Roger Callahan had suggested that if both therapist and patient showed strong/strong responses, one could account for this by treating both as being reversed around the same issue. I therefore extrapolated that, if both therapist and patient were tested separately, they would both show the normal reversal pattern of weak to positive and strong to negative statements.

2. In present EvTFT protocol, this strong/strong, non-polarized muscle response is treated as an *issue specific psychological reversal* (PR). The reversal is usually treated by both the patient/client and the therapist either rubbing their respective NLR areas or doing TAB at the side of hand while affirming, "I deeply accept myself even though I have this problem, its cause. . . ."

3. This positioning for muscle-testing is used in applied kinesiology and taught by Callahan and Diamond.

4. As taught by The BDB Group, the therapist takes a position 90 degrees to either side of the patient.

5. Some therapists frequently find themselves ignoring information from their patient in much the same way that the patient was ignored when having difficulty in early years. For example, the child that tells a parent about abuse is called a liar or ignored and then is ignored by their therapist. This is clearly a transferential/counter transferential issue.

GLOSSARY

acupoints The series of points which interconnect the acupuncture meridian system. Also known as acupuncture points, they are used for treatment in traditional Chinese medicine. The acupoints may function as signal amplifiers or transformers, and show a lower level of electrical impedance compared to non-acupoint skin surface.

acupuncture meridian system (AMS) A complex network that circulates the subtle energy of the chi influence throughout the body. Acupuncture meridian points are located on the AMS.

alarm point A diagnostic indicator originating in traditional Chinese medicine and used in EvTFT in conjunction with muscle testing. Each of the 12 main meridians have an associated alarm point generally located on or near the organ for which it is named. The alarm points for the two vessels are the same as their treatment points.

algorithm A predetermined treatment sequence used for a specific problem or emotional upset in thought field therapy.

applied kinesiology (AK) A subspecialty of chiropractic developed by George J. Goodheart, Jr., DC. It incorporates the use of manual muscle-testing and the acupuncture meridian system as diagnostic indicators. AK addresses neuromuscular functioning relative to structural, chemical, and mental components impacting physiologic regulation.

belief related block (BRB) A type of interference that reflects a negative self belief, which impedes successful treatment. It is characterized by reversed or non-polarized muscle responses to specific test statements such as, "It is safe to be over this problem . . . " and, "It is unsafe to be over this problem. . . ."

blocks An overall class of treatment disruptions that are both a physical and psychological manifestation of an individual's state of being. When present, they help sustain self-defeating attitudes and behaviors, thus preventing positive change from either taking place or being maintained.

brief energy correction (BEC) A procedure used to correct reversed or non-polarized muscle-test responses to the hand over head polarity check. The BEC uses the touch and breathe (TAB) treatment with a sequence of steps from the basic unswitching technique used in AK. The BEC can be used as a treatment for neurologic disorganization and is an ideal initial intervention when polarity problems arise early in treatment.

chi A concept originating in traditional Chinese medicine referring to various forms of essential life forces. Close to the Western interpretation as "energy," chi can be described as "that which influences," and a manifestation of matter and energy at the point of convergence. There are many types of chi, each with a definite form of energy with a specific direction, quality, function, or purpose.

contact directed diagnosis-patient (CDdx-p) A specific method of EvTFT diagnosis whereby the sequential bio-energy information about the patient's disturbed thought field is obtained as he or she is muscle tested while touching their meridian alarm points. This is a form of therapy localization used in AK.

contact directed diagnosis-therapist (CDdx-t) A specific method of EvTFT diagnosis derived from CDdx-p. However, with CDdx-t, the sequential bio-energy information about the patient's disturbed thought field is obtained as the *therapist* touches his or her own meridian alarm points, while muscle testing the patient who is attuned to the disturbed thought field.

elater (E) A construct hypothesized to be a micro-state, energy catalyst that influences the experience of *positive* emotions and sensations when attuned to specific thought fields. Like perturbations, elaters are detectable with EvTFT diagnostic methods and are treatment targets when positive thoughts, emotions, and feelings are connected to self-sabotaging behaviors.

emotional signaling mechanism (ESM) A hypothetical energy-based signaling mechanism that controls the total of the human emotional experience. Conceptually the ESM consists of a combination of elaters, perturbations, and harmonizers that influence the entire range of positive, negative, and profound emotions.

energy disrupter Any influence that corrupts the muscle-testing procedure and results in a polar reversal or non-polarized response. Such influences may be in the form of thought or toxin-like environmental substances.

energy psychology The sum of psychotherapeutic approaches that specifically utilize bio-energy systems for diagnosis and treatment of emotional and behavioral problems.

eye-roll Also called the ground to sky eye-roll, this treatment concludes an EvTFT session when the SUD or SUE level is 0 or 1. It is also used as part of a rapid stress reduction algorithm.

frequency resonance coherence (FRC) The hypothesis that EvTFT brings resonating frequencies of human energy fields into coherence whereby the resulting shifts in the field allows for changes in emotion and thought.

future performance imagery index (FPII) The FPII is an EvTFT assessment and treatment technique that uses a 1 to 7 point scale to assess how clearly the patient can imagine himself or herself successfully and comfortably being in or performing in a future situation. When a patient reports a score below 7, additional treatment is required.

generalized psychological reversal (GPR)   A global or systemic interference to treatment, the GPR is considered a predominant or first-degree psychological reversal in the hierarchy because treatment cannot progress successfully when a patient exhibits GPR. It is evidenced by weak muscle response to the positive statement "I want to be happy," and a strong muscle response to the negative statement "I want to be unhappy." Correction is also indicated when a patient demonstrates a strong/strong non-polarized muscle response to the same statements. Previously known as a Massive PR.

holon   The whole, or sub-set of a larger treatment, which consists of a treatment sequence of meridians, followed by the integration sequence, and ending with a repeat of the treatment sequence for a particular thought field. Diagnosed thought fields may involve single or multiple holons with varying amounts of meridians requiring treatment.

indicator muscle (IM) A muscle or muscle group that is used to gauge differences in strength in response to different stimuli.

integration sequence (ISq)   The ISq consists of nine sequential steps "sandwiched" in between an initial treatment sequence (TxSq) and the repetition of that same treatment sequence (i.e., TxSq → Isq → TxSq). The process appears to access, integrate, and balance different areas of the brain relative to the thought field, perhaps also facilitating neurologic organization. The ISq is performed with fingertips touching both collarbone treatment points (K-27) and using TAB.

issue–specific psychological reversal (issue–specific PR)   A psychological reversal that pertains to the specific issue or problem being addressed. It is evidenced by a weak response to the statement, "I want to be over this problem . . . " and a strong muscle response to, "I want to keep this problem. . . ." Correction of this issue-specific PR is also required when a patient shows a strong/strong non-polarized muscle response to the same statements. Previously known as a Specific PR.

muscle-testing   A method of exerting a small amount of physical force against a resisting muscle or muscle group in order to make a diagnostic determination.

neurolymphatic reflex area (NLR)   The neurolymphatic reflex area, sometimes referred to as the "sore spot," is used to help flush body toxins that may be contributing to reversals or non-polarized responses when muscle-testing. The NLR area is the only non-meridian related site used in EvTFT treatment.

neurologic organizer treatment (NOTx)   A treatment for neurologic disorganization developed by The BDB Group. It is an amalgam of the over energy correction popularized by Wayne Hook, and expanded breathing patterns used in AK. The NOTx is routinely recommended for use before studying, writing, and creative activities, any practice or performance activity, and as needed to maintain neurologic organization.

neurologic disorganization (ND)   A concept used in applied kinesiology that refers to the disorganization of the nervous system. According to Walther (1988), "it appears to result from afferent receptors sending conflicting information for interpretation by the central nervous system"(p. 147). ND is also known as "switching."

non-polarized muscle response   A non-differentiated muscle response (either weak/ weak or strong/strong) to opposing statements, or to the hand over head polarity check, when muscle tested. All non-polarized muscle responses need to be corrected before diagnosis can continue.

perturbations (P)   A construct hypothesized by Roger Callahan to be a micro-state, energy catalyst that causes the experience of *negative* emotions. This operational material resides in the thought field and creates the uncomfortable and undesirable emotional and somatic states when attuned to the thought field. Ps are described as the fundamental energy-generating structures that determine and influence underlying brain chemistry and hormonal response, as well as neurological, cognitive, emotional, and behavioral correlates usually associated with negative emotions. Ps are hypothesized to correlate with specific meridians.

polarity   A condition of physical and psychological being that reflects an energetic positive or negative state. The positive or negative manner in which a body reacts to magnetic, electric, or other fields (e.g., thought fields, energy fields of substances) is discernable with muscle testing. In EvTFT, a properly polarized person will muscle test strong to true statements and positive thoughts and emotions, and weak to false statements and negative thoughts and emotions. The hand over head test is a measure of polarity without attunement to any particular thought field.

process-specific psychological reversal (process-specific PR)   A type of psychological reversal (PR) that becomes evident during the process (i.e., in mid-treatment) of diagnosing and treating a thought field, and inhibits complete resolution of the problem. It is identified via muscle testing when a patient's muscle response is weak to, "I want to be *completely* over this problem . . . " and strong to, "I want to keep *some* of this problem. . . ." It was previously called a mini-PR.

psychological reversal (PR)   A type of energetic block which, when present, serves to maintain self-defeating attitudes and behaviors and impedes effective treatments for correcting or healing. PR is usually indicated by a reversed or non-polarized response to muscle test statements. They may be present in generalized, issue-specific, process-specific, belief related, and recurrent forms.

recurrent psychological reversal   A less common form of psychological reversal that is found in cases where a successfully treated problem returns sometime after treatment was completed. It is characterized by a weak muscle response to the statement, "I want to be over this problem once and for all," and a strong muscle response to, "I want this problem to keep coming back." A non-polarized muscle response to these statements also warrants treatment for correction, which involves rubbing the NLR area and saying (three times), "I deeply accept myself, even though this problem has come back." Clinically, the recurrent PR is more frequent in cases involving addictions and obsessive-compulsive disorders.

self muscle-testing   The process by which a therapist can perform manual muscle testing on oneself, either for self-diagnosis or as a surrogate for their patient.

simplified collarbone breathing (SCB)   A treatment for neurologic disorganization developed by The BDB Group. It is an amalgam of the collarbone breathing treatment popularized by Roger Callahan, and expanded breathing patterns used in AK. With SCB the collarbone treatment points (K-27) are lightly touched as the person repeats a structured breathing exercise with specified finger and knuckle placements. The SCB is routinely recommended for use before studying, writing, and creative activities, any practice or performance activity, and as needed to maintain neurologic organization.

subjective units of distress (SUD)   A scaling method whereby a person can subjectively rate his or her level of emotional distress on a scale of 0 to 10, where 0 represents an absence of emotional distress (or a neutral feeling) and 10 represents the highest level of distress. It is a modification of the 0–100 point scale introduced by Joseph Wolpe.

subjective units of elation or enjoyment (SUE) A scaling method introduced by John Diepold for use in the treatment of elaters as developed by The BDB Group. Similar in concept and operation to the SUD scale, levels of pleasure or elation are subjectively rated on a scale of 0 to 10, where 0 indicates no pleasure or enjoyment (or neutral) and 10 indicates the highest degree of pleasure or enjoyment the person can derive.

surrogate testing   A muscle testing arrangement in which a designated person takes the place of the patient for the purposes of diagnosis and treatment.

therapy localization   A diagnostic procedure found in applied kinesiology in which the patient touches a specific area of the body as he or she is being muscle tested, thus localizing the immediate area of dysfunction. Therapy localization has become synonymous with the term diagnosis in thought field therapy and is mainly used in EvTFT diagnostic methods to determine which meridians are involved when the patient is attuned to a particular thought field.

thought directed diagnosis (TDdx)   A bio-energetic extension of the contact directed diagnostic methods in which imagery and thought are used to guide diagnosis. With TDdx the sequential bio-energy information about meridian involvement to the thought field is obtained via manual muscle testing but without the need for either the patient or therapist to physically touch the meridian alarm points.

thought field   A hypothetical construct introduced by Roger Callahan. Thought fields can be characterized as an invisible, non-physical structure in space (i.e., an energetic field) that binds energetically encoded information into a cohesive arrangement. It is hypothesized that this energetic bridge between thought, memory, and emotional experience reaches beyond conscious awareness; and is conjectured to contain energetic information about real, imagined, or remembered experiences that have a direct effect on an individual's physical, emotional, and energetic state of being.

touch-and-breathe (TAB)   A gentle, mindful, and natural treatment used in lieu of tapping on meridian points to facilitate the flow of energy and/or chi influence along the acupuncture meridians. With TAB, the patient is invited to lightly touch the prescribed treatment sites along the acupuncture meridians with 1 to 4 fingers as he or she takes one complete respiration while attuned to the thought field.

traditional Chinese medicine (TCM)   The medical practices developed over the past 5000 years by Chinese practitioners. Acupuncture is a part of TCM.

treatment point(s)   Specific acupuncture meridian points that are used in the EvTFT treatment process in conjunction with the touch-and-breathe method. With the exception of the triple heater and the small intestine meridians, EvTFT treatment points are located exclusively either at the beginning or ending points of a particular meridian or vessel. EvTFT currently uses 14 treatment points. Also called acupoints.

treatment sequence (TxSq) The succession of one or more meridian treatment points derived via the EvTFT diagnostic process that constitutes the first and last parts of a holon.

unknown block (UB) A type of block (e.g., belief, thought field) that manifests during treatment of a thought field that neither the patient nor therapist can identify. In order for treatment to proceed the UB must be corrected. To do so the UB becomes an unknown thought field that is diagnosed and treated. After treatment of the UB, continued treatment of the targeted thought field can resume.

BIBLIOGRAPHY

American heritage dictionary of the English language (4th ed.). (2000). Boston: Houghton Mifflin.

American Psychiatric Association. (2000). *Diagnostic and statistical manual of mental disorders* (4th ed., text rev.). Washington, DC: Author.

American Psychological Association. (1992). Ethical principles of psychologists and code of conduct. Washington, DC: Author.

Becker, R. O. (1990). *Cross currents: The perils of electropollution, the promise of electromedicine.* New York: Putnam.

Bandler, R. O, & Grinder, J. (1975). *Patterns of the hypnotic techniques of Milton H. Erickson, M.D.* (Vol. 1). Cupertino, CA: Meta.

Becker, R. O., & Seldon, G. (1985). *The body electric: Electromagnetism and the foundation of life.* New York: Morrow.

Bender, S. S., Lange, G., Steffener, J., Bergmann, U., Grand, D., Liu, W., & Bly, B. M. (2000). *Imaging violence: Post traumatic stress disorder, eye movement desensitization and reprocessing, and functional magnetic resonance imaging.* (This study was supported by seed-grant funds from the Violence Institute of New Jersey, Index no. 103772). University of Medicine and Dentistry of New Jersey-Newark.

Bernstein, J. (1991). *Quantum profiles.* Princeton, NJ: Princeton University Press.

Bibby, C. (Ed.) (1967). *The essence of T. H. Huxley: Selections from his writings.* New York: St. Martin's Press; London: Macmillan.

Blaich, R. M. (1988). Applied kinesiology and human performance. In *Collected papers of the International College of Applied Kinesiology* (pp. 7–15). Shawnee Mission, KS: International College of Applied Kinesiology.

Bohm, D. (1980). *Wholeness and the implicate order.* London: Routledge & Kegan Paul.

Bohm, D., & Hiley, B. (1993) *The undivided universe: An ontological interpretation of quantum theory.* New York: Routledge.

Britt, V., Diepold, J. H., Jr., & Bender, S. S. (1998). *Thought field therapy comprehensive workshop: Training manual.* Montclair, NJ. Authors.

Britt, V., Diepold, J. H., Jr., & Bender, S. S. (2000). *Thought field therapy comprehensive workshop: Training manual* (2nd rev. ed.). Montclair, NJ: Authors.

Britt, V., Diepold, J. H., Jr., & Bender, S. S. (2002). *Thought field therapy comprehensive workshop:; Training manual* (4th rev. ed.). Montclair, NJ. Authors.

359

Callahan, R. J. (1981). Psychological reversal. In *Collected papers of the International College of Applied Kinesiology* (pp. 79–96). Shawnee Mission, KS: International College of Applied Kinesiology.

Callahan, R. J. (1985). *Five-minute phobia cure: Dr. Callahan's treatment for fears, phobias and self-sabotage.* Wilmington, DE: Enterprise.

Callahan, R. J. (1990). *The rapid treatment of panic, agoraphobia, and anxiety.* Indian Wells, CA: Author.

Callahan, R. J. (with Perry P.) (1991). *Why do I eat when I'm not hungry? How to use your body's own energy system to treat food addictions with the revolutionary Callahan techniques.* New York: Doubleday.

Callahan, R. J. (1992). *Special report #1: The cause of psychological problems: Introduction to theory.* Indian Wells, CA: Author.

Callahan, R. J. (1995). *The anxiety → addiction connection: Eliminate your addictive urges with TFT (thought field therapy).* Indian Wells, CA: Author.

Callahan, R. J. (1996). *Psychological reversal: Forms and treatments.* Presented material for diagnostic trainees in the Callahan techniques. Indian Wells, CA: Author.

Callahan, R. J. (1998). *Callahan techniques thought field therapy: Manual for diagnosis step A.* Indian Wells, CA: Author.

Callahan, R. J., & Callahan, J. (1996). *Thought field therapy and trauma: Treatment and theory.* Indian Wells, CA: Authors.

Callahan, R. J. (with Trubo, R.). (2001). *Tapping the healer within: Using thought field therapy to instantly conquer your fears, anxieties, and emotional distress.* Lincolnwood, IL: Contemporary Books.

Carlson, E., & Putnam, F.W. (1993). *Manual for the dissociative experiences scale.* Towson, MD: Sidran Press.

Childre, D., & Martin, H. (with Beech, D.) (1999). *The heartmath solution.* San Francisco: HarperCollins.

Cho, Z.-H. (1998). New findings of the correlation between acupoints and corresponding barin cortices using functional MRI. *Proceedings of the National Academy of Sciences, 95,* 2670–2673.

Chu, J. A., & Bowman, E. S. (2000). Trauma and dissociation: 20 years of study and lessons learned along the way. *Journal of Trauma and Dissociation, 1*(1), 5–20.

Conable, K. M., & Hanicke, B. T., (1987). Inter-examiner agreement in applied kinesiology manual muscle testing. *Selected Papers of the International College of Applied Kinesiology.* Shawnee Mission: KS: ICAK.

Craig, G., & Fowlie, A. (1997). *Emotional freedom techniques: The manual.* The Sea Ranch, CA: Author. Retrieved August 5, 2003, from http://www.emofree.com/EFTmanl.pdf

Davies, P.C.W., & Brown, J.R. (1986). *The ghost in the atom.* Cambridge, U.K.: Cambridge University Press.

Dennison, P., & Dennison, P. (1994). *Brain gym.* Ventura, CA: Edu-Kinesthetics.

Dennison, P, Dennison, P., & Teplitz, J. (1994). *Brain gym for business.* Ventura, CA: Edu-Kinesthetics.

Diamond, J. H., Jr. (1979). *Behavioral kinesiology.* New York: Harper & Row.

Diamond, J. H., Jr. (1980). *The collected papers of John Diamond, MD* (Vol. 2). Valley Cottage, NY: Archaeus.

Diamond, J. H., Jr. (1985). *Life energy: Using the meridians to unlock the hidden power of your emotions.* New York: Paragon House.

Diamond, J. H., Jr. (1988). *Life-energy analysis: A way to cantellation.* New York: Archaeus.

Diepold, J. H., Jr. (1998, November). *Touch and breathe (TAB): An alternative treatment approach with meridian-based psychotherapies.* Paper presented at the Innovative and Integrative Approaches to Psychotherapy conference. Edison, NJ.

Diepold, J. H., Jr. (2000). Touch and breathe (TAB): An alternative treatment approach with meridian-based psychotherapies. *Traumatology: The International Journal of Innovations in the Study of the Traumatic Process and Methods for Reducing, Preventing, and Eliminating Related Human Suffering, 6*(2), Article 4. Retrieved May 18, 2003, from http://www.fsu.edu/~trauma/v6i2a4.html

Diepold, J. H., Jr. (2002). Thought field therapy: Advancements in theory and practice. In F. Gallo (Ed.), *Energy psychology in psychotherapy* (pp. 3–34). New York: Norton.

Diepold, J. H., Jr., & Goldstein, D. (2000). *Thought field therapy and QEEG changes in the treatment of trauma: A case study.* Moorestown, NJ: Author.

Dubrov, A. P., & Pushkin, V. N. (1982). *Parapsychology and contemporary science.* New York: Consultants Bureau.

Durlacher, J. V. (2000). *Freedom from fear forever: The acu-power way to overcoming your fears, phobias, and inner problems* (Rev. Ed.). Tempe, AZ: Van Ness.

Eddington, A. (1958). *The philosophy of physical science.* Ann Arbor: University of Michigan Press.

Eden, D. (with Feinstein, D.) (1998). *Energy medicine.* New York: Jeremy P. Tarcher/Putnam.

Figley, C. R., & Carbonell, J. (1995). *The "active ingredient" project: The systematic clinical demonstration of the most efficient treatments of PTSD, a research plan.* Tallahassee, FL: Florida State University Psychosocial Stress Research Program and Clinical Laboratory.

Fisher, S., & Greenberg, R. P. (Eds.). (1997). *From placebo to panacea: Putting psychiatric drugs to the test.* New York: Wiley.

Fleming, T. (1996). *Reduce traumatic stress in minutes: The tapas acupressure technique (TAT) workbook.* Torrance, CA: Author.

Frost, R. (2002). *Applied kinesiology: A training manual and reference book of basic principles and practices.* Berkeley, CA: North Atlantic Books.

Furman, M. E. (2002). Grounding energy psychology in the physical sciences. In F. Gallo (Ed.), *Energy psychology in psychotherapy* (pp. 368–386). New York: Norton.

Furman, M. E., and Gallo, F. P. (2000). *The neurophysics of human behavior: Explorations at the interface of the brain, mind, behavior, and information.* Boca Raton: CRC Press.

Gallo, F. (1994a). *Thought field therapy level 1 (and associated methods): Training manual.* Hermitage, PA: Author.

Gallo, F. (1994b). *Thought field therapy level 2 (and associated methods): Training manual.* Hermitage, PA: Author.

Gallo, F. (1999). *Energy psychology: Explorations at the interface of energy, cognition, behavior, and health.* Boca Raton, FL: CRC.

Gallo, F. (2000). *Energy diagnostic and treatment methods.* New York: Norton.

Gallo, F. (Ed.) (2002). *Energy psychology in psychotherapy.* New York: Norton.

Gallo, F., & Vincenzi, H. (2000). *Energy tapping.* Oakland, CA: New Harbinger.

Gallo, F. P., & Vincenzi, H. (2000). *Energy tapping: How to rapidly eliminate anxiety, depression, cravings, and more using energy psychology.* Oakland, CA: New Harbinger Publications.

Gendlin, E. T. (1962). *Experiencing and the creation of meaning: A philosophical and psychological approach to the subjective.* New York: Free Press of Glencoe. Reprinted (1997) by Evanston, IL: Northwestern University Press.

Gendlin, E. T. (1996). The use of focusing in therapy. In J. K. Zeig (Ed.), *The evolution of psychotherapy* (pp. 197–210). New York: Brunner/Mazel.

Gerber, R. (1988). *Vibrational medicine: New choices for healing ourselves.* Santa Fe, NM: Bear.

Gillispie, C. C. (1960). *The edge of objectivity: An essay in the history of scientific ideas.* Princeton, NJ: Princeton University Press.

Goodheart, G.J. (1987). *You'll be better.* Geneva, OH: Author.

Hannaford, C. (1995). *Smart moves: Why learning is not all in your head.* Arlington, VA: Great Ocean.

Hartung, J. G., & Galvin, M. D. (2003). *Energy psychology and EMDR: Combining forces to optimize treatment.* New York: Norton.

Hawkins, D. R. (1995). *Power vs. force: The hidden determinants of human behavior.* Sedona, AZ: Veritas.

Hofstadter, D. (1979). *Gödel, Escher, Bach: An eternal golden braid.* New York: Basic Books.

Hover-Kramer, D. (2002). *Creative energies: Integrative psychotherapy for self-expression and healing.* New York: Norton.

Jacobs, G. E. (1981). Applied kinesiology: An experimental evaluation by double blind methodology. *Journal of Manipulation and Physical Therapeutics, 4*(3), 141–145.

Jarrett, L. S. (1999). *Nourishing destiny: The inner tradition of Chinese medicine.* Stockbridge, MA: Spirit Path Press.

Jiyu-Kennett, R., & MacPhillamy, Rev. D. (1979). *The book of life.* Mt. Shasta, CA: Shasta Abbey Press.

Kaptchuk, T. J. (1983). *The web that has no weaver: Understanding Chinese medicine.* New York: Congdon and Weed.

Kendall, H. O., & Kendall, F. M. P. (1949). *Muscles: Testing and function.* Baltimore: Williams & Wilkins.

Kluft, R. P., & Fine, C. G. (Eds.) (1993). *Clinical perspectives on multiple personality disorder.* Washington, DC: American Psychiatric Press.

Koestler, A. (1967). *The ghost in the machine.* New York: Macmillan.

Korzybski, A. (1980). *Science and sanity: An introduction to non-Aristotelian systems and general semantics* (4th ed.). Lakeville, CT: International Non-Aristotelian Library Publishing Company.

Kuhn, T. S. (1957). *The Copernican revolution: Planetary astronomy in the development of western thought.* Cambridge, MA: Harvard University Press.

Kuhn, T. S. (1964). A function for thought experiments. In R. Taton & I. B. Cohen (eds.), *Mélanges Alexandre Koyré* (Vol. 2), *L'aventure de l'esprit* (pp. 307–334). Paris: Hermann.

Kuhn, T. S. (1996). *The structure of scientific revolutions* (3rd ed.). Chicago and London: University of Chicago Press.

Lambrou, P., & Pratt, G. (2000). *Instant emotional healing: Acupressure for the emotions.* New York: Broadway Books.

Lambrou, P. T, Pratt, G. P., & Chevalier, G. (2001).Report on preliminary investigation of physiological correlates of a thought energy therapy. In *Proceedings of the eleventh annual conference of the International Society for the Study of Subtle Energy & Energy Medicine* (pp. 29–41). Boulder CO: ISSSEEM.

Lazarus, A.A., & Lazarus, C.N. (1991). *Multimodal life history inventory.* Champaign, IL: Research Press.

Levy, S.L, & Lehr, C. (1996). *Your body can talk: How to use simple muscle testing to learn what your body needs and knows.* Prescott, AZ: Hohm Press.

MacPhillamy, Rev. D. (1979). In Jiyu-Kennett, R., & MacPhillamy, Rev. D. (1979). *The book of life* (Book II). Mt. Shasta, CA: Shasta Abbey Press.

Monti, D. A., Sinnott, J., Marchese, M., Kunkel, E. J. S., & Greeson, J. M. (1999). Muscle test comparisons of congruent and incongruent self-referential statements. *Perceptual and Motor Skills,* 88, 1019–1028.

Medical Economics Company (2001). *Physicians' Desk Reference.* Montvale, NJ: Author.

Nambudripad, D. (1993). *Say goodbye to illness.* Buena Park, CA: Delta.

Newton, M. (2002). *Journey of souls: Case studies of life between lives* (5th rev. ed.). St. Paul, MN: Llewellyn.

Nims, L. (2001). *BSFF training manual: Behavioral and emotional system elimination training for resolving excess emotion: Fear, anger, sadness, trauma.* Orange, CA: Author.

Oschman, J. L. (2000). *Energy medicine: The scientific basis.* Leith Walk, U.K.: Churchill Livingstone/Harcourt.

Penfield, W. (1969). Consciousness, memory, and man's conditioned reflexes. In K. H. Pribram (Ed.), *On the biology of learning* (pp. 127–168). New York: Harcourt, Brace.

Porkert, Manfred. *The theoretical foundations of Chinese medicine: Systems of correspondence.* Cambridge, MA: MIT Press, 1974.

Pribram, K. H. (Ed.). (1969). *On the biology of learning.* New York: Harcourt, Brace.

Putnum, F. W. (1989). *Diagnosis and treatment of multiple personality disorder.* New York: Guilford Press.

Rapp, D.J. (1989). *The impossible child: In school–at home* (2nd ed.). Buffalo, NY: Practical Allergy Research Foundation.

Reisman, J. M. (1976). *A history of clinical psychology.* New York: Irvington.

Rochlitz, S. (1997). *Allergies and candida: With the physicist's rapid solution.* New York: Human Ecology Balancing Sciences.

Rosenthal-Schneider, I. (1980). *Reality and scientific truth: Discussions with Einstein, von Laue, and Planck.* Detroit, MI: Wayne State University Press.

Ross, C. A. (1989). *Multiple personality disorder: Diagnosis, clinical features, and treatment.* New York: Wiley.

Salzinger, K. (2002). What if all psychologists understood each other? *Monitor on Psychology,* 33, 27.

Schwartz, G. E., & Russek, G. (1997). Dynamical energy systems and modern physics: Fostering the science and spirit of complementary and alternative medicine. *Alternative Therapies,* 3(3), 46–56.

Sheldrake, R. (1988), *The presence of the past: Morphic resonance and the habits of nature.* Rochester, VT: Park Street.

Sheldrake, R. (1995). A *new science of life.* Rochester, VT: Park Street.

Spiegel, M., & Spiegel, D. (1978). *Trance and treatment: Clinical uses of hypnosis.* New York: Basic Books.

Spira, J. L. (Ed.). (1996). *Treating dissociative identity disorder.* San Francisco: Jossey-Bass.

Thie, J. (1979). *Touch for health: A practical guide to natural health using acupuncture touch and massage to improve postural balance and reduce physical and mental pain and tension.* (Rev. ed.). Marina del Ray, CA: DeVorss.

Tiller, W. A. (1997). *Science and human transformation: Subtle energies, intentionality, and consciousness.* Walnut Creek, CA: Pavior.

Tiller, W. A., Dibble, W. E., & Kohane, M. J. (2001). *Conscious acts of creation: The emergence of a new physics.* Walnut Creek, CA: Pavior.

Tsuei, J. J. (1996). Scientific evidence in support of acupuncture and meridian theory: I. Introduction. *IEEE Engineering in Medicine and Biology Magazine, 15*(3). Retrieved August 5, 2003, from http://www.healthy.net/scr/Article.asp?Id=1087

van der Hart, O, & Brown, P. (1992). Abreaction re-evaluated. *Dissociation, 5*(3), 127–140.

van der Kolk, B. A. (1994). The body keeps the score: Memory and the evolving psychobiology of posttraumatic stress. *Harvard Review of Psychiatry, 1,* 253–265.

Versendaal, D. A., & Versendaal-Hoezee, D. (1993). *Contact reflex analysis and designed clinical nutrition.* Jenison, MI: Hoezee Marketing.

Voll, R. (1975). Twenty years of electro acupuncture diagnosis in Germany: A progress report. *American Journal of Acupuncture, 3,* 7–17.

Voll, R. (1978). Electroacupuncture according to Voll. *American Journal of Acupuncture, 6,* 5–15.

Walker S. (1990). The triangle of health: once more with feeling. *Digest of Chiropractic Economics,* May/June, 16–25.

Walker, S. (1992). Ivan Pavlov, his dog, and chiropractic. *The Digest of Chiropractic Economics,* March/April, 34–46.

Walther, D. S. (1981). *Applied kinesiology. Vol. 1: Basic procedures and muscle testing.* Pueblo, CO: Systems DC.

Walther, D. S. (1988). *Applied kinesiology: Synopsis.* Pueblo, CO: Systems DC.

Webster's encyclopedic unabridged dictionary. (1996). New York: Gramercy.

Webster's new world dictionary of the American language: College edition. (1966). New York: World.

Weiss, B. L. (1988). *Many lives, many masters.* New York: Simon & Schuster.

Weiss, B. L. (1992). *Through time into healing.* New York: Simon & Schuster.

Wells, S., Polglase, K., Andrews, H. B., Carrington, P., & Baker, A. H. (in press). Evaluation of a meridian-based intervention, emotional freedom techniques (EFT), for reducing specific phobias of small animals. *Journal of Clinical Psychology.*

Whisenant, W. F. (1994). *Psychological kinesiology: Changing the body's beliefs.* Kailua, HI: Monarch Butterfly Press.

Wise, A. (1995). *The high-performance mind: Mastering brainwaves for insight, healing, and creativity.* New York: Putnam.

Woollerton, H., & McLean, C. J. (1979). *Acupuncture energy in health and disease: A practical guide for advanced students.* Wellingsborough, U.K.: Thorsons.

Worsley, J. R. (1993). *Traditional Chinese acupuncture: Meridians and points.* Boston: Element Books.

Young, A. M. (1984). *The foundations of science: The missing parameter.* San Francisco: Robert Briggs.

Young, J. (1999). *Cognitive therapy for personality disorders: A schema-focused approach* (3rd ed.). Sarasota, FL: Professional Resource Press.

Young, J.E. (1994). *Cognitive therapy for personality disorders: A schema focused approach.* Sarasota, FL: Professional Resource Press.

INDEX

abandonment, 50, 111–12, 274–75
abreaction, 212–13
abuse, history of
  in case examples, 260–62, 270–71, 274–
    75, 276–80
  and dissociative disorders, 205
  and muscle testing, 56, 68
academic performance, 72
ACTH. *see* adrenocorticotropic hormone
active information, 117–19
active meridian alarm point, 153–54
acupoints
  antenna effect, 84, 87–88, 90
  and electrical signals, 35
  finger-tapping, 5, 7, 80–82
  as frequency modulators, 88
Acu-POWER, 147
acupuncture meridian system (AMS)
  antenna properties, 84, 88–89, 90
  and Callahan techniques™, 4–5
  and chi/prana pump, 316
  and emotions, 3
  and muscle testing, 51–52
  research, 35–36
  treatment points, 132–33
  yin and yang, 37–38
  see also conception vessel; governing ves-
    sel; meridians
addictions
  and cluster technique, 214
  and elaters, 180–84
  home treatment, 175–76
  and PRs, 106, 113
  treatment points, 47, 50
ADHD. *see* attention deficit hyperactivity dis-
    order
adjunctive therapy, EvTFT as
  case consultations, 244–45
  cautions, 8, 207
  and elaters, 10
  uses, 8, 241–44
  see also integration

adolescents, 61–62, 243, 304
  performance case, 267–68
adrenal glands, 92
adrenocorticotropic hormone (ACTH), 92
affirmations
  and BRBs, 108–12
  and Callahan techniques™, 9, 102
  and chi, 3
  for children, 242–43
  and elaters, 183–84, 337
  in flowcharts, 330, 332
  if *versus* though, 110
  mirroring, 104
  in PR protocol, 187–88
  and PRs, 102–6
  repetitions of, 104
  uses, 102
  wording, 103
  in worksheets, 333, 337
Agar, W. E., 27
AK beginning-and-ending techniques,
    81
alarm points
  active, 153–54
  description, 38–39
  in diagnosis, 164–65
  and DID, 209
  in flowchart, 331*f*
  locations, 39–41, 47*f*, 48*t*
alcoholics, children of, 50
alertness, 91
algorithm-based therapy, 5
algorithms
  clinical study, 304
  defined, 230
  and diagnosis, 232–34, 293
  and dissociative disorders, 209
  for elaters, 184
  and emotions, 236, 237*t*
  extended trauma, 275–76
  9G treatment, 134
  in incest survivor, 274–75

algorithms (*cont.*)
  last resort, 238
  and muscle-testing, 234, 235–36
  treatment with, 234–38, 304
  and unconscious mind, 300
  uses, 232–33
  see also emotional freedom technique
allergens, 113, 175–76, 216–21
allergies, 237*t*
allergy elimination technique, 217–18
alpha waves, 140
alters, 205. *see also* resources
American Psychological Association (APA)
  on abreaction, 213
  on ethics, 10, 55, 240
AMS. *see* acupuncture meridian system
Anderson, G., 85
Andrews, H. B., 305
anger
  algorithms, 237*t*
  family of origin case, 251–53
  and FPII, 194
  in marriage and family therapy, 243–44
  phantom pain case, 262–64
  treatment points, 46, 47
  variations of, 45, 234
animal electricity, 20
anma arts, 85–87
anorexia. *see* eating disorders
antenna effect, 84, 87–88, 90
anxiety
  algorithms, 232, 237*t*
  and breathing, 93
  Callahan techniques™, 5
  in delusional disorder, 248–49
  and EvTFT, 8
  in family therapy, 244
  home treatment, 175–76
  in incest survivor, 274–75
  and performance issues, 196, 267–68
  and self-healing, 226
  treatment sequences, 292
apex problem, 178–79, 251
aphasia, 69
appliances (household), 216
applied kinesiology
  alarm points, 38–41, 47*f*, 48*t*
  muscle testing, 2–3, 51–53 (*see also* muscle testing)
  NLR, 44
  therapy localization, 3
Aristotle, 23
arm swing, 69
arthritis, 226–29
Aspect, A., 322
athletes, 72, 265–68
attention deficit hyperactivity disorder (ADHD), 272–74
auric sheaths, 300–301

autonomic nervous system, 87–88
awkwardness, 69

Baker, A. H., 305
Bandler, R. O., 135
baseball metaphor, 319–20
basic protocol
  apex problem, 178–79
  diagnosis, 164–66 (*see also* diagnosis)
  DID modifications, 210–12
  for energy disrupters, 219–22
  flowcharts, 329–32
  home treatment, 175–76
  next session, 175
  preparation, 162–64, 329*f*
  unchanged SUD, 170–73
  variations, 166–74
    CDdx-p, 166–67
    CDdx-t, 167–68
    TDdx, 168–69
Basic Unswitching Procedure, 78
BDB Group
  on blocks, 98–101
  diagnostic approach, 147
  on ethics, 240
  EvTFT method, 8–10
  flowcharts, 329–32
  mission, 310–11
  neurologic organization, 71–79
  origins, xv–xviii
BEC. *see* brief energy correction
Becker, R. O., 20–22, 35, 97, 217, 219
bedridden patients, 8, 226–29
Beech, D., 283
beginning-and-ending technique, 134
behaviors
  and dynamical energy, 296–97
  learned, transmission of, 26–27
  self-defeating, 10, 180–84, 241
belief-related blocks (BRBs)
  affirmations, 108–12
  in basic protocol, 164, 170–73
  and Callahan techniques™, 9
  diagnosis of, 107–8
  diagnosis protocol, 186–90
  in DID, 211–12
  examples, 325–26
  in flowchart, 332
  record keeping, 144
  types, 108–12
beliefs
  core, 111, 127
  and pain management, 202–3
Bell, J., 322
Bender, S. S., x, xvi–xvii, 319–23
Berkeley, G., 319
Bernstein, J., 21–22, 319
bitterness, 46
bladder meridian
  alarm points, 47*f*, 48*t*

and CDdx-p, 154
emotions, 46, 449*t*
in EvTFT, 42
eye injury, 92
in TCM, 36, 39
and trauma, 234
treatment points, 47*f*, 48*t*
and yang meridians, 91–92
Blaich, R., 3, 68, 69, 71, 75
blocks
and algorithms, 234
belief-related, 106–14
causes, 113–14
unknown (preverbal), 112–14, 171–73,
190–92
criteria-related, 106
defined, 98–101
diagnosis, 186–92
to peak performance, 196–98
polarity patterns, 97–98
see also belief-related blocks; psychological
reversalss
bodily sensations, 103, 251–53
body
Chinese measurements, 39
and electric fields, 89–91
as semiconductor, 22
Bohm, D., 115, 117, 124–27, 289, 307–8, 311
Bowman, E. S., 204
brain
beliefs about, 13–14
and FRC, 285–86
heart connection, 285–86
imaging of, 25–26, 304, 310 (*see also* magnetic resonance imaging)
one-sided activity, 135–36
Brain Gym, 54
brain hemispheres, 135
brain-wave patterns, 304
BRB. *see* belief-related blocks
breathing
and acute anxiety, 93
and chi, 86–87, 90
and DID, 93
and intention, 91, 203–4
and pain management, 93, 203–4
piezoelectric effect, 89–91
see also simplified collarbone breathing
treatment; Touch-And-Breathe
bridges, fear of, 259–60
brief energy correction (BEC)
in flowchart, 329
steps, 78–79, 333, 337
uses, 70
Britt, V., x, xvii–xviii
Brown, J. R., 306, 322
Brown, P., 213
Bruner, J. S., 12
Buddhism, 85–87
buzzing, 252

Callahan, J., 4–5, 67, 99, 116, 118, 230, 251
Callahan, R. J., ix, 3–4, 7, 41, 67, 69, 71, 75,
80, 81, 84, 99, 116, 132, 133–34, 146,
147, 153, 178–79, 217, 221, 230, 232,
236, 283, 293, 304, 305
Callahan techniques[TM]
and affirmations, 9, 102
algorithm, 238
and AMS, 4–5
diagnosis, 146–47
eye roll, 139–40
finger tapping, 5, 7, 80–85
gamut point, 116, 121
and perturbations, 127
and research, 304
terminology, 116, 121
and unconscious mind, 300
Carbonell, J., 7–8, 241, 304
carpets, 219
Carrington, P., 305
case consultations, 244–45
case examples
ADHD child (parent of), 272–74
child drowning witness, 247–48
delusional disorder, 248–49
depression, 246
DID, 260–62, 274–75
eating disorders (elaters), 253–54, 264–65
enuresis, 276–80
ethnic prejudice, 271–72
gagging, 268–69
heights, 259–60
MRI refusal, 249–50
nail biting, 258–59
negative belief cluster, 270–71
OCD, 257–58
pill swallowing, 254–56
PTSD, 251–53, 256–57, 262–64, 274–75
rape victim, 275–76
sexual attraction (inappropriate, elaters),
265
sport performance, 265–68
suicidal ideation (elaters), 250–51
surrogate use, 259–60, 260–62, 276–80
catatonic victim, 275–76
causes
of blocks, 113–14
of pain, 200–202
of performance issues, 196–97
perturbations as, 119–20
of TDdx efficacy, 158–59
unconscious, 103, 111–12
of unknown blocks, 191
cautions
and dissociative patients, 207, 211, 212–13
eye injury, 92
and muscle testing, 56
and surrogacy, 227
see also permission
CDdx-p. *see under* contact directed diagnosis

CDdx-t. *see under* contact directed diagnosis
cells, 22, 35–36, 97
change, 12–14
chaos theory, 89
Chapman, F., 44
Chevalier, G., 304
chi
    in AMS, 316
    and breath, 86–87, 90
    definition, 32–33
    in EvTFT, 9
    excess of, 88
    forms, 33–34
    and FRC, 286–89
    and harmonizers, 130
    and muscle testing, 90–91
    research, 3, 36
    reservoirs (*see* conception vessel; governing
        vessel)
    translation of, 25
childhood, 197. *see also* abuse, history of
Childre, D., 283, 285, 289
children
    and algorithms, 233
    and allergens, 218
    car accident case, 250–51
    and contact directed diagnosis, 156
    drowning witness case, 247–48
    EvTFT in, 8, 242–43
    muscle testing, 61–62
    SUD level, 139
    surrogate testing, 226–29
Chinese medicine. *see* acupuncture meridian
        system; traditional Chinese medicine
chi/prana pump, 316
Cho, Z.-H., 36
Chu, J. A., 204
circulation/sex meridian
    alarm points, 47*f*, 48*t*
    emotions, 49*t*, 50
    in EvTFT, 43
    in OCD case, 257–58
    in TCM, 37, 40
    treatment points, 47*f*, 48*t*
Clausius, R., 115
claustrophobia, 304
clumsiness, 69, 237*t*
cluster technique, 214–15, 270–71
cognitive behavioral therapy, 309–10
cognitive clarity, 148–49, 206
cognitive therapy, 102, 207, 241
coherence. *see* frequency resonance coher-
        ence
collarbone breathing treatment, 75–76, 258.
        see also simplified collarbone breath-
        ing treatment
collarbone treatment points, 136–37, 140
communication
    and blocks, 98
    of emotions, 45

interdisciplinary approach, 308–10
intergenerational transmission, 23–25
    muscle testing as, 56–57
    by phone, 226–29, 232
    yes/no muscle responses, 152
compliance, 92, 176
comprehensive algorithm, 238
compulsions, 180–81, 264–65. *see also* obses-
        sive-compulsive disorder
computers, 216
conception vessel
    alarm/treatment points, 39, 47*f*, 48*t*
    and BRBs, 110
    description, 35, 38
    emotions, 49*t*, 50
    in EvTFT, 44
    and FRC, 286
    meridian connection, 291–94
confidentiality, 240
connection related BRB, 326
connective tissue, 89
consciousness, 298–302
Constable, K. M., 53–54
construction sites, 219
consultations, 244–45
contact directed diagnosis
    patient (CDdx-p), 153–55, 160, 166–67
    therapist (CDdx-t), 155–57
contact reflex analysis, 54
container technique, 214
control BRB, 325
control issues, 50
cooperation, 151–53
core beliefs, 111, 127
cosmetics, 216–19
counter transference
    energetic basis, 319–23
    and muscle testing, 56, 57, 320–21
courage, 47
Craig, G., 7, 147, 184, 233, 238, 283, 293
current of injury, 21

Dale, H., 26
Darwin, C., 27
Davies, P. C. W., 306, 322
decision-making, 46, 47
deep-level reversals. *see* belief-related blocks
defectiveness, 111–12
Delacato, C. H., 69
deltoid muscle, 57–62
deltrons, 291, 312–16
delusional disorder, 248–49
Dennison, P., 54
depression
    algorithms, 237*t*
    case example, 246
    and dynamical energy systems, 296
    and performance issues, 196
    suicide ideation case, 250–51
    treatment points, 50

deprivation BRB, 326
deservedness BRBs
  assessment of, 111
  description, 110
  in DID case, 260–62
  in protocol, 171
despair, 50
diagnosis
  alarm points, 38–41, 47*f*, 48*t*
  versus algorithms, 232–34, 292–93
  with algorithms, 234
  of blocks, 186–92
  of BRBs, 107–8
  contact directed, 153–57, 166–68
  disrupter identification, 219–21
  of elater problems, 180–84
  in flowcharts, 329, 330, 332
  intuition, 164
  meridian-based, 156–47
  and ND, 69–71
  of nonpolarized response, 192–93
  of performance problems, 196–98
  in protocol, 164–66
  of PRs, 186–90
  in psychotherapy, 145–46
  sequence, 160
  TFT *versus* EvTFT, 9
  and therapy localization, 41
  thought directed, 157–60
  see also muscle testing; surrogacy
Diagnostic and Statistical Manual of Mental Disorders (DSM-IV), 145–46, 204
Diamond, J., xviii, 2–3, 7, 46, 49n, 52, 54, 57–58, 90–91, 99, 146, 304
Dibble, W. E., 11, 291, 301, 308, 313
DID. *see* dissociative identity disorder
Diepold, J. H., Jr., x, xv–xvi, xvii
disgust, 46
disrupters (energy), 215–22, 329*f*
dissociation
  and incest history, 274–75
  and SUD reporting, 263
  visual kinesthetic, 304
dissociative disorders
  basic considerations, 207–8
  cautions, 211, 212–13
  EvTFT usefulness, 205–7, 208–9
  incest survivor case, 274–75
  preliminaries, 207–8
  therapy, 208–10
dissociative identity disorder (DID)
  and breathing, 93
  case examples, 260–62
  cautions, 207, 212–13
  therapy, 209–12
distance
  healing at, 322 (*see also* surrogacy)
  and morphic resonance, 28
distress. *see* emotional upsets; subjective
    units of distress

documentation, 140–44, 163–64
Dogen Zenji, 86
dogma, 15–17
DSM-IV, 145–46, 204
D-space, 301
Dubois-Reymond, E., 21
Dubrov, A. P., 285
Durlacher, J. V., xviii, 57–58, 84, 99, 102, 106, 107, 147
dyes, 216–18
dynamical energy systems, 6, 294–98

eating disorders
  anorexia, 46
  case example, 253–54
  compulsive eating, 264–65
  and elaters (eating in-orders), 180–84, 214
ECT. *see* energy consciousness therapy
Eddington, A., 309–10
Eden, D., 56–57, 85, 137
EDxTM. *see* energy diagnostic and treatment methods
EFT. *see* emotional freedom technique
ego states
  fusion of, 206, 208
  in incest survivor, 274–75
EID. *see* eyes into distortion
Einstein, A., 307
elaters
  and cluster technique, 214
  compulsive eating case, 264–65
  description, 127–28
  and dynamical energy systems, 296–98
  inappropriate attraction case, 265
  muscle testing, 183–84
  and nail biting case, 258–59
  and self-sabotage, 10, 180–81
  worksheet, 337–39
elation. *see* subjective units of elation
electric current
  and acupoints, 35
  and finger-tapping, 83–85, 89–91
  as life force, 21
  and mind-body interface, 312–16
electroencephalogram, quantitative (QEEG), 304, 310
electromagnetic fields, 216, 217–19, 283
electromagnetic resonance, 90
electromagnetism, 313*f*, 315
electronic devices, 216
elevators, 259–60, 310
embarrassment
  algorithms, 237*t*
  and dynamical energy systems, 296
  and performance issues, 196
  treatment points, 50
  triggering act, 149–50
EMDR. *see* eye movement desensitization and reprocessing
emergency treatment, 232, 275–76

emotional exhaustion, 46
emotional freedom technique (EFT)
    clinical studies, 305
    and elaters, 184
    finger tapping, 7
    mechanism of action, 292–93
    order of treatment, 238
emotional signaling mechanism (ESM), 9,
        127–28. *see also* elaters; harmonizers;
        perturbations
emotional upsets
    and algorithms, 236
    and FRC, 283–84, 288
    and self-healing, 226
emotion-meridian correlations, 234
emotions
    as abstraction, 24
    and algorithms, 236
    attachment to, 151
    and brain evolution, 13–14
    and dissociative disorders, 205, 208
    and dynamical energy systems, 296
    as energy constructs, 7
    as energy transformation, 11
    EvTFT effect, 213
    individual differences, 45, 234
    and meridians, 45–50, 49*t*, 234
    and muscle testing, 2–3
    and pain management, 202
    and performance issues, 196
    in referential frame, 312–15
    see also elaters; perturbations
empathy, 109
empowerment, 229, 243
energy
    defined, 284
    dynamic systems, 6, 294–98
    forms of, 284
    in interpersonal interaction, 319–23
energy consciousness therapy, ix
energy diagnostic and treatment methods
        (EdxTM), ix, 7, 147
energy disrupters, 215–22, 329*f*
energy forces
    and emotions, 11
    and history of medicine, 19–22
    lines of, 17–18
    release of, 88, 275
    shen, 34
    and thoughts, 4, 11
    von Mayer work, 19
    see also chi
energy psychology
    definition, 1–2
    roots, ix, 26–28
    see also mechanism of action
energy psychotherapy, 2, 5–6
energy systems, dynamical, 6, 294–98
energy toxins. *see* toxins
enjoyment. *see* elaters
enuresis, 276–80

epinephrine, 92
epoxies, 219
ER. *see* eye-roll
Erasistratus, 19–20
ESM. *see* emotional signaling mechanism
ethics
    BDB recommendations, 10, 240
    and expertise, 8
    and surrogacy, 227
    touching patients, 55
ethnic prejudice, 271–72
evolution
    and acquired characteristics, 27
    of brain, 13–14
evolving thought field therapy (EvTFT)
    acceptance path, 303
    as adjunctive therapy (*see* adjunctive
            therapy)
    at a distance, 322 (*see also* surrogacy)
    as first line intervention, 241
    limitations, 8, 206–7
    origins, 2–3
    overview, 6–8
    as paradigm shift, 11–17
    terminology, 115–20, 141*t*
    versus TFT, 8–10
    workshops (*see* BDB group)
    see also energy psychology
exhibitionism, 182
explicate order, 124–27, 289–90
extended trauma algorithm, 275–76
external reality, 315*f*, 319
eye contact, 57
eye movement desensitization and reprocess-
        ing (EMDR), 131, 207, 304
eye-roll (ER). *see* ground to sky eye-roll
eyes
    injury warning, 92
    new eyeglasses, 219
    and sensory input, 135
eyes into distortion (EID), 133–34

family of origin, 251–52
family therapy, 233, 243–44
family tragedy case, 247–48
Faraday, M., 17–18, 97
fear
    of abandonment, 50, 274–75
    and affirmations, 103
    and BRBs, 109
    of heights, 259–60, 304
    of injury, 50
    loss of self (BRB), 326
    of pills, 254–56
    side effects, 103
    of touch, 226–29, 232
    treatment points, 46–47, 50
fields
    concept of, 18–19
    information-storing, 28
    location of, 28

morphic resonance, 27–28
in TFT, 116–17
field shifting, 9, 285
Figley, C. R., 7–8, 241, 304
Fine, C. G., 204
fingers
    as indicator muscle, 62–64
    phantom pain case, 262–64
    self-muscle testing, 222–25
finger tapping
    in Callahan techniques™, 5, 7, 80–85
    and chaos theory, 89
    description, 80–85
    and electric current, 89–91
    in 9G treatment, 134
    imagined, 82
    versus TAB, 80, 92–93
first line intervention, 233, 241
Fisher, S., 341
five minute phobia cure, 230
flashbacks
    and affirmations, 103
    after sexual assault, 251–53
    after stressful year, 253–54
    amputated finger case, 262–64
    in dissociative disorders, 212, 213, 260–62
    in drowning witness, 247–48
    in incest survivor, 274–75
    privacy, 205
    in stalker victim, 256–57
Flavell, J. H., 308
Fleming, T., 7, 322
flowcharts, 329–32
fluorescent lighting, 219
fMRI. *see* functional magnetic resonance imaging
follow-up
    for consultations, 245
    in next session, 174
    and TAB, 92
foods, 216–18
force(s)
    lines of, 17–18
    von Mayer work, 19
    see also energy forces
formaldehyde, 218, 268–69
Fowlie, A., 7, 147, 184, 233, 238, 293
FPII. *see* future performance imagery index
FRC. *see* frequency resonance coherence
freedom, 121
frequency modulation, 88
frequency resonance coherence (FRC)
    diagram, 290
    and info-energy exchange, xxiii
    and relief, 6
    and TAB, 85
    as underlying mechanism, 9, 283–89
    and yin and yang, 38
Freud, S., 57
Frost, R., 216
frustration, 46, 196

fugue, 204
functional magnetic resonance imaging (fMRI), 136
Furman, M., 309
future belief related blocks
    description, 108–9
    in phantom digit pain case, 262–64
    in protocol, 170
    in suicide ideation case, 250–51
future performance imagery index (FPII)
    ADHD parent case, 272–74
    description, 193–94
    in gagging case, 268–69
    in protocol, 174
    purpose, 10
    stalker victim case, 256–57
    and TAB, 93
    use, 194–96

9G. *see* nine gamut (9G) treatments
gagging, 268–69
gait irregularity, 69
Galen, 20
gall bladder meridian
    alarm points, 47f, 48t
    emotions, 46, 49t
    in enuresis case, 276–80
    in EvTFT, 43
    in TCM, 36, 39
Gallo, F. P., ix–x, xvi, xvii, 1–2, 5, 7, 52, 57–58, 79, 82, 100, 102, 106, 107, 118, 136, 147, 214, 216, 233, 236, 309
Galvani, L., 20–21
Galvin, M. D., x
gamut point
    and Callahan techniques™, 116, 121
    versus collarbone point, 136–37
    in integration sequence, 137–38
    location, 133–36
gate control theory, 83–84
gender factors, 56
Gendlin, E. T., 149
generalized PRs
    correction, 103–5
    description, 100
    in DID, 211
    in flowchart, 330f
    in incest survivor, 274–75
    in protocol, 163
    in stalker victim case, 256–57
generations, 23–25, 28, 114
genetics, 26–27, 114
Gerber, R., xviii, 32, 283
Gillispie, C. C., 17–19, 22, 29, 115–16
glands
    adrenal, 92
    pituitary, 46, 92
    thymus, 3
Goldstein, D., 285, 304
Goodheart, G. J., Jr., ix, 2, 3, 41, 51–52, 83, 84, 90, 133–34, 226

governing vessel
  alarm point, 40, 47f, 48t
  and BRBs, 108, 109
  description, 35, 38
  emotions, 49t, 50
  in EvTFT, 43
  and FRC, 286
  meridian connection, 291–94
  treatment point, 47f, 48t
Greenberg, R. P., 341
Greeson, J. M., 53
grief, 50, 249–50
Grinder, J., 135
ground to sky eye-roll (ER)
  cases
  description, 139–40
  and elaters, 184
  in flowchart, 331–32
  in protocol, 169–70, 173–74
  steps, 334, 338
group sessions
  and algorithms, 232–33
  family therapy, 244
guilt
  algorithms, 237t
  in DID case, 260–62
  and dynamical energy system, 296
  in incest survivor, 274–75
  and memories, 206
  treatment points, 50

handicapped patients, 8, 156, 162, 226–29
hand over head polarity test, 156, 162
hands
  alarm points, 47f, 48t
  and elaters, 183
  in EvTFT, 55, 58, 63–64
  finger tapping (see finger tapping)
  palm up and palm down, 95
  and self-muscle testing, 222–25
Hanicke, B. T., 53–54
Hannaford, C., 135, 218
hardware stores, 219
harmonizers, 128–30, 294
Hartung, J. G., x
Hawkins, D. R., 54
health care setting
  emergencies, 232, 233
  fear of pills, 254–56
  MRI refusal case, 249–50
  oncology patients, 23
heart. see pericardium
heart/brain connection, 285–86
HeartMath, Institute of, 283, 285–86
heart meridian
  alarm points, 47f, 48t
  emotions, 49t, 50
  in EvTFT, 43
  and FRC, 285–86
  in TCM, 37, 39
  treatment points, 47f, 48t

heart rate variability, 305
heights, 259–60, 304
Helmholtz, H., 21
heredity, 26–27, 114
Herrick, J., 14
high spirit-self, 312
Hiley, B. J., 115, 117, 124–27, 289, 308, 311
Hippocrates, 19
holarchy, 121
holograms, 25–26, 123
holons, 121–24
home treatment
  for children, 243
  SCB as, 274–75
  testing for, 175–76
  worksheets, 333–35, 337–39
hopelessness, 50
Hover-Kramer, D., x
Hume, D., 319
humming, 134–35, 138
hydration, 68
hypertonicity, 215–22
hypervigilance, 46
hypnosis, 207
hypotheses, 281–82

imagery, 157–60, 194, 220
imagined-Touch-And-Breathe (i-TAB),
  92–93
implicate order, 124–27, 289–90
incest, 274–75
indicator muscle
  fingers as, 63–64
  response calibration, 60–61
  selection of, 57–58, 86
individual differences
  and disrupters, 218
  in emotions, 45, 234
  law of individuality, 102–3
  in treatment sequences, 292
infants, 226–29
inferiority, 50
information
  and dynamical energy systems, 294–98
  in fields, 26–28
  and FRC, 288
  intergenerational transmission, 28
  as mind-body bridge, 117–19
injury, fear of, 50
Institute of HeartMath, 283, 285–86
integration
  of ego states, 206, 208
  of EvTFT and psychotherapy, 239–42 (see
    also adjunctive therapy)
integration sequence (ISq)
  algorithm table, 237
  description, 137–38
  in flowchart, 331–32f
  steps, 334
  in worksheets, 334, 338
intelligence BRB, 326

intention
    and breath, 91, 203–4
    and reality, 315*f*
    and spirit-self, 315
interdisciplinary approach, 308–10
intergenerational transmission, 23–25, 28,
    114
intestine meridians
    alarm points, 47*f*, 48*t*
    and BRBs, 109–10, 111, 112–13
    emotions, 49*t*, 50
    in EvTFT, 43
    and issue-specific PRs, 164
    and PRs, 104, 105
    in TCM, 37, 40
    treatment points, 47*f*, 48*t*
intuition, 157–159, 165
ISq. *see* integration sequence
issue-specific PRs
    correction, 105
    description, 100
    in DID, 211
    and elaters, 183
    in flowchart, 330*f*
    in protocol, 164
i-TAB. *see* imagined-Touch-And-Breathe

Jacobs, G. E., 54
Jarrett, L., 32–33, 34
jealousy, 50
jet lag, 226, 237*t*
Jiyu-Kennett, R., 85, 86, 87
Jung, C., 299

Kaptchuk, T., 32, 45, 46, 49n
Kendall, F. P., 51–52
Kendall, H. O., 51–52
kidney meridian
    alarm points, 47*f*, 48*t*
    as catalyst, 136–37
    in comprehensive algorithm, 238
    emotions, 46, 49*t*
    in EvTFT, 43
    and eye-role, 140
    versus gamut point, 136–37
    in integration sequence, 137–38
    in TCM, 36–37, 39
    treatment points, 47*f*, 48*t*
Kim B. H., 35
Kluft, R. P., 204
Koestler, A., 14, 117, 121, 125
Kohane, M. J., 11, 291, 301, 308, 313
Korzybski, A., 24–25, 45, 102–3
Kuhn, T., 12–14, 25
Kunkel, E. J. S., 53

Lamarck, J. B. de, 26–27
Lambrou, P. T., 5, 36, 84, 233, 238, 293, 304
language
    of affirmations, 102–3
    for children, 242–43

chi symbol, 32–33
for DID patients, 211–12
for emotions, 45
limitations, 23–25
preverbal causes, 103
though *versus* if, 110
transpositions, 69
see also terminology
lasers, 82
Lashley, K., 26
laundry products, 216–19
law of individuality, 102–3
law of non-identity, 102–3
learning, 27–28
left brain, 135–36
left/right confusion, 69
Lehr, C., 221
Levy, S., 221
life energy, 3
light, 219
lines of force, 17–18
liver meridian
    emotions, 47, 49*t*
    in EvTFT, 43
    in TCM, 37, 39
    treatment/alarm points, 47*f*, 48*t*
loneliness BRB, 325
love pain, 237*t*
Luber, M., xvii
lung meridian
    alarm points, 47*f*, 48*t*
    emotions, 49*t*, 50
    in EvTFT, 43
    in MRI refusal case, 249–50
    in TCM, 37, 39
    treatment points, 47*f*, 48*t*
lymphatic system. *see* neurolymphatic reflex

McDougall, W., 26–27
McLean, C. J., 33–34, 38, 92, 137, 286, 302
MacLean, P., 14
MacPhillamy, D., 85, 86, 87
magnetic resonance imaging (MRI)
    impact, 25–26
    and phobias, 233, 250
    refusal case, 249–50
    see also fMRI
magnetism, 21
magnetoelectricism, 315
managed care, 7–8, 15
Mann, F., 52
Mappa, N., 304
mapping, 208
Marchese, M., 53
marriage therapy, 233, 243–44
Martin, H., 283, 285, 289
massage, 82, 93
mathematics, 135–36
Maxwell, J. C., 18–19
measurements, 39. *see also* subjective units of
    distress; subjective units of elation

mechanism of action
  dynamical energy systems, 294–98
  elusiveness, 24
  FRC, 283–89
  hypotheses, 281–82
  and sequence, 282–83, 289–94
  spirit and consciousness, 298–302
  of TAB, 316
mechanists, 20
mediation, 3
medication
  as disrupter, 219
  fear of, 254–56
  research status, 341
Melzack and Wall gate control theory, 83–84
memories
  in DID patients, 209, 212–13
  in drowning witness, 247
  and dynamical energy systems, 294
  erasing, 206
  in sports case, 267–68
  and thought field switch, 150
meridians
  alarm points, 38–41, 47f, 48t (see also alarm
      points)
  electrical resistance, 284–85
  and emotions, 45–50, 234, 449t
  extraordinary, 35
  and FRC, 285–86, 290
  and information-bearing signals, 288
  interconnections, 291–94
  main, 36–38
  major, 34–35, 132
  and mudras, 87–93
  and muscle testing, 52
  as transducers, 22
  treatment points, 47f, 48t (see also treat-
      ment points)
  and yin and yang, 37–38
Mesmer, F. A., 21
metacognition, 69
metals, 219
mind-body interface
  bridge, 117
  diagrams, 314
  levels, 312–16
  and morphic resonance, 26–28
  and polarity, 97
  space of, 18–19
  transduction, 22
mind clearing, 57, 58
mind direction. see intention
mirroring, 104
Monti, D. A., 53
morphic resonance, 27–28
Motoyama, H., 36
MRI. see magnetic resonance imaging
mudras
  description, 85–87
  and meridians, 87–93

muscle testing
  and algorithms, 234, 235–36
  for BRBs, 108, 109, 111, 112, 170–73
  in Callahan techniques™, 5
  cautions, 56
  and chi, 90–91
  of children, 61–62
  in DID patients, 210
  early work, 51–53
  and elaters, 183–84
  and emotions, 2–3
  and energy disrupters, 218–19, 220–22
  and eye contact, 57
  in flowcharts, 329–31
  and FRC, 288–89
  and gender, 56
  hydration testing, 68
  for known blocks, 186
  and meridians, 52
  for ND, 69–71
  permission, 55–56, 162, 163
  and polarity, 95–98
  preparation, 54–56, 58–59, 162, 329f
  pressure estimation, 59
  in protocol, 162–74
  for PRs, 100–101, 186
  in PTSD case, 251–53
  response calibration, 60–61, 60–63
  reverse response, 65, 78
  on self, 222–25
  and shirt, 67
  shoulder problems, 57–58, 62–63
  subjectivity, 52, 53–54, 57
  at SUD level, 176–78
  therapist attitude, 56–57
  therapy localization, 41
  time factors, 221
  and transference, 3, 56, 57, 319–23
  trouble shooting, 64–67
  validation, 53–54
  see also indicator muscle; nonpolarized re-
      sponses; strong/strong response; weak/
      weak response

nail biting, 258–59
Nambudripad, D., 54, 217–18
Nambudripad allergy elimination technique,
  54, 217–18
nasal congestion, 237t
ND. see neurologic disorganization/switching
neck problems, 57–58, 62–63, 226–29
nerve impulse, 21–22
neurolinguistic programming, 135
neurologic disorganization (ND)
  description, 68–69
  diagnosis, 69–71
  home treatment, 175–76
  in protocol, 173
  and rubbing, 93
  and TAB, 93

neurologic organizer treatment (NOTx)
  description, 70–72, 76–78
  and DID patients, 212
  in enuresis case, 276–80
  in flowchart, 329
  and formaldehyde case, 268–69
  incest survivor case, 274–75
neurolymphatic reflex (NLR)
  in enuresis surrogacy case, 276–80
  and generalized PRs, 103–4, 163
  location, 44, 47f, 48t
  in PTSD/dissociation case, 274–75
  and recurrent PRs, 106
  and unknown blocks, 113
neurons, 35–36
Newton, M., 301
Nietzsche, F., 13
Nims, L., 7
nine gamut (9G) treatments, 133–36
NLR. see neurolymphatic reflex
nonpolarized responses
  and BRBs, 107
  correction, 78
  description, 96–97
  diagnosis, 192–93
  and energy disrupters, 215–22
  in flowchart, 329
  and switching, 68
notation, 141t
NOTx. see neurologic organizer treatment
novelty effect, 16
nutrition, 3, 54

objectors, in DID, 211
obsessive-compulsive disorder (OCD)
  algorithms, 237t
  case example, 257–58
  and elaters, 181
  and genetics, 114
  home treatment, 175–76
  and PRs, 106
  in sexual attraction case, 265
  treatment points, 50
odors, 268–69
oncology patients, 23
option BRB, 326
order. see implicit order; integration sequence;
    sequence; treatment sequence
Oschman, J. L., 89–90
Ostwald, W., 22, 23

pain management
  algorithms, 237t
  amputated digit, 262–64
  assessment, 200–202
  breathing through, 203–4
  Chinese appendectomy, 30–31
  gate control theory, 83–84
  home treatment, 175–76
  limiting beliefs, 202–3

TAB role, 93
  treatment points, 50
pancreas. see spleen/pancreas meridian
panic disorders
  algorithms, 237t
  in case example, 271–72
  and home treatment, 175–76
  and self healing, 226
Paracelsus, P., 20, 97
paradigms
  and communication, 24–25
  definition, 12
  shifting, 13–14
parents, 61–62
  of ADHD child, 272–74
patients
  apex problem, 178–79
  limiting beliefs, 202–3
  permission, 55–56, 151–53, 162, 163
  physically disabled, 8, 156, 162, 226–29
  privacy, 205
  and PRs, 102
  respect for, 23, 205
  and tapping versus TAB, 92
  see also therapist-patient rapport; touching
patterns
  of behavior, 28
  brain-waves, 304
  previous treatment, 274–75
  recognition of, 26
Pearlman, R., 84
pectoral muscles, 57–58, 62
Penfield, W., 26, 29
perfectionism, 50
performance issues
  blocks, 196–98
  evaluation index, 10
  and FPII, 194
  home treatment, 175–76
  and neurologic organization, 72
  and self-healing, 226
  sports cases, 265–68
  as therapy indication, 8
  treatment points, 47
performing arts, 72
perfume, 216–19
pericardium, 257–58
permission
  and DID, 211
  in flowcharts, 329, 330
  from parents, 61–62
  to start work, 151–53, 163
  for surrogacy, 227
  to touch, 55–56, 162
personality disorders, 181
personality-self, 312–13
perturbations
  and Callahan techniques™, 4, 127
  defined, 118
  subsumption of, 120–24

PET. *see* positron emission tomography
phantom pain, 262–64
phobias
    algorithm treatment, 231, 237*t*
    and BRBs, 108, 109
    claustrophobia, 304
    clinical studies, 304, 309–10
    elevators, 259–60, 310
    five minute cure, 230
    and FPII, 194
    and genetics, 114
    in health care setting, 233
    heights, 259–60, 304
    and morphic resonance, 28
    and self-healing, 226
phonon spectrum, 90
physical changes, 24
physical disability, 8, 156, 162, 226–29
physical D-space, 301
physical R-space, 300–301
physical sensations, 103, 251–53
    phantom pain, 262–64
physics
    and distance healing, 322–23
    fields, 18–19
    human model, 312–16
    lines of force, 17–18
    research issues, 306
    terminology, 284
piezoelectric effect, 83–85, 89–91
pituitary gland, 46, 92
placebo effects, 16
play therapy, 242–43
polarity
    and biological reversals, 99
    and BRBs, 107
    and formaldehyde, 268
    and FRC, 288
    hand over head test, 156, 162
    measures of, 95–97
    and mind-body interface, 97
polarity check, 329*f*
polarity reversal
    definition, 98
    and energy disrupters, 220–21
Polglase, K., 305
Porkert, M., 33
positron emission tomography (PET), 310
possibility BRB, 326
Postman, L., 12
posttraumatic stress disorder (PTSD)
    and abreaction, 212–13
    algorithms, 237
    case examples, 251–53, 256–57, 274–75
    and elaters, 181–82
    and EvTFT, 8, 310
    phantom pain case, 262–64
postural changes, 209
powerlessness, 46, 50, 181
powerlessness BRB, 326
PRs. *see* psychological reversalss

Pratt, G. P., 5, 36, 84, 233, 238, 293, 304
prejudice, 271–72
pressure, 59, 66
pressure holding, 82
Pribram, K., 26, 29
privacy, 205
problems
    background information, 149
    causes, 103
    thoughts about, 4
    tuning into, 148–49, 163
process-specific BRBs, 110–11
process-specific PRs
    correction, 105–6
    description, 100–101
    in DID patients, 211
    in flowchart, 332*f*
    record keeping, 144
    testing for, 169–70
    and unknown blocks, 192
procrastination, 214
protocols
    algorithm method, 235
    basic (*see* basic protocol)
    for block diagnosis, 186–92
    for clinical trial, 309–10
    for disrupter identification, 219–21
    for dissociative disorders, 204–13
    for elater-related problems, 184
    nonpolarized response diagnosis, 192–93
    pain management, 200–204
    for performance issues, 196–200
    PR diagnosis, 186–90
    surrogate use, 228
psychological reversalss (PRs)
    affirmations, 102–6
    algorithm treatment, 231
    corrections, 101–6
    definition, 99
    diagnosis protocol, 186–90
    in DID, 211–12
    and energy toxins, 217
    flowchart, 330
    and FRC, 288
    and genetics, 114
    in protocol, 163, 164, 174
    record keeping, 144
    in therapist, 67
    types, 99–101
    see also blocks
psychopharmacology, 341
psychoses, 46
psychotherapy
    dogma, 15–17
    with EvTFT, 239–42
    interdisciplinary cooperation, 308–10
    paradigm shift need, 15
    and TAB, 91–93
    traditional diagnosis, 145–46
    unifying theory, 22–25
    see also energy psychotherapy

PTSD. *see* posttraumatic stress disorder
Pulos, L., xvi
puppets, 242–43
Pushkin, V. N., 285
Putnam, F. W., 204

qi. *see* chi
quantitative electroencephalogram (QEEG), 304, 310
quantum field theory, 284
quantum theory, 117–20, 284, 306, 322

radio wave metaphor, 28
rage, 46, 237*t*, 251–53
rape, 182, 275–76
Rapp, D., 218
rapport. *see* therapist-patient rapport
reading, 69, 72
  self-help literature, 15
reality, 315*f*, 319
record keeping, 140–44, 163–64
recurrent PRs, 101, 144, 174
reframing, 205
regeneration, 97
relaxation procedure, 237*t*
releases, 55
religion, 56
research
  versus clinical results, 341
  dogma about, 16–17
  future directions, 305–11
  limitations, 23, 24–25, 28–29
  in physics, 306
  studies, 304–5
resistance
  electrical, 284–85
  to muscle testing, 60
  terminology for, 94–95
  to traditional therapy, 181
  unconscious aspect as, 151–52
  see also blocks; psychological reversalss
resonance. *see* frequency resonance coherence
resources, 205–6, 208–13
respect, 23, 205
responsibility, 50
responsibility BRB, 111, 325
reversal
  of actions, 69
  double, 320
  of muscle response, 65, 78
  of polarity, 98 (*see also* polarity reversal)
  of words/letters, 69
  see also psychological reversals
reversal of body morality, 3, 4, 5, 99. *see also* psychological reversals
right brain, 135–36
risk, 109
Rochlitz, S., 268
Rogers, C., 103
Rosenthal-Schneider, I., 307

Ross, C. A., 204
R-space, 300–301, 301
rubbing
  and NLR, 93
  and PRs, 103–4, 106, 163
  versus tapping, 82
  in unknown blocks, 113
Russek, G., 284, 294–95

sadism, 182
sadness, 50
safety
  and abuse survivors, 274
  eye injury, 92
  sense of, 56
safety BRBs
  assessment and correction, 111, 171
  in delusional disorder case, 248–49
  description, 109–10
  in DID case, 260–62
  in phantom digit pain case, 262–64
  in stalker victim case, 256–57
  in suicide ideation case, 250–51
Salzinger, K., 308–9
scale. *see* subjective units of distress; subjective units of elation
SCB. *see* simplified collarbone breathing treatment
Schwartz, G. E., 284, 294–95
seasons, 221
secondary gains, 182, 202
self
  negative emotions toward, 205
  three levels, 312–16
  treatment points, 47, 50
self acceptance, 103
self assurance, 47
self-care, 92, 209. *see also* home treatment
self-condemnation, 110
self-defeating behavior, 10, 180–84, 241
self-diagnosis, 226
self-esteem, 108, 110
self-healing
  algorithms, 233
  in medical history, 19–20, 21
  uses, 226
self-help literature, 15
self-muscle testing, 222–25
self trust BRB, 325
semiconductors, 22, 89
sensory input, 102, 135, 268–69
sequence
  in diagnosis, 5, 160
  and holons, 123
  of TAB, in DID patients, 212
  of treatment, 289–90
sex, 244. *see also* circulation/sex meridian
sexual abuse, 260–62, 271–72, 274–75
sexual arousal, continual, 72
sexual assault, 251–53, 275–76
sexual attraction, 265

sexual meridian, 257–58. *see also* circulation/
    sex meridian
shame
    BRBs, 110
    and dynamical energy system, 296
    in incest survivor, 274–75
    and memories, 206
    and performance issues, 196
    treatment points, 50
Shapiro, F, xvii
Shelden, G., 35
Sheldrake, R., 27–28, 114, 191, 294, 299,
    301
shen, 34, 302
shirt, 67, 218
shopping centers, 219
shoulder problems, 57–58, 62–63
siblings, 197
side effects, 103
Siegal, B., 23
simplification, 28–29
simplified collarbone breathing treat-
    ment(SCB)
    description, 73–75
    and DID, 212
    in flowchart, 329
    and incest survivor case, 274–75
    and ND, 70–71
Sinnott, J., 53
sleep, 69, 274–75
smells, 268–69
sore spot. *see* neurolymphatic reflex
soul-self
    of patient, 312, 313
    of therapist, 316
sound spectrum, 90
spacetime, 313–16
speech, 69
Spiegel, D., 140
Spiegel, M., 140
Spira, J. L., 204
spirit, 301–2
spirit-self, 312, 315
spleen/pancreas meridian
    in ADHD parent case, 272–74
    alarm point, 47*f*, 48*t*
    emotions, 47, 49*t*
    in EvTFT, 43
    in TCM, 37, 39
    treatment points, 47*f*, 48*t*
sports, 8, 265–67
stalker, 256–57
stomach meridian
    alarm points, 47*f*, 48*t*
    emotions, 46, 49*t*
    in EvTFT, 43
    in gagging case, 269
    in TCM, 36, 39
    treatment points, 47*f*, 48*t*
stress, 8, 91, 232–33

string loops, 291, 293–94
string theory, 293
stroke victim, 257–58
strong/strong response
    and BRBs, 108
    description, 66–67
    in DID patients, 212
    in enuresis case, 276–80
    in OCD case, 257–58
    and therapist, 66, 283
    and transference, 320
subjective units of distress (SUD)
    and BRBs, 107, 111, 112
    and children, 242
    in cluster technique, 215
    description, 138–40
    and dissociation, 263
    failure to drop, 170–72
    and holons, 123
    muscle testing, 176–78
    rating points, 331–32*f*
    record keeping, 144, 163, 169, 174
    single point drops, 68–69, 170, 173
    in surrogate testing, 229
    unknown block indicator, 190
    verification, 177
subjective units of elation (SUE)
    and children, 242
    description, 183–84
    in cluster technique, 215
    in elater approach, 183–84
    and surrogate testing, 229
    unknown block indication, 190
subsumption, 120–24
SUD. *see* subjective units of distress
SUE. *see* subjective units of elation
suicide, 181–82, 251–51, 274–75
superstring theory, 293–94
surrogacy, 8, 226–29
    cases, 259–60, 260–62, 276–80
swallowing, 254–56
switching, 150–51. *see also* neurologic disorga-
    nization
synergy, 291–92
Szent-Gyorgyi, A., 22, 97

talk therapy, 241–42, 243
TCM. *see* traditional Chinese medicine
TDdx. *see* thought directed diagnosis
telephone
    therapy by, 226–29, 232
    as trigger, 256–57
terminology
    of Callahan techniques™, 116, 121
    of EvTFT, 115–30, 141*t*
    impact of, 23–24
    of physics, 284
    for resistance, 94–95
    in TFT, 115–17
    treatment point notation, 132–33

TFT. *see* thought field therapy
theories, 281–82
therapist
  in contact directed diagnosis, 155–57
  expertise of, 8
  mind clearing, 57
  in muscle testing, 56–57, 61
  PRs, 67, 283
  soul-self, 316
  as surrogate, 227
therapist-patient rapport
  (counter)transference, 319–23
  as emphasis, 206–7
  as energy, 159, 240
  physics viewpoint, 315–16
therapy
  algorithm-based, 5
  apex problem, 178–79
  cluster technique, 214–15
  diagnostic method, 4–5
  of elaters, 180–84
  flowcharts, 329–32
  holons, 121–24
  permission to start, 152–53, 163
  by phone, 226–29, 232
  for psychological reversalss, 101–6
  variables, 289–90
  see also basic protocol; integration se-
      quence; protocols; psychotherapy;
      treatment sequence
therapy localization, 3, 41
Thie, J., 54, 68
thought directed diagnosis (TDdx), descrip-
      tion of, 157–60, 168–69
thought experiments, 307–8
thought field(s)
  clustered, 214–15
  definitions, 4, 116–17, 118, 148–49
  and DID, 210–11
  and dissociative disorders, 205–6
  and FRC, 288–89, 290
  and holons, 122
  and language, 102
  and pain, 202
  primary, 149–50
  selection, 149–51
  shifting, 9
  switching, 150–51
  targeting, 148–51, 330*f*, 331*f*
  and unconscious, 298–302
thought field therapy (TFT)
  basic premises, 1
  Callahan techniques^TM, 4–5
  comparative study, 304
  description, ix
  versus EvTFT, 8–10
  fields in, 116–17
  origins, ix
  sources, xviii
  see also evolving thought field therapy

thought(s)
  about problem, 4
  and brain evolution, 13–14
  definition, 307–8
  research on, 24
thymus gland, 3
thyroid meridian. *see* triple heater meridian
Tiller, W., xviii, 2, 11, 87–88, 89, 90, 91, 203,
      281, 283, 291, 301, 308, 312–16
time factors
  and DID, 209
  and dogma, 16
  and holons, 123
  and muscle testing, 221, 288–89
  for paradigm shift, 15
  and performance issues, 196
  and research studies, 23
  seasons, 221
  and space, 313–16
  and trauma, 123, 206
  treatment sequence, 212, 289–90
Touch-And-Breathe (TAB)
  advantages, 91–93
  antenna effect, 83–85, 87–89, 90
  bilateral, 203, 212
  and BRBs, 109–10, 112–13
  and CDdx-p, 153–54
  and CDdx-t, 157
  description, 9, 93
  in DID patients, 209, 212
  and elaters, 183, 337–38
  versus finger tapping, 7, 80, 92–93
  in flowcharts, 330
  and FRC, 85
  in homework, 333–34, 337–38
  imagined (i-TAB), 92–93
  implementation, 93
  mechanism of action, 316
  and meridians, 87–93
  and mudras, 86–87
  and ND, 71–72, 78
  and NLR, 93
  origins, 82–83
  and pain, 203, 262–64
  and PRs, 104, 105
  sequence, 212
  and surrogate testing, 228
  and TDdx, 1559–160
  see also breath
Touch for Health, 54, 68
touching
  of DID patients, 210
  fear of, 226–29, 232
  issues, 55–56, 162
toxins
  contact with, 113
  diagnosing, 54
  as energy disrupters, 216
  in flowchart, 329
  frequency, 217

toxins (*cont.*)
  home treatment, 175–76
  types, 216
traditional Chinese medicine
  anatomy measurement, 39
  Buddhism, 85–87
  description, 31–34
  main meridians, 37–38
  yin and yang, 32
  see also acupuncture meridian system
training, 8, 61
transducers, 22
transference
  energetic basis, 319–23
  and muscle testing, 3, 56, 57, 320–21
trauma
  and abreaction, 212–13
  algorithms, 234, 237*t*
  and BRBs, 109
  comparative study, 304
  and dissociative disorders, 205
  and FPII, 194
  immediate aftermath, 232, 233–34
  lifetime *versus* incident, 206
  memory of, 148, 150
  and muscle testing, 56
  and pain, 201–2
  and personality self, 313
  recent *versus* old, 123
  response persistence, 120
  and self-healing, 226
  thought field switching, 150–51
  treatment points, 46, 92, 234
traumatic incident reduction, 304
treatment points
  control issues, 50
  for courage, 47
  for decision-making, 46, 47
  for depression, 50
  in EFT, 238
  and emotions, 45–50, 49*t*
  locations, 41–44, 47*f*, 48*t*
  majors, 132
  and majors, 132
  notation, 132–33
  in pain management, 203
  for PRs or blocks, 186–90
  for trauma, 46, 92, 234
treatment sequence (TxSq)
  algorithm table, 237
  definition, 132
  in flowchart, 331–32*f*
  versus holon, 121
  as issue, 282–83, 289–94
  in negative belief cluster, 270–71
  in PTSD cases, 262–64
  in sports cases, 265–68
triggers
  in cases, 256–57, 274–75
  elimination of, 252
  and thought fields, 149–50

triple heater meridian
  alarm points, 47*f*, 48*t*
  emotions, 49*t*, 50
  in EvTFT, 43
  and 9G treatment, 133, 136
  in TCM, 37, 40
  treatment points, 47*f*, 48*t*
Trubo, R., 75, 133, 304, 305
trust, 109, 111
Tsuei, J. J., 86–87
Tudor, T., xvi, 305, 341
"tuning in"
  to enjoyment, 183
  in PR diagnosis protocol, 187–90
  to problems, 148–49, 163
twitching, 252
TxSq. *see* treatment sequence

unconscious mind, 103, 111–12, 298–302
unknown blocks
  description, 112–14
  diagnosis, 190–92
  and energy toxins, 217
  in family therapy, 244
  in flowchart, 332*f*
  in protocol, 171–72
  in sports case, 265–67
unknown entities, 244
unworthiness, 50

van der Hart, O., 213
variables, 289–90
vengeance, 50
verification
  of affirmations, 104, 105, 106
  in flowcharts, 330
  of SUD level, 177, 331–32*f*
Versendaal, D. A., 54
Versendaal-Hoezee, D., 54
Vesalius, A., 20
vessels. *see* conception vessel; governing
  vessel
Vincenzi, H., ix, 233
violent crime, 182. *see also* sexual assault
visualization, 157–60
visual kinesthetic dissociation, 304
vitalists, 20, 21
Voll, R., 35, 285
Volta, A., 21
von Mayer, J. R., 39
vulnerability, 50, 109

Walker, S., 54
Walther, D., 2, 3, 38, 41, 51–52, 53–54, 75,
  83, 84, 90, 133–34, 135–36, 136–37
water, 68
wavicles, 284
weak/weak response, 64–66, 108, 212
Weiss, B. L., 301
Wells, S., 305
Whisenant, W. F., 46, 49n

willpower, 50, 326
Wise, A., 130, 140
Witmer, L., 306
Wolpe, J., 138
Woollerton, H., 33–34, 38, 92, 137, 286, 302
words
    power of, 23–24
    transpositions, 69

worksheets, 333–35, 337–39
worry, 47
Worsley, J. R., 37–38
worthlessness, 50, 108, 110
Wundt, W., 308

yin and yang, 32, 37–38, 91–92
Young, J., 107